Public Health in the 21st Century

snova
New York

Public Health in the 21st Century

The Role of Reactive Oxygen Species in Health and Disease
Kuladip Jana, PhD (Editor)
2024. ISBN: 979-8-89113-283-2 (Hardcover)
2024. ISBN: 979-8-89113-330-3 (eBook)

Interdisciplinary Perspectives on Occupational Safety and Health
Mehmed Zahid Çögenli, PhD (Editor)
2023. ISBN: 979-8-89113-085-2 (Hardcover)
2023. ISBN: 979-8-89113-120-0 (eBook)

Critical Care and COVID-19
Salim Surani (Editor)
Syed Anjum Khan, MD (Editor)
Reena Shah (Editor)
2023. ISBN: 979-8-88697-940-4 (Hardcover)
2023. ISBN: 979-8-88697-969-5 (eBook)

Barakoa (Masks) During COVID-19: Malevolent Pathogens and Pandemic Responses in Kenya After 600 Days
Stephen M. Magu, PhD (Editor)
2022. ISBN: 978-1-68507-798-3 (Hardcover)
2022. ISBN: 979-8-88697-014-2 (eBook)

Encyclopedia of Public Health (22 Volume Set)
Arnold Aboubacar (Editor)
Marguerita Hoyle (Editor)
2022. ISBN: 978-1-68507-015-1 (Hardcover)
2022. ISBN: 979-8-88697-084-5 (eBook)

More information about this series can be found at
https://novapublishers.com/product-category/series/public-health-in-the-21st-century/

Anne Winter
Editor

Healthcare Coverage

Legislation, Outcomes and Universal Coverage

snova
New York

NOTICE TO THE READER

Library of Congress Cataloging-in-Publication Data

ISBN: 979-8-89113-564-2

Published by Nova Science Publishers, Inc. † New York

Contents

Preface

More than 27 million people in the United States are uninsured, and even for some who do have insurance, it is not enough to insulate them from the significant cost of getting healthcare. Chapter 1 examines seven bills to improve Americans' healthcare and coverage. Chapter 2 looks at a proposal to transition our healthcare system to a national single-payer model where no patient is denied necessary medical care.

Chapter 1

Legislation to Improve Americans' Healthcare Coverage and Outcomes*

Committee on Energy and Commerce

Wednesday, January 8, 2020
House of Representatives, Subcommittee on Health,
Committee on Energy and Commerce,
Washington, DC.

The subcommittee met, pursuant to call, at 10:04 a.m., in room 2322, Rayburn House Office Building, Hon. Anna G. Eshoo (chairwoman of the subcommittee) presiding.

Members present: Representatives Eshoo, Engel, Matsui, Sarbanes, Schrader, Kennedy, Cárdenas, Welch, Ruiz, Dingell, Kuster, Kelly, Barragán, Blunt Rochester, Pallone (ex officio), Burgess (sub-committee ranking member), Upton, Shimkus, Guthrie, Griffith, Bilirakis, Long, Bucshon, Brooks, Mullin, Hudson, Carter, Gianforte, and Walden (ex officio).

Also present: Representatives Doyle and Soto.

Staff present: Austin Flack, Staff Assistant; Waverly Gordon, Deputy Chief Counsel; Stephen Holland, Health Counsel; Saha Khaterzai, Professional Staff Member; Zachary Keita, Intern; Aisling McDonough, Policy Coordinator; Meghan Mullon, Staff Assistant; Samantha Satchell, Professional Staff Member; Kimberlee Trzeciak, Chief Health Advisor; Rick Van Buren, Health Counsel; Madison Wendell, Intern; C. J. Young, Press

* This is an edited, reformatted and augmented version of Hearing before the Subcommittee on Health, of the Committee on Energy and Commerce, House of Representatives, One Hundred Sixteenth Congress, Second Session, Serial No. 116–85, dated January 8, 2020.

In: Healthcare Coverage
Editor: Anne Winter
ISBN: 979-8-89113-564-2

Secretary; Nolan Ahern, Minority Professional Staff Member, Health; S. K. Brown, Minority Press Assistant; William Clutterbuck, Minority Staff Assistant; Tyler Greenberg, Minority Staff Assistant; J. P. Paluskiewizc, Minority Chief Counsel, Health; Brannon Rains, Minority Legislative Clerk; and Kristen Shatynski, Minority Professional Staff Member, Health.

Ms. ESHOO. Good morning, everyone.

The Subcommittee on Health will now come to order. I just want to note that we will be recessing the hearing for an all-Member classified briefing today on Iran and Iraq at 1:00, so, if needed, we will return and continue the hearing once the briefing is complete.

The Chair now recognizes herself for 5 minutes for an opening statement.

Opening Statement of Hon. Anna G. Eshoo, a Representative in Congress from the State of California

I want to welcome our witnesses and thank them for being here, and the Chair wishes all of the members, everyone that is in the room, those that are here to observe, a blessed new year to each one of you and to your families.

Last year, our subcommittee was remarkably productive. We held 19 hearings and passed 31 bills, all of which had some bipartisan support, and today we will continue that progress by examining seven bipartisan bills to improve Americans' healthcare and coverage.

Our first panel will deal with three bills, important bills, that aim to prevent the single greatest tragedy a family can experience: the death of a child. Among developed nations, the United States has one of the highest infant mortality rates. For every 1,000 live births in our country, nearly 6 babies will not live to see their first birthday.

The Healthy Start Reauthorization Act of 2019 introduced by Representatives Tim Ryan and Anthony Gonzalez invests $135 million annually to improve birth outcomes in high-risk communities by providing services to women and families before, during, and after pregnancy. The Healthy Start program has been proven to reduce rates of low birth weights, preterm births, and prenatal opioid exposure.

We will also consider the Scarlett's Sunshine on Sudden Unexpected Death Act introduced by Representatives Gwen Moore and Tom Cole. We are honored today to have with us Scarlett's mother, Stephanie Zarecky. A warm welcome to you, Ms. Zarecky.

This is what I would consider an unimaginably difficult day for you because it is the third anniversary of Scarlett's unexplained death, so we are very grateful to you, and know that you are surrounded by a full room of people that care deeply about this and that you are here to inform us, and we will pay close attention to what you instruct us relative to action.

No family should suffer the death of a child without knowing why, yet over 400 children and 3,600 infants die each year from unexplained causes. We will honor these children today by considering the Scarlett's Sunshine Act, which provides funding to improve data collection and death scene investigations related to unexpected deaths and promotes safe sleep practices.

The third bill is the School-Based Allergies and Asthma Management Program Act introduced by Representatives Steny Hoyer and David Roe. Children should be able to go to school feeling secure that their school can handle an asthma attack or an allergic reaction. This is not the case today. The legislation preferentially awards children's asthma treatment grants to States whose public schools have plans for managing asthma—I like the sound; that is all right, let them fuss; it sounds good—for managing asthma and allergy triggers in emergencies.

With our second panel, we are going to consider four bills that close damaging gaps in health insurance coverage. The first is the Comprehensive Immunosuppressive Drug Coverage for Kidney Transplant Patient Act—mouthful, that is a mouthful—introduced by Representatives Ron Kind and our own Dr. Burgess.

While Medicare covers a lifetime of dialysis, kidney transplant recipients currently lose their Medicare coverage 36 months after transplant. It doesn't make sense. Without Medicare coverage for needed immunosuppressive drugs, transplant patients risk losing their new kidney. The legislation closes that gap by continuing coverage for kidney transplant recipients, which a nonpartisan HHS analysis found would save 375 kidney transplants each year.

The Ensuring Lasting Smiles Act, introduced by Representatives Collin Peterson and Denver Riggleman, requires health plans to cover medically necessary dental services related to a patient's congenital anomaly. About 4 percent of children in the United States are born with congenital anomalies such as cleft palate, and health plans systematically delay claims for dental-related procedures to treat them. This practice leaves families in debt from high out-of-pocket costs despite their paying for their health insurance that really should cover medically necessary procedures.

And the final two bills reform core pieces of the Medicare and Medicaid programs. And I am not going to go into them, but the Protecting Patients

Transportation Care Act was introduced by Buddy Carter—two members of this subcommittee, Buddy Carter and Tony Cárdenas. And we will have an excellent conversation about that, because Medicaid's coverage of transportation to health services is a lifeline for patients, especially those that live in rural or underserved areas.

And the final bill, introduced by Representatives Raul Ruiz and Jackie Walorski, updates the Part B enrollment process for the first time in 50 years.

So today's hearing, I would say, is bursting with commonsense legislation that will improve the health and the care for every American from the youngest to the oldest, and I am proud to help advance these bills and continue our record of bipartisan productivity in the new year.

[The prepared statement of Ms. Eshoo follows:][1]

Prepared Statement of Hon. Anna G. Eshoo

Good morning and welcome to the Health Subcommittee's first hearing of the new year.

Last year, our subcommittee was remarkably productive. We held 19 hearings and passed 31 bills, all of which had some sort of bipartisan support.

Today, we will continue that progress by examining seven bipartisan bills to improve Americans' healthcare and coverage.

Our first panel will deal with three bills that aim to prevent the single greatest tragedy a family can experience—the death of a child.

Among developed nations, the U.S. has one of the highest infant mortality rates. For every 1,000 live births in the United States, nearly 6 babies will not live to see their first birthday.

The Healthy Start Reauthorization Act of 2019 introduced by Representatives Tim Ryan and Anthony Gonzalez invests $135 million annually to improve birth outcomes in high-risk communities by providing services to women and families before, during, and after pregnancy.

The Healthy Start program has been proven to reduce rates of low birth weights, preterm births, and prenatal opioid exposure.

We will also consider the Scarlett's Sunshine on Sudden Unexpected Death Act introduced by Representatives Gwen Moore and Tom Cole.

---

[1] Text of the proposed legislation has been retained in committee files and also is available at https://docs.house.gov/Committee/Calendar/ByEvent.aspx?EventID=110355.

We're honored to hear testimony from Scarlett's mother, Stephanie Zarecky. Thank you, Ms. Zarecky, for joining us on an unimaginably difficult day for you— the third anniversary of Scarlett's unexplained death.

No family should suffer the death of a child without knowing why, yet over 400 children and 3,600 infants die each year from unexplained causes.

We will honor these children today by considering the Scarlett's Sunshine Act, which provides funding to improve data collection and death scene investigations related to unexpected deaths and promotes safe sleep practices.

The third bill is the School-Based Allergies and Asthma Management Program Act introduced by Representatives Steny Hoyer and David Roe.

Children should be able to go to school feeling secure that their school can handle an asthma attack or an allergic reaction. This is not the case today.

This legislation preferentially awards children's asthma treatment grants to States whose public schools have plans for managing asthma and allergy triggers and emergencies.

With our second panel, we will consider four bills that close damaging gaps in health insurance coverage.

I'm proud to be an original cosponsor on the first bill, the Comprehensive Immunosuppressive Drug Coverage for Kidney Transplant Patient Act introduced by Representative Ron Kind and Dr. Michael Burgess.

While Medicare covers a lifetime of dialysis, kidney transplant recipients currently lose their Medicare coverage 36 months after transplant. Without Medicare coverage for needed immunosuppressive drugs, transplant patients risk losing their new kidney.

The legislation closes that gap by continuing coverage for kidney transplant recipients, which a nonpartisan HHS analysis found would save 375 kidney transplants each year.

The Ensuring Lasting Smiles Act introduced by Representatives Collin Peterson and Denver Rigglemen requires health plans to cover medically necessary dental services related to a patient's congenital anomaly.

About 4 percent of children in the U.S. are born with congenital anomalies such as cleft palate, and health plans systematically delay claims for dental-related procedures to treat them.

This practice leaves families in debt from high out-of-pocket costs despite their paying for health insurance that should cover medically necessary procedures.

Our final two bills reform core pieces of the Medicare and Medicaid programs.

The Protecting Patients Transportation to Care Act introduced by Representatives Buddy Carter and Tony Cárdenas requires States to offer a nonemergency medical transportation benefit. Our committee also heard from Representative Sanford Bishop about this legislation during our Members Day panel.

Medicaid's coverage of transportation to health services is a lifeline for patients, especially those who live in rural or underserved areas.

Finally, the BENES Act introduced by Representatives Raul Ruiz and Jackie Walorski updates the Part B enrollment process for the first time in 50 years.

It requires Medicare to notify people nearing eligibility about their rights and responsibilities, protecting beneficiaries from a lifetime of financial penalties for failure to enroll promptly.

Today's hearing is bursting with commonsense legislation that will improve the health and care for every American, from the youngest to the oldest among us.

I'm proud to advance these bills and to continue our record of bipartisan productivity in the new year.

* * *

Ms. ESHOO. The Chair now recognizes the ranking member of our subcommittee for 5 minutes for his opening statement, Dr. Michael Burgess.

Opening Statement of Hon. Michael C. Burgess, a Representative in Congress from the State of Texas

Mr. BURGESS. And I thank the Chair, and we are considering seven bills this morning. We might call them the Magnificent Seven since they are the first bills to be considered in our health subcommittee this year. And these are bills designed to provide access to medical services or medicines for different American patients.

I am appreciative of the inclusion of H.R. 5534, the Comprehensive Immunosuppressive Drug Coverage for Kidney Transplant Patients Act of 2019. This is something where I have worked for nearly 10 years to try to effect. Congress enacted legislation in 1972 to allow certain individuals with end-stage renal disease to be covered under Medicare. It was the first time that individuals under the age of 65 became eligible to enroll in Medicare because of a medical condition.

Medicare beneficiaries with end-stage renal disease are about 1 percent of the total Medicare enrollment, but they are 7 percent of Medicare spending. These patients are incredibly ill. They often have numerous other costly chronic conditions.

A kidney transplant is an investment that the Government makes into the patient's future. Medicare pays for the patient's kidney transplant if they have this end-stage renal disease benefit, and that transplant should be a solid investment in the future health of that patient. Unfortunately, that investment is lost, and the patient's health will take a turn for the worst, if they cannot get their immunosuppressive drugs and then ultimately reject the kidney transplant. We should protect that investment.

Currently, Medicare covers only immunosuppressive drugs for 36 months. However, these patients require these immunosuppressives for the rest of their lives. H.R. 5534 directly addresses that problem by extending Medicare coverage of immunosuppressive drugs past 36 months for patients who do not obtain health coverage elsewhere. This is a policy that has the support from patients and transplant surgeons, and it is something the kidney community has been behind for years.

In July, I attended the launch of President Trump's Advancing American Kidney Health Initiative, which aims to improve care and foster innovation to benefit kidney patients across the country. This policy, H.R. 5534, aligns with the goals of the administration. In fact, both the Centers for Medicare and Medicaid Services Office of the Actuary and the Office of the Assistant Secretary for Planning and Evaluation at Health and Human Services have published reports on the benefits of extending Medicare coverage for immunosuppressive drugs, which includes financial savings for the Medicare program.

There is momentum. We can make a difference in the lives of kidney patients, and H.R. 5534 is a critical component of that effort as it will improve patient adherence to an immunosuppressive regimen and help ensure that patients can maintain their transplant and avoid future kidney-related complications.

Other bills are part of this hearing, and they include efforts to improve access to different types of care. For example, Representative Carter's bill, H.R. 3935, would continue the requirement that State Medicaid programs provide coverage of nonemergency transportation to medically necessary services.

Other bills such as H.R. 2477, the BENES Act, are well intentioned, and we want our health system working better for individuals, but we also know from the Congressional Budget Office that this particular bill comes with a significant cost. People may avoid late enrollment penalties, but we want to make sure that, in trying to ease enrollment, we do not harm the integrity of the enrollment processes.

H.R. 2271, the Scarlett's Sunshine on Sudden Unexpected Death Act, aims to improve the investigation of sudden unexpected deaths amongst infants and children. This bill has a goal similar to that of the Preventing Maternal Deaths Act, which was signed into law in the last Congress, and that would help States equip themselves to identify and address the causes of these tragedies.

H.R. 4801 will reauthorize the Healthy Start Program at the Health Resources and Services Administration, and it is also imperative in improving health outcomes for American mothers and children.

On the topic of children's health, 2468, the School-Based Allergies and Asthma Management Program Act, would equip schools to better handle asthma and allergies among students. Ten percent of children have asthma. Our schools must be better prepared to handle that growing population.

So, Madam Chair, I am glad we are looking at these bills today, and we had an agreement to consider them all before the subcommittee, and I hope other bills that we requested to be part of this hearing are soon under consideration.

I want to thank all of our witnesses for being here today and sharing their information with us, and I will yield back.

[The prepared statement of Mr. Burgess follows:]

Prepared Statement of Hon. Michael C. Burgess

Thank you, Madame Chair. Today we are considering seven bills that will help provide access to medical services or medicines for different American patients. I am most appreciative of the inclusion of H.R. 5534, the Comprehensive Immunosuppressive Drug Coverage for Kidney Transplant Patients Act of 2019, a policy that I have championed for nearly a decade.

Congress enacted legislation in 1972 to allow certain individuals with end-stage renal disease (ESRD) in Medicare, which was the first time that individuals under age 65 became eligible to enroll in Medicare because of a medical condition. Medicare beneficiaries with ESRD account for roughly 7 percent of Medicare fee-for-service spending, but only make up 1 percent of total Medicare enrollment. These patients are incredibly ill and often have numerous other costly chronic conditions.

A kidney transplant is an investment that the Government makes into the patient's future. Medicare pays for the patient's kidney transplant if they have the ESRD benefit, and that transplant should be a solid investment in the future health of that patient. Unfortunately, that investment is lost and the patient's health takes a turn for the worse if they cannot get their immunosuppressive drugs and reject their kidney transplant. We should protect that investment.

Currently, Medicare only covers immunosuppressive drugs for 36 months; however, these patients require these drugs for the rest of their lives. H.R. 5534 directly addresses that problem by extending Medicare coverage of immunosuppressive drugs past 36 months for patients that do not obtain healthcare coverage elsewhere. This is a policy that has the support from everyone from patients to transplant surgeons, and it is something that the kidney community has coalesced behind for years. In July, I attended the launch of President Trump's "Advancing American Kidney Health" Initiative, which aims to improve care and foster innovation to benefit kidney patients across the country. My policy, H.R. 5534, aligns with the goals of the administration. In fact, both the CMS Office of the Actuary and the Office of the Assistant Secretary for Planning and Evaluation at HHS have published reports on the benefits of extending Medicare coverage of immunosuppressive drugs, which include financial savings for the Medicare program.

There is momentum to make a difference in the lives of kidney patients, and H.R. 5534 is a critical component of this effort as it will improve patient adherence to immunosuppressive drugs and help to ensure that patients can maintain their transplant and hopefully avoid future kidney-related health care complications.

The other bills that are part of this hearing include efforts to improve patient access to different types of care. For example, Rep. Buddy Carter's bill, H.R. 3935, would continue the requirement that State Medicaid programs provide coverage of nonemergency transportation to medically necessary services. Other bills, such as H.R. 2477, the BENES Act, are well intentioned and we want our healthcare system to work better for individuals, but we know from the Congressional Budget Office that this particular bill has a cost. People may avoid late enrollment penalties, but we want to make sure that in trying to ease enrollment we do not harm the integrity of the enrollment process.

H.R. 2271, the Scarlett's Sunshine on Sudden Unexpected Death Act, aims to improve the investigation of sudden unexpected deaths among infants and children.

This bill has a goal similar to that of the Preventing Maternal Deaths Act, which was signed into law in December 2018, and would help States equip themselves to identify and address the causes of these tragedies. H.R. 4801, which would reauthorize the Healthy Start program at the Health Resources and Services Administration, is also imperative in improving healthcare outcomes for American mothers and children.

On the topic of children's health, H.R. 2468, the School-Based Allergies and Asthma Management Program Act, would equip schools to better handle asthma and allergies among students. According to the Centers for Disease Control and Prevention, 10 percent of children have asthma. Our schools must be prepared to handle that growing population so that children will be safe in school.

I am glad that we are looking at these bills today, as we had an agreement to consider them all before the subcommittee, but I do hope that the other bills we requested be a part of this hearing are considered soon. Thank you for all our witnesses for being here today, and I look forward to the discussion.

* * *

Ms. ESHOO. The gentleman yields back. I have the fullest intention to break our first-year record, so I look forward to more and more bills being heard, taken up, acted upon.

It is a pleasure to recognize the chairman of the full committee, Mr. Pallone, for his opening statement for 5 minutes.

Opening Statement of Hon. Frank Pallone, Jr., a Representative in Congress from the State of New Jersey

Mr. PALLONE. Thank you, Madam Chair.

Today, the Health Subcommittee continues its bipartisan work to improve health outcomes and healthcare coverage. Our first panel will examine three bills to improve health outcomes for babies and children.

The first bill, H.R. 2271, the Scarlett's Sunshine on Sudden Unexpected Death Act, will improve investigations, data collection, surveillance, and research into sudden unexpected infant death and sudden unexpected death in childhood. It also includes critical support for families who face these unimaginable tragedies. As the author of the Sudden Unexpected Death Data Enhancement and Awareness Act, which was signed into law by President Obama in 2014, I have long supported this cause, and I am glad we are taking further steps today.

The subcommittee will also examine H.R. 4801, the Healthy Start Reauthorization Act, which will enhance programs that support perinatal health, reduce infant mortality, and improve longterm health outcomes. Despite serving communities that have much higher rates of infant mortality, Healthy Start grantees have shown their ability to bring their community's overall infant mortality rate below the national average, demonstrating the program's success and the need to expand and strengthen it.

In rounding out the first panel, the subcommittee will review H.R. 2468, the School-Based Allergies and Asthma Management Program Act, a bill that will provide incentives for schools to help prevent and treat asthma and allergy-related emergencies.

Now, our second panel will examine four bills that improve health insurance coverage. H.R. 2477, the BENES Act, will provide individuals approaching Medicare eligibility with critical information about the Medicare enrollment process. This commonsense notice will empower people to make better choices about their healthcare coverage and avoid costly lifetime late enrollment penalties, and it will also eliminate harmful gaps in Medicare coverage.

We will also discuss H.R. 5534, the Comprehensive Immunosuppressive Drug Coverage for Kidney Transplant Patients Act. This bill removes the 36-month limit on Medicare coverage of immunosuppressive drugs after a kidney transplant surgery. Those who are fortunate enough to receive the kidney transplant rely on this medication for the rest of their lives, so it is important that Medicare offers the coverage necessary to protect the incredible gift of life that a transplant brings.

We also discuss H.R. 1379, the Ensuring Lasting Smiles Act, which requires all individual and group market health plans to cover medically necessary treatment resulting from congenital abnormalities. About 3 percent of American children are born with congenital abnormalities or birth defects that affect the way they look, develop, or function, and often for the rest of their lives.

So these children require serious medical treatment that is often not covered by health plans either because it is deemed cosmetic or because the treatment involves dental services. However, this treatment is critically important and medically necessary, particularly for children with serious dental anomalies.

Our witness today, Kevin Koser, will tell us about his family's longstanding struggles to get his son Kannon's medical treatment covered, and H.R. 1379 would ensure that children like Kannon get the treatment they need.

And finally, we will consider H.R. 3935, the Protecting Patients Transportation to Care Act, which will ensure that some of the most vulnerable Americans will continue to be able to access the care they need through Medicaid regardless of where they live.

These bills make important strides to improving health outcomes and health coverage. I agree with Chairwoman Eshoo, who said that these are—this is a group of very commonsense, rational proposals, and I look forward to the witnesses' testimony. Thank you, Madam Chair, and I yield back.

[The prepared statement of Mr. Pallone follows:]

Prepared Statement of Hon. Frank Pallone, Jr.

Today, the Health Subcommittee continues its bipartisan work to improve health outcomes and healthcare coverage.

Our first panel will examine three bills to improve health outcomes for babies and children. The first bill, H.R. 2271, the Scarlett's Sunshine on Sudden Unexpected Death Act, will improve investigations, data collection, surveillance, and research into sudden unexpected infant death and sudden unexpected death in childhood. It also includes critical support for families who face these unimaginable tragedies. As the author of the Sudden Unexpected Death Data Enhancement and Awareness Act, which was signed into law by President Obama in 2014, I have long supported this cause, and I am glad we are taking further steps today.

The subcommittee will also examine H.R. 4801, the Healthy Start Reauthorization Act, which will enhance programs that support perinatal health, reduce infant mortality, and improve long-term health outcomes. Despite serving communities that have had much higher rates of infant mortality, Healthy Start grantees have shown their ability to bring their communities' overall infant mortality rate below the national average, demonstrating the program's success and the need to expand and strengthen it.

Rounding out the first panel, the subcommittee will review H.R. 2468, the School-Based Allergies and Asthma Management Program Act, a bill that will provide incentives for schools to help prevent and treat asthma- and allergy-related emergencies.

On our second panel we will examine four bills that improve health insurance coverage. H.R. 2477, the BENES Act, will provide individuals approaching Medicare eligibility with critical information about the Medicare enrollment process. This commonsense notice will empower people to make better choices about their health care coverage and avoid costly, lifetime late enrollment penalties. It will also eliminate harmful gaps in Medicare coverage.

We will also discuss H.R. 5534, the Comprehensive Immunosuppressive Drug Coverage for Kidney Transplant Patients Act. This bill removes the 36-month limit on Medicare coverage of immunosuppressive drugs after a kidney transplant surgery. Those who are fortunate enough to receive a kidney transplant rely on this medication for the rest of their lives, so it's important that Medicare offers the coverage necessary to protect the incredible gift of life a transplant brings.

We will also discuss H.R. 1379, the Ensuring Lasting Smiles Act, which requires all individual and group market health plans to cover medically necessary treatment resulting from congenital abnormalities. About 3 percent of American children are born with congenital abnormalities or birth defects that affect the way they look, develop, or function, often for the rest of their lives.

These children require serious medical treatment that is often not covered by health plans, either because it is deemed "cosmetic," or because the treatment involves dental services. However, this treatment is critically important and medically necessary, particularly for children with serious dental anomalies. Our witness today, Kevin Koser, will tell us about his family's longstanding struggles to get his son Kannon's medical treatment covered. H.R. 1379 would ensure that children like Kannon get the treatment they need.

We will also consider H.R. 3935, the Protecting Patients Transportation to Care Act, which will ensure that some of the most vulnerable Americans will continue to be able to access the care they need, through Medicaid, regardless of where they live.

These bills make important strides to improve health outcomes and health coverage. I look forward to the witnesses' testimony and now yield the remainder of my time.

* * *

Ms. ESHOO. The gentleman yields back.

It is a pleasure to recognize the ranking member of the full committee, our friend from Oregon, Mr. Walden, for his 5 minutes.

Opening Statement of Hon. Greg Walden, a Representative in Congress from the State of Oregon

Mr. WALDEN. Thank you, Madam Chair, and welcome to everyone in the new year, and a good group of bills before us today in our first hearing of the new year.

As you know, at today's hearing, we will have the opportunity to review initiatives intended to advance public health and wellness in children as well as other proposals affecting the Medicare and Medicaid programs.

H.R. 2271, the Scarlett's Sunshine on Sudden Unexpected Death Act, works to improve current efforts to further understand both sudden unexplained infant death and sudden unexplained death in childhood.

I would like to thank Stephanie Zarecky for being here today, the mother of Scarlett for whom the bill is named, for being here to share Scarlett's story. It is really important.

Circumstances surrounding these unfortunate tragedies are oftentimes not fully understood, which makes determining the causes of sudden deaths of infants and children very challenging. H.R. 2271, as you know, would improve the comprehensiveness and standardization of child infant death investigations.

As someone who has lost a child, I can't imagine the added heartache of a child's death being without any explanation. My hope is this legislation will find answers to those questions, and more importantly, prevent deaths in the future.

In addition to H.R. 2271, we will review H.R. 4801, the Healthy Start Reauthorization Act, which reauthorizes grants to State and local organizations to provide services and support that reduce infant mortality and improve pregnancy outcomes.

We will also review H.R. 2468. That is the School-Based Allergy and Asthma Management Program Act. This bill authorizes the Department of Health and Human Services in making asthma-related grants to give preferences to a State with comprehensive school-based allergy and asthma management programs and include on-site personnel trained in the administration of allergy and asthma rescue medications.

We will also review H.R. 1379, the Ensuring Lasting Smiles Act, which will ensure that children with congenital anomalies have their medically necessary treatment covered by private insurance. Last year, I met with Dr. Keith Krueger, a surgeon in central Oregon, about this issue and heard the frustrations of his patients and their parents who had to fight too hard just to get the treatment covered.

So I think my colleagues on both sides of the aisle would agree that the language in this bill could be improved to avoid any unintended consequences, but I do believe we should fix this issue and give patients the peace of mind that their care will be covered.

We will also review H.R. 3935. That is the Protecting Patients Transportation to Care Act, which codifies in statute the non-emergency medical transportation benefits for the States, which has the odd distinction of being a mandatory benefit that is not in the statute but instead established through regulation.

So I am glad we are having a hearing on this bill, as it is critical we hear from States and communities served by this benefit as to how it is working and what value it brings to the Medicaid program.

Next, there is H.R. 2477, the BENES Act, which seeks to better align enrollment under Medicare Part B. The bill also seeks to provide more outreach to those eligible for Medicare Part B to sign up as soon as an individual is eligible and attempts to mitigate enrollment penalties for those who do not sign up in time.

The version of the bill we are considering today and what has been reported out of Ways and Means are both improvements over previously introduced versions, and I look forward to negotiating the language if the majority chooses to proceed with the markup, Madam Chair.

Finally, we will review H.R. 5534, which Dr. Burgess has championed for years. It is a great example of how Medicare rules can be nonsensical—not what he has championed, but what he wants to fix. Individuals who have received a kidney transplant require immunosuppressive drugs for the rest of their life in order to minimize the risk of their immune system rejecting the kidney.

Unfortunately, Medicare currently only provides payment for immunosuppressive drugs for 3 years, while providing coverage for a lifetime of dialysis treatments. So Medicare will currently pay for dialysis, pay for a transplant, pay for the drugs for 3 years, and then stop paying, so patients are more likely to lose their transplanted kidney, and then guess what, Medicare goes back to paying for dialysis, will pay for a new transplant and 3 more years of drug coverage.

Extending immunosuppressive drug coverage for the lifetime of kidney patients is a cost-effective way for the Federal Government to improve clinical outcomes for those with end-stage renal disease. Despite decades of legislative efforts and supporting clinical data, extending coverage for immunosuppressive drugs has not been passed into law. Though I am pleased we are reviewing this bill today, hopefully, we can change that in this year.

So together these are really important pieces of legislation, Madam Chair, and I look forward to hearing from our witnesses and working with you going into the new year.

And also, just as a note, I have to go down to the other subcommittee. We have two subcommittees meeting simultaneously. So some of us you will see come and go.

And so thanks for having this important hearing today, and I yield back the balance of my time.

[The prepared statement of Mr. Walden follows:]

Prepared Statement of Hon. Greg Walden

At today's hearing, we will have the opportunity to review initiatives intended to advance public health and wellness in children as well as other proposals affecting the Medicare and Medicaid programs.

H.R. 2271, the Scarlett's Sunshine on Sudden Unexpected Death Act, works to improve current efforts to further understand both sudden unexplained infant death (SUID) and sudden unexplained death in childhood (SUDC). I'd like to thank Stephanie Zarecky, the mother of Scarlett Pauley, who the bill is named after, for being here today to share Scarlett's story. The circumstances surrounding these unfortunate tragedies are oftentimes not fully understood, which makes determining the causes of sudden deaths of infants and children very challenging. H.R. 2271 would improve the comprehensiveness and standardization of child and infant death investigations. As someone who has lost a child, I can't imagine the added heartache of a child's death being without any explanation. My hope is this legislation will help us find those answers and prevent those deaths in the future.

In addition to H.R. 2271, we will review H.R. 4801, the Healthy Start Reauthorization Act, which reauthorizes grants to State and local organizations to provide services and supports that reduce infant mortality and improve pregnancy outcomes.

We will also review H.R. 2468, the School-Based Allergies and Asthma Management Program Act. This bill authorizes the Department of Health and Human Services in making asthma-related grants to give preference to a State with comprehensive school-based allergy and asthma management programs that include on-site personnel trained in the administration of allergy and asthma rescue medications.

We will also review H.R. 1379, the Ensuring Lasting Smiles Act, which would ensure children with congenital anomalies have their medically necessary treatment covered by private health insurance. Last year I met with Dr. Keith Krueger, a surgeon in central Oregon, about this issue and heard the frustrations of his patients— and their parents—who had to fight too hard just to get their treatment covered. I think my colleagues on both sides of the aisle would agree that the language in this bill could be improved to avoid any unintended consequences, but I do believe we should fix this issue and give patients the peace of mind that their care will be covered.

We will also review H.R. 3935, the Protecting Patients Transportation to Care Act, which codifies in statute the Nonemergency Medical Transportation benefit for States, which has the odd distinction of being a mandatory benefit that is not in the statute but instead established through regulation. I am glad that we are having a hearing on this bill as it is critical that we hear from States and the communities served by the this benefit as to how it is working and what value it brings to the Medicaid program.

Next, there is H.R. 2477, the BENES Act, which seeks to better align enrollment under Medicare Part B. The bill also seeks to provide more outreach to those eligible for Medicare Part B to sign up as soon as an individual is eligible and attempts to mitigate enrollment penalties for those who do not sign up in time. The version of the bill we are considering today and what has been reported out of Ways and Means are both improvements over previously introduced versions and I look forward to negotiating the language if the majority chooses to proceed to a markup.

Finally, we will review H.R. 5534, which Dr. Burgess has championed for years and is a great example of how Medicare rules can be nonsensical. Individuals who have received a kidney transplant require immunosuppressive drugs for the rest of their life in order to minimize the risk of their immune system rejecting the kidney. Unfortunately, Medicare currently only provides payment for immunosuppressive drugs for 3 years while providing coverage for a lifetime of dialysis treatments. So, Medicare will currently pay for dialysis, pay for a transplant, pay for the drugs for 3 years and then stop paying so patients are more likely to lose their transplanted kidney and then guess what? Medicare goes back to paying for dialysis, will pay for a new transplant and then 3 more years of drug coverage.

Extending immunosuppressive drug coverage for the lifetime of kidney patients is a cost-effective way for the Federal Government to improve clinical outcomes for those with End-Stage Renal Disease. Despite decades of legislative efforts and supporting clinical data, extending coverage for immunosuppressive drugs has not been passed into law. But I am pleased we are reviewing this bill today and hopefully we can change that this year.

Taken together these bills demonstrate this committee's commitment to addressing improved health outcomes in children and Medicare beneficiaries, and I look forward to hearing from our witnesses on these initiatives.

* * *

Ms. ESHOO. Thank you. The gentleman yields back.

The Chair reminds Members that, pursuant to committee rules, all Members' written openings statements shall be made part of the record.

Now I would like to introduce our witnesses for our first panel. First, our collective thanks to each one of you. Ms. Stephanie Zarecky, she is the mother of Scarlett Pauley and the public relations manager of the SUDC Foundation. Welcome to you. Thank you very much.

Dr. Lee Beers is president-elect of the American Academy of Pediatrics. Welcome to you. It is lovely to see you.

And Mr. Kenneth Mendez, it is great to see you, president and CEO of the Asthma and Allergy Foundation of America.

So we are all grateful for your testimony today. We look forward to hearing it. I think you are all familiar with the lights. Maybe Ms. Zarecky isn't, but green is go, yellow means red is coming up, and then we stop, OK.

So let me call on Ms. Zarecky first. You are recognized. You have 5 minutes, and we look forward to hearing your testimony.

And again, we are really indebted to you for traveling to us. And, as I said in my opening statement, this is a tough day, but just think of how you are optimizing your time and instructing us so that others hopefully will not have to bear the sorrow that you have. So you are recognized for 5 minutes.

Statements of Stephanie Zarecky, Mother of Scarlett Pauley, and Ambassador Program and Public Relations Manager, SUDC Foundation; Lee Beers, M.D., President-Elect, American Academy of Pediatrics; and Kenneth Mendez, President and Chief Executive Officer, Asthma and Allergy Foundation of America

Statement of Stephanie Zarecky

Ms. ZARECKY. Thank you. I thank the committee for inviting me today. I also thank Representatives Moore, Herrera Beutler, and Cole for introducing Scarlett's Sunshine Unexpected Death Act in the House of Representatives and Senators Casey and Isakson for their leadership in the Senate. I know this issue is one that the chairman and Ms. Moore in particular have cared about and worked on for many years.

As grateful as I am, I hope you will understand why I wish I weren't here. This legislation is named after my daughter Scarlett Lillian Pauley, and I am here because she cannot be. Today is the third anniversary of the worst day of my life, the day when the girl you see with big blue eyes and an angelic face left this Earth when she was just 16 months old. Scarlett lit up the world from the moment she entered it. She loved to read. Her favorite book was "Barnyard Dance!" by Sandra Boynton. Her face would light up when I would read it to her as she sat on my lap and my husband, Ryan, would do a dance that matched each line.

Scarlett also loved music. Her favorite song was "You Are My Sunshine" which is the inspiration for the legislation's name.

Scarlett loved to smile. She was known for her serious face, which led many to think she didn't like them, but we always knew it was just because she was studying them. Once she learned how much she loved to smile and to make others smile, Scarlett was never happy until she could get everyone around her smiling.

Scarlett loved life and made the most of her short one. January 7, 2017, Scarlett came down with a mild cold and had a slightly elevated temperature. Three years and approximately 16 hours ago, Scarlett enjoyed her bath and a final performance of "Barnyard Dance!" I nursed her to sleep, gave her warm cheeks some final kisses and put her in her crib. Three years and 11 hours ago, I checked on her, as parents often do, before heading to bed. I opened the door to her room, expecting to hear the sweet noises of her sleeping peacefully.

If you have children, I am sure you remember holding your breath waiting for your child to take their next one. If it took a bit too long, your heart would sink into your stomach until you heard that next sweet inhale and your heart bounced back to your chest. Three years and approximately 11 hours ago, that next breath never came for Scarlett.

The next hour is a blur of EMTs, police officers, ambulances, sitting on the bathroom floor praying to God for a miracle, a police car ride to the hospital, and being escorted into a room of doctors and nurses, one of whom I recall wiped away tears as we entered.

Three years and 10 hours ago, a doctor told us there was nothing more they could do and my Scarlett, the very reason for every beat of my heart and every breath I took, was gone.

To this day, we do not know what took Scarlett from us. We agonized for 5 months and 6 days waiting for the results of her autopsy. Even participating in research being conducted at New York University on deaths like Scarlett's did not give us answers as to why she is not here. Scarlett's death is considered sudden unexplained death in childhood, or SUDC. SUDC is a category of death in children between the ages of 1 and 18 that remains unexplained after a thorough investigation, including an autopsy.

At this time, we do not know what causes SUDC, how to predict it, or how to prevent it. Since losing Scarlett, we have been blessed with our second daughter, Eliana. She is the one making the noise in the back. Because we don't know what happened to Scarlett, we live every day in fear we will lose Eliana as well. We also don't know that it won't happen to your children or grandchildren.

According to the Centers for Disease Control and Prevention, SUDC occurs in about 400 children in the U.S. each year, but because of the lack of a specific way to record sudden and unexplained deaths in children that have been thoroughly investigated, it is impossible to know how widespread the problem is. And there are more than 3,600 infants lost annually to sudden unexpected infant death, or SUID, which is the sudden death of an infant under 1 year of age that when first discovered did not have an obvious cause.

Research into the potential causes of SUDC and SUID is desperately needed. Facilitating and standardizing data collection and analysis, as this legislation seeks to do, is an essential step in one day preventing these tragedies. Losing a child is the single greatest pain we could ever imagine, and to be without answers as to why magnifies it exponentially.

We read parenting books, followed all recommended safe sleep guidelines, and made sure Scarlett received good medical care. Yet we still lost our healthy, thriving, precious baby girl. It is an unimaginable tragedy no parent should have to live with, and there are thousands of us who do it every day.

We have done far too little for far too long to try to stop these tragedies. We have to change that in memory of all the children who are deeply loved and dearly missed, and for the future of all children.

Scarlett's Sunshine on Unexpected Death Act will help us take steps to solve this medical mystery and prevent future deaths, and I thank the committee for their support of it.

[The prepared statement of Ms. Zarecky follows:]

* * *

I thank the Committee for inviting me today. I also thank Representatives Moore, Hererra Beutler and Cole for introducing Scarlett's Sunshine on Unexpected Death Act in the House of Representatives and Senators Casey and Isakson for their leadership in the Senate. I know this issue is one the Chairman and Ms. Moore, in particular, have cared about and worked on for many years.

As grateful as I am, I hope you will understand why I wish I weren't here. This legislation is named after my daughter, Scarlett Lillian Pauley, and I am here because she cannot be. Today is the third anniversary of the worst day of my life – the day when the girl you see with big, blue eyes and an angelic face left this earth when she was just 16 months old.

Scarlett lit up our world from the moment she entered it. She loved to read. Her favorite book was *Barnyard Dance* by Sandra Boynton. Her face would light up when I would read it to her as she sat on my lap, and my husband Ryan would do a dance that matched each line. Scarlett also loved music. Her favorite song was "You are My Sunshine," which is the inspiration for the legislation's name.

Scarlett loved to smile. She was known for her "serious face," which led many to think she didn't like them. But we always knew it was just because she was studying them. Once she learned how much she loved to smile and make others smile, Scarlett was never happy until she could get everyone around her smiling.

Scarlett loved life and made the most of her short one.

January 7th, 2017 Scarlett came down with a mild cold and had a slightly elevated temperature.

Three years and approximately 16 hours ago, Scarlett enjoyed playing in her bath and a final performance of *Barnyard Dance*. I nursed her to sleep, gave her warm cheek some final kisses and put her in her crib.

Three years and 11 hours ago, I checked on her as parents often do before heading to bed. I opened the door to her room, expecting to hear the sweet noises of her sleeping peacefully. If you have children, I'm sure you remember holding your breath waiting for your child to take their next one. If it took a bit too long, your heart would sink into your stomach until you heard that next sweet inhale and your heart bounced back to your chest. Three years and approximately 11 hours ago, that next breath never came for Scarlett.

The next hour is a blur of EMTs, police officers, ambulances, sitting on the bathroom floor praying to God for a miracle, a police car ride to the hospital and being escorted into a room of doctors and nurses, one of whom I recall wiped away tears as we entered.

Three years and 10 hours ago, a doctor told us there was nothing more they could do and my Scarlett, the very reason for every beat of my heart and every breath I took, was gone.

To this day, we do not know what took Scarlett from us. We agonized for five months and six days waiting for the results of her autopsy. Even participating in research being conducted at New York University on deaths like Scarlett's did not give us answers on why she is not here.

Scarlett's death is considered Sudden Unexplained Death in Childhood, or SUDC. SUDC is a category of death in children between the ages of 1 and 18 that remains unexplained after a thorough investigation, including an autopsy. At this time, we do not know what causes SUDC, how to predict it or how to prevent it.

Since losing Scarlett, we have been blessed with our second daughter, Eliana. Because we don't know what happened to Scarlett, we live every day in fear we will lose Eliana as well. We also don't know it won't happen to your children or grandchildren.

According to the Centers for Disease Control and Prevention, SUDC occurs in about 400 children in the U.S. each year, but because of the lack of a specific way to record sudden and unexplained deaths in children that have been thoroughly investigated, it is impossible to know how widespread the problem is. And there are more than 3,600 infants lost annually to Sudden Unexpected Infant Death, or SUID, which is the sudden death of an infant under one year of age that, when first discovered, did not have an obvious cause.

Research into the potential causes of SUDC and SUID is desperately needed. Facilitating and standardizing data collection and analysis as this legislation seeks to do is an essential step in one day preventing these tragedies.

Losing a child is the single greatest pain we could ever imagine. And to be without answers as to why magnifies it exponentially. We read parenting books, followed all recommended safe sleep guidelines and made sure Scarlett received good medical care. Yet, we still lost our healthy, thriving, precious baby girl. It is an unimaginable tragedy no parent should have to live with, and there are thousands of us who do it every day.

We have done far too little for far too long to try to stop these tragedies. We have to change that, in memory of all the children who are deeply loved and dearly missed and for the future of all children.

Scarlett's Sunshine on Unexpected Death Act will help us take steps to solve this medical mystery and prevent future deaths, and I thank the Committee for their support of it.

* * *

Ms. ESHOO. We thank you. I want to recognize our colleague, Congressman Mike Doyle, that is here. Ms. Zarecky is represented by Congressman Doyle, and the reason that he hasn't spoken up yet is because he is not a member of our subcommittee.

We have these funny rules around here, but he will be recognized, but it is after members of the committee are—we finish recognizing them, but we welcome Congressman Doyle to the subcommittee and for your testimony.

I now would like to recognize Dr. Lee Beers. Again, the president-elect of the American Academy of Pediatrics. Welcome to you, and you have 5 minutes for your testimony.

Statement of Lee Beers, M.D.

Dr. BEERS. Wonderful. Good morning, Chairwoman Eshoo, Ranking Member Burgess, and members of the subcommittee. My name is Dr. Lee Beers, and I am a pediatrician and president-elect of the American Academy of Pediatrics.

First, thank you, Ms. Zarecky, for your powerful testimony.

I am here today officially representing the AAP, a nonprofit professional medical organization of over 67,000 pediatricians, pediatric medical subspecialists, and pediatric surgical specialists.

Thank you for holding this hearing today on a number of bills to improve health outcomes. Today I will speak to two of them, the Scarlett's Sunshine on Sudden Unexpected Death Act and the Healthy Start Reauthorization Act. The AAP strongly supports both pieces of legislation. Together, these bills will help reduce infant mortality, prevent sudden unexpected infant and child death, and promote healthy child development.

I will first discuss opportunities to address sleep-related infant deaths and other unexplained child deaths through the AAP-endorsed Scarlett's Sunshine on Sudden Unexpected Death Act.

In the 1990s AAP recommended that babies sleep on their back and partnered with government agencies on a successful Back to Sleep campaign. These efforts initially led to a substantial declined in sudden unexplained infant deaths. However, we have seen little progress in over a decade, and persistent racial and ethnic disparities remain.

To make additional progress, we need better information on the circumstances surrounding sleep-related death and other unexplained child death and to better promote what we already know about keeping children safe.

Scarlett's Sunshine would help improve and standardize death scene investigations and autopsies and would provide training on best practices. In addition, the bill would expand the vital work of child death review teams. It would help promote evidence-based, safe infant sleep, including providing safe sleep products like cribs and play yards to low-income families.

Finally, the bill would authorize funding for parent support services like grief and bereavement counseling. I vividly remember the first time I consoled a grieving father in the emergency department after losing his infant son to a sleep-related death. The lack of answers or services for this family left me feeling helpless and angry.

Scarlett's Sunshine would help us better understand and prevent these and similar tragedies while better supporting affected families. I urge the committee to advance this legislation as written.

I also thank the committee for advancing the Safe Sleep for Babies Act, which would ban dangerous inclined sleepers and crib bumpers. The full House passed that bill last year, and we urge the Senate to pass it without delay.

The AAP also strongly supports the Healthy Start Reauthorization Act of 2019. In the United States, the infant mortality rate fell by 14 percent between 2007 and 2017. Healthy Start has played a critical role in this success by working to ensure that women living in communities with higher than average infant mortality rates have access to early prenatal, post partum, and infant care.

However, despite a declining infant mortality rate nationally, significant inequities persist in infant birth outcomes. In fact, infants born to non-Hispanic Black, Native American, Alaskan Native, and Pacific Islander mothers all experience higher than average rates of mortality.

Maternal mortality is also a serious ongoing crisis in the United States. According to the CDC, the national rate of maternal mortality has more than doubled since 1987. Alarmingly, Black women, Native Americans, and Alaska Natives are 2 to 3 times more likely to experience pregnancy-related deaths regardless of socioeconomic status.

These staggering statistics on maternal health and infant mortality illustrate the importance of reauthorizing Healthy Start. As a pediatrician right here in Washington, DC, I have seen firsthand the need for and the positive impact of programs like Healthy Start.

Mothers, infants, and families greatly benefit from the connection to resources that may not otherwise be available to them, including healthcare services like prenatal care, enabling services like case management, and public health services such as immunizations.

The Healthy Start Program has positively impacted families and communities throughout the United States and here in DC. For instance, in 2015, Healthy Start reduced infant mortality rates among program participants compared to the national rate. Despite its success, this program has not been renewed since 2013.

The Healthy Start Reauthorization Act of 2019 would not only reauthorize this essential program for 5 years, it also makes key updates, including explicit consideration of social determinants of health. We know that negative social influences can impact physical health, social, emotional development, and educational achievement throughout the life span.

Healthy Start is a much-needed program that works in reducing preterm birth, infant mortality, and maternal mortality. We urge its swift reauthorization.

Thank you for the opportunity to be here today, and I look forward to answering any questions you may have.

[The prepared statement of Dr. Beers follows:]

Statement of Lee Beers, MD, FAAP, on behalf of the American Academy of Pediatrics, before the U.S. House of Representatives, Committee on Energy and Commerce, Health Subcommittee, "Legislation to Improve Americans' Health Care Coverage and Outcomes," January 8, 2020

Good morning. Chairwoman Eshoo, Ranking Member Burgess, and members of the subcommittee, it is my pleasure to be here today to address vitally important legislation to advance and protect child health. My name is Dr. Lee Beers and I am a pediatrician and the president-elect of the American Academy of Pediatrics (AAP). I am here today officially representing the AAP, a non-profit professional medical organization of over 67,000 pediatricians, pediatric medical subspecialists, and pediatric surgical specialists across the United States. In addition, I am an Associate Professor of Pediatrics at Children's National Hospital here in Washington, DC, where I serve as the Medical Director of Community Health and Advocacy in the Child Health Advocacy Institute. I also co-direct the Early Childhood Innovation Network, a local collaborative that works to promote the healthy development of young children who are exposed to early childhood adversity.

Thank you for holding this hearing today on a number of bills to improve health outcomes and coverage. Today, I will speak to two of them: the Scarlett's Sunshine on Sudden Unexpected Death Act (H.R. 2271) and the Healthy Start Reauthorization Act (H.R. 4801). The AAP strongly supports both pieces of legislation. Together these bills will help reduce infant mortality, prevent sudden unexpected infant death, and promote healthy child development.

Scarlett's Sunshine on Sudden Unexpected Death Act

I will first discuss policy opportunities to address sleep-related infant and child deaths through the Scarlett's Sunshine on Sudden Unexpected Death Act. The AAP endorsed this important bipartisan legislation as a key component of a comprehensive federal policy agenda to protect more children and prevent more families from the tragedy of losing a child. This is an issue of critical importance to the Academy, and we appreciate the Committee's ongoing efforts to prevent and address these fatalities through this and other related legislation.

Sudden unexpected infant deaths (SUID) are those occurring among infants younger than one year of age where the cause of death is not obvious before investigation, often occurring during sleep. Sudden unexplained death in childhood (SUDC) refers to the death of a child older than 12 months, which remains unexplained after a thorough case review. The Centers for Disease Control and Prevention (CDC) estimates that in 2017 there were approximately 3,600 SUID cases, and that SUDC affected approximately 243 children between 1 and 4 years of age.[2]

In the 1990s, the AAP introduced its revised safe sleep guidelines recommending supine—on the back—sleep positioning. The AAP also partnered with government agencies on the successful Back to Sleep campaign.

These efforts generated a major public health advance in the form of a substantial decline in SUID, from over 150 SUID cases per 100,000 live births in 1990 to 93.4 SUID cases per 100,000 live births in 2017.[3] However, we have seen very little progress in reducing SUID in a decade or more, and these numbers remain unacceptably high. There also remain large disparities in the incidence and prevalence of SUID and SUDC based on race and ethnicity, with disproportionately high rates among black and Native American families. This is a significant public health issue necessitating a multifaceted approach to best understand the problem and effectively address it.

As a pediatrician, I know that questions related to sleep are at the top of any new parent's list when they come to see me. The guidance I give parents is critical to promoting safe sleep practices, but it alone will not suffice. Parents want to know why I am making these safe sleep recommendations, and to understand why they are so important 100 percent of the time when frankly, they may be receiving differing advice from family members or feeling so desperately tired they think, "I'll bring my baby in bed with me just this one time." We need to better understand why infants and young children continue to die during sleep, and how we can prevent it through policy reform and revised clinical practice and anticipatory guidance. Scarlett's Sunshine offers a major opportunity to make significant progress in reducing sleep-related deaths. I'd like to highlight key provisions of the bill that the AAP believes are essential to this work.

Scarlett's Sunshine would authorize $8 million annually to improve and standardize death scene investigations and autopsies, and $2 million annually

---

[2] See https://www.cdc.gov/sids/data.htm#suid-chart.

[3] https://www.cdc.gov/sids/data.htm#suid-chart.

to support training to implement those approaches. This would entail new guidance for better data reporting on circumstances surrounding SUID and SUDC, and grants to states to support the completion of comprehensive and standardized death scene investigations and autopsies. Because progress has plateaued on reducing sleep-related fatalities, it's vital that we better understand risk factors to prevent future deaths. We need to know if the problem is that we still are not reaching enough families with education about safe sleep, if that education needs to be reframed to address different cultural or socio-economic considerations, if infants are in particular unsafe sleep environments such as an inclined sleeper or a crib with bumpers and soft bedding, or if yet another factor is still contributing to sleep-related deaths. This approach would help us better understand SUID and SUDC, ultimately enabling pediatricians like me to best tailor our guidance to families to prevent these tragedies.

In addition, the bill would support the vital work of child death review teams. Pediatricians around the country serve on child death review teams, which can operate either locally or statewide. This is essential work that studies the sentinel events of unexpected child deaths to understand how to prevent such fatalities in the future. Unfortunately, these teams often operate with little to no funding support, and the scope and breadth of their work varies significantly nationwide. Scarlett's Sunshine would authorize $15 million annually for states and localities to build capacity to review 100 percent of all infant and child deaths. The bill's provision to enhance the CDC's National Fatality Review Case Reporting System would draw upon these efforts and further support evidence-based policymaking to prevent child deaths.

The bill also would take critical steps to better meet families' needs in preventing and responding to sleep-related deaths. The authorization of $5 million annually for the promotion of evidence-based safe infant sleep would support prevention approaches including home visits, public education campaigns, and the provision of safe sleep products like cribs and play yards to low-income families. The AAP particularly appreciates the bill's clarity on the types of guidance and products these grants would provide, to ensure they adhere to safe sleep guidelines. It's critical that these resources only promote the use of safe sleep environments, especially given the proliferation of untested and often dangerous sleep-related products, including crib bumpers, inclined sleepers, and in-bed sleepers. In addition, we strongly appreciate that the bill would authorize $1 million annually for parent support services, like grief and bereavement counseling. Losing a child is the deepest grief a parent can imagine, and these are essential services to help them in their time of need.

I still remember like it was yesterday—twelve years ago, when pregnant with my own son-consoling a father in the emergency department who was cradling his infant son, who had just been lost to Sudden Unexplained Infant Death. And then, the feelings of helplessness, and even anger, I felt afterwards when despite our best efforts, our team was unable to identify timely and accessible grief counseling for this unimaginably suffering family.

I'd like to also note that the AAP strongly supports the Committee's leadership in advancing legislation this year to ban dangerous crib bumpers and inclined sleepers like the recalled Rock 'n Play. We appreciate that the full U.S. House advanced these policies together in the *Safe Sleep for Babies Act* (H.R. 3172), and we continue to urge the Senate to pass that legislation without delay. The enactment of Scarlett's Sunshine will build on the Committee's leadership in preventing infant and child fatalities, and we urge the Committee to advance this important legislation as written.

Healthy Start Reauthorization Act of 2019

I will now turn to the Healthy Start Reauthorization Act of 2019. In the United States, infant mortality – defined as the death of a child before his or her first birthday – has been declining. Nationally, the infant mortality rate fell by 14 percent between 2007 and 2017.[4] Since 1991, Healthy Start has played a critical role in this effort to reduce infant mortality rates across the country. Healthy Start aims to improve birth outcomes by working to ensure that women living in communities with infant mortality rates at least 1.5 times the national average have access to early prenatal, postpartum, and infant care. It serves women of reproductive age, pregnant women, postpartum mothers, and infants and families from birth until the child is 18 months old. Each family enrolled in the program receives a comprehensive assessment that considers physical and behavioral health, employment, housing, domestic violence risks, and more. While known for the prenatal care it provides, the program also offers many other support services like case management, home visiting services, parenting skill-building, transportation, child-care, and breast feeding and nutrition support, to name a few, as well as provider training.

[4] Kamal R, Hudman J, and McDermott D. "What do we know about infant mortality in the U.S. and comparable countries?" *Peterson Center on Healthcare and the Kaiser Family Foundation Health System Tracker*. Published on October 18, 2019. Accessed on December 30, 2019. Accessed from: https://www.healthsystemtracker.org/chart-collection/infant-mortality-u-s-compare-countries/#item-.

However, despite recent reductions in the national infant mortality rate, significant inequities unfortunately remain. The mortality rate for infants born to non-Hispanic black mothers is more than twice as high as that for infants born to non-Hispanic white mothers.[5] Non-Hispanic black mothers also have the highest rates of preterm birth and low birth weight among all racial and ethnic groups.[6] Moreover, the mortality rate remains higher than average for infants born to Native American, Alaska Native, and Pacific Islander mothers.[7] These rates are evidence of worrisome infant health disparities and deserve our attention. Healthy Start attempts to alleviate this problem through providing intensive and culturally sensitive parent support. In addition to reducing infant mortality rates overall, Healthy Start aims to reduce racial and ethnic disparities among birth outcomes. The prevalence of these infant health inequities underscores the continued need for Healthy Start programs in vulnerable communities.

Maternal mortality is also a serious, ongoing crisis in the United States. According to the CDC, the national rate of maternal mortality has more than doubled between 1987 and 2016.[8] Alarmingly, black women, Native Americans, and Alaska Natives are two to three times more likely to experience pregnancy-related deaths regardless of socioeconomic status. Studies indicate that more than half of these deaths are preventable.[9] Again, these staggering statistics illustrate the importance of reauthorizing Healthy Start. Along with improving infant health outcomes, Healthy Start seeks to reduce maternal mortality rates and improve women's health before, during, and after pregnancy.

As a pediatrician in Washington, DC with a focus on community pediatrics, I have seen firsthand the need for and the positive impact of programs like Healthy Start. My experience is that every family wants the best for their child but sometimes doesn't have the support they need to ensure their child grows up in a safe and stable home with access to quality education.

---

[5] Ely DM, Driscoll AK. Infant mortality in the United States, 2017: Data from the period linked birth/infant death file. *National Vital Statistics Reports*, vol 68 no 10. Hyattsville, MD: National Center for Health Statistics. 2019.

[6] Ely DM, Driscoll AK.

[7] Ely DM, Driscoll AK.

[8] US Centers for Disease Control and Prevention. Pregnancy Mortality Surveillance System. Updated on October 10, 2019. Accessed on December 30, 2019. Accessed from: https://www.cdc.gov/reproductivehealth/maternal-mortality/pregnancy-mortality-surveillance-system.htm.

[9] US Centers for Disease Control and Prevention. Vital Signs: Pregnancy-related Deaths. Updated on May 7, 2019. Accessed on December 30, 2019. Accessed from: https://www.cdc.gov/vitalsigns/maternal-deaths/.

Mothers, infants, and families greatly benefit from the connection to resources that may not otherwise be available to them, including health care services such as prenatal care, enabling and social services such as case management and child care, and public health services such as immunization and health education. Healthy Start also supports provider training to help ensure that patients receive targeted and appropriate comprehensive services no matter where they receive their care.

Here in Washington, DC, there are great inequities in access to needed prenatal care and wide disparities in birth outcomes. For example, according to a Perinatal Health and Infant Mortality Report issued in April 2018 by the DC Department of Health, for the period covering 2006 through 2016, the percentage of preterm births for non-Hispanic Black mothers was double the percentage for White mothers, which can lead to long term negative health and educational outcomes for children. In addition, the percentage of preterm births was nearly three times higher for women who did not receive prenatal care compared to women who entered prenatal care in their 1st trimester. During 2015-2016, 52 percent of non-Hispanic black mothers entered prenatal care in the 1st trimester compared to 86 percent of non-Hispanic white mothers and 64 percent of Hispanic mothers, highlighting the impact that poor access to prenatal care can have on infant health.

The Healthy Start program is working and has impacted families and communities throughout the United States. In 2015, Healthy Start reduced infant mortality rates among Healthy Start program participants to 5.2 infant deaths per 1,000 live births – lower than the national rate of 5.96. That same year, 68.3 percent of Healthy Start participants initiated prenatal care during the first trimester. Healthy Start also helps remove barriers to accessing health care. It helps eligible women and children enroll in Medicaid or private insurance, and in 2014 over 92 percent of program participants had some form of health insurance, further increasing their access to critical health services.

Despite its success, this program has not been reauthorized since 2013. The Healthy Start Reauthorization Act of 2019 would not only reauthorize this essential infant and maternal health program for another five years, it would also provide a necessary increase in the authorized appropriations level.

This bill also makes key changes and updates to the program, including explicit consideration of social determinants of health. The AAP wholeheartedly supports this update to the program, as we know that negative environmental influences can lead to adverse health outcomes in birth, childhood, and across the lifespan, negatively affecting physical health, socioemotional development, and educational achievement. We know that poverty, a key determinant of health, has a profound effect on indicators such as birth weight and infant mortality.[10] Child poverty also influences genomic function and brain development, mediated by exposure to toxic stress,[11] a condition characterized by "excessive or prolonged activation of the physiologic stress response systems in the absence of the buffering protection afforded by stable, responsive relationships."[12] These impacts on child brain development begin prenatally. As such, it is crucial that Healthy Start formally recognizes these challenges and supports providers in addressing them as it continues to deliver services.

This reauthorization of Healthy Start also encourages grant applicants to collaborate with local communities in the development of their projects. As a pediatrician who works with multi-disciplinary partners in the local community, including parent run organizations, I cannot emphasize enough how important it is to collaborate with local organizations and leaders when developing programs and initiatives that will provide services in a local community. This is crucial in the development of quality and responsive programs and in gaining buy-in from participating providers and, most especially, those who will receive services.

For all these reasons, the AAP supports the reauthorization of the Healthy Start program. It is a much-needed program that works in reducing preterm birth, infant mortality, and maternal mortality. If we want to continue to improve the lives of mothers and babies across the country, Congress must reauthorize Healthy Start immediately.

Thank you for the opportunity to be here today. We look forward to working with the subcommittee to quickly advance these two important bills for child health.

---

[10] AAP Policy Statement. Poverty and Child Health in the United States. COUNCIL ON COMMUNITY PEDIATRICS. Pediatrics Apr 2016, 137 (4) e20160339; DOI: 10.1542/peds.2016-0339. https://pediatrics.aappublications.org/content/137/4/e20160339.

[11] Boyle CA, Boulet S, Schieve LA, et al. *Trends in the prevalence of developmental disabilities in US children, 1997-2008. Pediatrics. 2011;127(6):1034–1042pmid:21606152.*

[12] Garner AS, Shonkoff JP; Committee on Psychosocial Aspects of Child and Family Health; Committee on Early Childhood, Adoption, and Dependent Care; Section on Developmental and Behavioral Pediatrics. *Early childhood adversity, toxic stress, and the role of the pediatrician: translating developmental science into lifelong health. Pediatrics. 2012;129(1). www.pediatrics.org/cgi/content/full/129/1/e224pmid:22201148.*

Ms. ESHOO. Thank you, Dr. Beers. I think you would be pleased to know that the subcommittee has addressed the issue of maternal mortality rates in our country, and that legislation now awaits the full committee.

It is a pleasure to—the floor. I am sorry. Big difference between the two. But we are on our way on that one. It is just a horrible statistic, shameful statistic in our country.

It is a pleasure to recognize Mr. Mendez for 5 minutes for your testimony. Welcome again and thank you.

Statement of Kenneth Mendez

Mr. MENDEZ. Thank you, Chairwoman Eshoo, Ranking Member Burgess, and members of the committee. I am Kenneth Mendez, president and CEO of the Asthma and Allergy Foundation of America, or AAFA. AAFA is the leading patient organization for Americans with asthma and allergies and the oldest asthma and allergy patient group in the world.

Thank you for inviting me to offer testimony in support of 2468, the School-Based Allergies and Asthma Management Program Act. This bipartisan bill is an important step in promoting health and even preventing death for the millions of American children living with asthma and with food allergies. First, I would like to give you some perspective on American children living with asthma and food allergies, and then I would like to tell you how this bill helps.

One in 13 American children have asthma. One in 13 have food allergies. This means that every school in the U.S. is likely to have children with these conditions. Imagine breathing through a straw filled with cotton and the fear you would feel knowing you weren't getting enough air to breathe. That is what it is like to have asthma.

About 3,600 people die every year from asthma in the U.S. For example, just last month, we heard about a 13-year-old Broadway star, Laurel Griggs, dying of an asthma attack. No one needs to die from asthma.

Here are some more statistics. Asthma is the most common chronic disease among children and major cause of childhood disability. Asthma is more common among children from low-income families and among Black and Hispanic children. Childhood asthma is one of the top reasons for missed school days, close to 13.8 million missed school days, and substantial economic costs through lost work days for caregivers.

Now, imagine having a life-threatening food allergy where accidental exposure to a known food allergen can trigger an allergic reaction that could kill you if you don't have life-saving epinephrine administered in the first few minutes of the reaction. That is what it is like to live with food allergies.

Food allergy deaths are relatively rare but are tragic and often preventable. Food allergy prevalence among children, along with related emergency department visits, have increased sharply over the past two decades. Food allergy prevalence among children increased by 50 percent, with peanut allergies more than tripling.

Schools can help by preparing to address emergency situations, promoting awareness among teachers and staff, and providing a safe and healthy school environment that minimizes asthma and allergy triggers.

AAFA issues a State honor roll looking at asthma and allergy policies related to schools. We have seen a great deal of progress over the years in many areas, with 15 States on our 2019 honor roll compared to 8 in 2013.

However, there are still too many gaps. For example, only 27 States require schools to have emergency protocols for asthma and only 36 require emergency protocols for anaphylaxis. Only 24 States require schools to maintain allergy and asthma incidents reports. Only 12 require indoor air quality management plans, and only 8 accept acceptable minimum standards for nurse-to-school ratios.

H.R. 2468 would help address these gaps by creating a grant-making preference in CDC's existing asthma grants program for those States that require all public secondary and elementary schools to have certain key measures in place as part of a comprehensive school-based allergy and asthma management program.

The bill has support from a number of major stakeholder organizations, including AAFA, the two major allergy, asthma, and immunology doctor organizations, the National Association of School Nurses, and other nonprofit patient organizations in the asthma and allergy community.

This bill is important because both asthma and food allergies present serious threats to health and children's learning, as well as posing enormous economic burdens on families and on the healthcare system.

This bill will help children be safe, healthy, and ready to learn. AAFA is grateful for the subcommittee's consideration of the bill, and we stand ready to help the committee in any way.

[The prepared statement of Mr. Mendez follows:]

Written Statement of Kenneth Mendez, President and CEO, Asthma and Allergy Foundation of America, U.S. House of Representatives Committee on Energy and Commerce, Subcommittee on Health, Hearing on "Legislation to Improve Americans' Health Care Coverage and Outcomes," January 8, 2019

Introduction

Chairwoman Eshoo, Ranking Member Burgess, and Members of the Subcommittee:

I am Kenneth Mendez, President and CEO of the Asthma and Allergy Foundation of America, or AAFA. AAFA is the leading patient organization for people with asthma and allergies, and the oldest asthma and allergy patient group in the world. Thank you for inviting me to offer testimony in support of H.R. 2468, the School-Based Allergies and Asthma Management Program Act.

This bipartisan bill is an important step in promoting health and learning for the 5.5 million American children living with asthma and the nearly 6 million American children with food allergies. Put differently, 1 in 13 children have asthma, and 1 in 13 have food allergies – meaning that every school in the U.S. is likely to have children with these conditions. The bill would create a preference within the Centers for Disease Control and Prevention's (CDC) existing asthma grant program for states that require schools to take a series of actions to address asthma and food allergy. AAFA strongly supports this legislation.

Background: Asthma and Allergy in Schools

Both asthma and food allergies present serious threats to children's health and learning.

Asthma is the most common chronic disease among children and a major cause of childhood disability.[13] In 2018, an estimated 8.5 million children under the age of 18 had ever been diagnosed with asthma, and 5.5 million were

[13] Ferrante G, Grutta SL. The burden of pediatric asthma. *Front Pediatr.* 2018; 6:186.

currently living with asthma, translating to about 1 in 13 children in the U.S. living with the condition.[14]

Among children, the highest rates of asthma are seen in those who are school-aged. Eight percent of children aged 5 to 11 years old were living with asthma in 2018, as were 9.9 percent of children aged 12-17.[15]

Asthma disproportionately affects children from low-income families. Poor children are more likely to have asthma, less likely to be able to manage symptoms, more likely to visit the emergency department, and more likely to be admitted to the hospital due to an uncontrolled episode.[16] In 2018, the asthma prevalence for children in poverty was 10 percent; the rate among children not in poverty was 6 percent.[17]

The U.S. also continues to see persistent racial disparities in asthma prevalence. Asthma remains far more common among black and Hispanic children (14 percent and 8 percent, respectively) than among white children (5.6 percent).[18]

Children with asthma miss far more school than those without the disease. One analysis found that school-aged children with asthma miss an additional seven million school days annually.[19] Research shows these asthma-linked absences have many adverse effects on children, including mental and social challenges as well as diminished academic performance.[20] In addition to

---

14 Centers for Disease Control and Prevention. Summary health statistics: National health interview survey, 2018. Centers for Disease Control and Prevention, National Center for Health Statistics. Accessed December 23, 2019.

15 Centers for Disease Control and Prevention. Summary health statistics: National health interview survey, 2018. Centers for Disease Control and Prevention, National Center for Health Statistics. Accessed December 23, 2019. https://ftp.cdc.gov/pub/Health_Statistics/NCHS/NHIS/SHS/2018_SHS_Table_C-1.pdf.

16 Al-Muhsen S, et al. Poor asthma education and medication compliance are associated with increased emergency department visits by asthmatic children. *Ann Thorac Med.* 2015;10(2):123-131.

17 Centers for Disease Control and Prevention. Summary health statistics: National health interview survey, 2018. Centers for Disease Control and Prevention, National Center for Health Statistics. Accessed December 23, 2019. https://ftp.cdc.gov/pub/Health_Statistics/NCHS/NHIS/SHS/2018_SHS_Table_C-1.pdf.

18 Centers for Disease Control and Prevention. Summary health statistics: National health interview survey, 2018. Centers for Disease Control and Prevention, National Center for Health Statistics. Accessed December 23, 2019. https://ftp.cdc.gov/pub/Health_Statistics/NCHS/NHIS/SHS/2018_SHS_Table_C-1.pdf.

19 Sullivan P, et al. School absence and productivity outcomes associated with childhood asthma in the USA. *J of Asthma.* 2017; 55(2).

20 Moonie S, Sterling DA, Figgs LW, et al. The relationship between school absence, academic performance, and asthma status. *J Sch Health*. 2008;78:140–148.

limiting in-school time, childhood asthma results in a 16 percent increase in missed work days for adult family members.[21]

Asthma among children has been shown to result in significant health resource utilization and both direct and indirect economic costs.[22] Asthma is the third-leading cause of hospitalization among children under the age of 15.[23] Overall, a recent analysis estimated the economic burden of childhood asthma in the U.S. to be $5.92 billion in direct healthcare costs.[24] Approximately 3,600 Americans die from asthma every year, and while asthma deaths among children are relatively rare, they are largely preventable.[25]

Food Allergy and Schools

Food allergies are an immune system response to food that can cause hives, asthma, difficulty breathing, vomiting, diarrhea, anaphylactic shock, and, in rare cases, death.[26]

Today, more than 5.6 million children in the U.S. are estimated to have a food allergy, and approximately 40 percent of children with a food allergy are allergic to more than one food.[27] Roughly 90 percent of childhood food allergies in the US are caused by eight foods: eggs, milk, peanuts, tree nuts,

---

[21] Sullivan P, et al. School absence and productivity outcomes associated with childhood asthma in the USA. *J of Asthma.* 2017; 55(2).

[22] Wang LY, Zhong Y, Wheeler L. Direct and indirect costs of asthma in school-age children. *Prev CH.R.on Dis*. 2005;2(1):A11.

[23] American Lung Association. Asthma & children fact sheet (2014). Available at www.lung.org/lung-health-and-diseases/lung-disease-lookup/asthma/learn-about-asthma/asthma-children-facts-sheet.html.

[24] Perry, R., Braileanu, G., Palmer, T. et al. The Economic Burden of Pediatric Asthma in the United States: Literature Review of Current Evidence. *PharmacoEconomics* (2019) 37: 155.

[25] Centers for Disease Control and Prevention, "AsthmaStats: Asthma as the Underlying Cause of Death." Available at https://www.cdc.gov/asthma/asthma_stats/documents/AsthmStat_Mortality_2001-2016-H.pdf.

[26] Food Allergies in Children. Johns Hopkins Medicine. Available at www.hopkinsmedicine.org/health/conditions-and-diseases/food-allergies-in-children.

[27] Gupta RS, Warren CM, Smith BM, Blumenstock JA, Jiang J, Davis MM, Nadeau KC. The Public Health Impact of Parent-Reported Childhood Food Allergies in the United States. *Pediatrics* 2018;142(6):e20181235.

soy, fish, shellfish, and wheat; sesame allergy now ranks a close ninth.[28,29] The CDC reports that since 1997, food allergy prevalence among children has increased by 50 percent,[30] with peanut allergies more than tripling in prevalence.[31] More recent data indicate that prevalence has continued to rise over the past decade.[32]

Childhood food allergies have serious impacts on health and wellbeing. A severe allergic reaction, or anaphylaxis, can be fatal if epinephrine treatment is not administered within minutes. Between 2005 and 2014, there was a nearly 200 percent increase in food allergy-related emergency department visits among children 5-17 years old.[33]

In addition to the health and economic costs, food allergies create social burdens on children and families. Parents often report that food allergies limit their children's participation in summer camp or social gatherings and hinder their ability to eat out or travel.[34,35] Children with food allergies are more likely to experience bullying, including bullying involving food-related threats.[36]

Like asthma, food allergies pose a major economic burden on families, the healthcare system, and society. The annual estimated cost of food allergies in the U.S. is $24.8 billion, including $4.3 billion in direct medical costs and $20.5 billion in costs experienced by the family, including out of pocket costs,

---

[28] Turke PW. Childhood food allergies: An evolutionary mismatch hypothesis. *Evol Med Public Health*. 2017;2017(1):154–160. Published 2017 Oct 4.

[29] Sicherer SH, Muñoz-Furlong A, Godbold JH, Sampson HA. US Prevalence of self-report peanut, tree nut, and sesame allergy: 11-year follow-up. *J Allergy Clin Immunol.* 2010;125(6): 1322-1326pmid:20462634.

[30] Jackson KD, Howie LD, Akinbami LJ. Trends in allergic conditions among children: United States,1997-2011. NCHS data brief, no 121. Hyattsville, MD: National Center for Health Statistics. 2013.

[31] *Id.*

[32] R. Gupta, C. Warren, J. Blumenstock, J. Kotowska, K. Mittal, B. Smith. OR078 The prevalence of childhood food allergy in the United States: an update. *Annals of Allergy, Asthma and Immunology* November 2017, Volume 119, Issue 5, Supplement, Page S11.

[33] Motosue MS, Bellolio Mf, Van Houten HK, Shah ND, Campbell Rl. Increasing emergency department visits for anaphylaxis, 2005-2014. *J Allergy Clin Immunol Pract*. 2017;5(1):171-175.e3.

[34] Herbert L, Shemesh E, Bender B. Clinical management of psychosocial concerns related to food allergy. *J Allergy Clin Immunol Pract.* 2016; 4(2):205-213.

[35] Bollinger ME; Dahlquist LM, Mudd K; Sonntag C, Dillinger L, McKenna K. The impact of food allergy on the daily activities of children and their families. *Ann Allergy Asthma Immunol*. 2006; 96:415-421.

[36] Lieberman JA, Weiss C, Furlong TJ, Sicherer M, Sicherer SH. Bullying among pediatric patients with food allergy. *Ann Allergy Asthma Immunol*. 2010 Oct;105(4):282-6.

lost labor productivity, and opportunity costs related to leaving or changing jobs.[37]

Children with food allergies have two to four times the risk of asthma or other allergic conditions, and children with both asthma and food allergies may be more likely to experience anaphylaxis and death when exposed to an allergen.[38]

What Schools Can Do

Schools can play an enormous role in supporting children's health. For children with asthma and allergies, schools can help families manage the condition; prepare to address emergency situations; promote awareness among teachers, parents, and children; and provide a safe and healthy school environment that minimizes asthma and allergy triggers.

For many years now, AAFA has developed a "State Honor Roll," which examines policies and programs related to asthma and food allergies in schools. Our 2019 Honor Roll report is attached for the record. To produce this analysis, we comb through changes in state law and regulations to determine if states are meeting 23 key standards; states that meet at least 18 of the 23 join the honor roll.

We have seen a great deal of progress over the years in many areas. Overall, there are now 15 states on our honor roll, compared to 8 in 2013.

However, there are still too many gaps. For example, only 27 states require schools to have emergency protocols for asthma, and only 36 require emergency protocols for anaphylaxis. Only 24 states require schools to maintain allergy and asthma incidence reports, and only 12 require schools to have indoor air quality management plans. And even though school nurses are often the backbone of school efforts to help children with asthma and food allergies, only 8 states set a minimum nurse-to-student ratio for schools.

---

[37] Gupta R, Holdford D, Bilaver L, Dyer A, Holl JL, Meltzer D. The economic impact of childhood food allergy in the United States. *JAMA Pediatr.* 2013 Nov;167(11):1026-31.

[38] Branum A, Lukacs S. Food allergy among U.S. children: Trends in prevalence and hospitalizations. NCHS data brief, no 10. Hyattsville, MD: National Center for Health Statistics. 2008. Available at https://www.cdc.gov/nchs/data/databriefs/db10.pdf.

H.R. 2468, the School-Based Allergies and Asthma Management Program Act

H.R. 2468 would help address these gaps by creating a preference in CDC's asthma grant program for states that require all public elementary and secondary schools to have:

- a nurse or other trained individual who can administer asthma or allergy medication onsite during all operating hours; and
- a comprehensive school-based allergies and asthma management program that
  - identifies all students with asthma or allergies;
  - establishes individual action plans;
  - educates school staff;
  - reduces environmental triggers of allergies and asthma; and
  - coordinates management of allergies and asthma with families and primary care providers.

The act has support from a number of major stakeholder organizations including AAFA, the American Academy of Allergy, Asthma and Immunology; the American College of Allergy, Asthma, and Immunology; the Allergy and Asthma Network; Food Allergy Research & Education; and the National Association of School Nurses.[39]

H.R. 2468 leverages CDC's National Asthma Control Program (NACP), an existing initiative that awards competitive grants to states for efforts aimed at reducing the number of asthma deaths, hospitalizations, and visits to the emergency room; reducing the number of missed school and workdays; and helping people with asthma be active without limitation.

While AAFA believes that CDC's NACP grant program should be expanded to all fifty states, H.R. 2468 would not directly increase spending for the program. Instead, it creates a preference within the existing NACP program. The CDC would establish the specific standards that would allow a state to qualify for the preference. As noted above, our own Honor Roll research has identified some serious gaps that this legislation would help

---

[39] American Academy of Allergy, Asthma & Immunology, "School-Based Allergies and Asthma Management Program Act (H.R. 2468)." Available at www.aaaai.org/Aaaai/media/MediaLibrary/PDF%20Documents/Advocacy/AAAAI-leave-behind-H.R.-2468-School-Based-Allergies-and-Asthma-Management-Act-FINAL.pdf.

address. For example, given the low number of states that set school nurse standards, it is important for states to require that someone – whether a nurse or other trained individual – be available during all operating hours to administer asthma or allergy medication. Similarly, the components of the school plan that H.R. 2468 establishes would help fill gaps in state requirements related to emergency protocols, indoor air quality, and other preparedness factors. AAFA would be pleased to further discuss our Honor Roll findings and methodology to help CDC develop their criteria. To strengthen their allergy and asthma programs, schools can draw upon many resources developed by stakeholders, including the SAMPRO program developed by the American Academy of Allergy, Asthma & Immunology (AAAAI) in collaboration with AAFA and other stakeholders.[40]

Conclusion

All parents want to send their kids to school knowing that they will be safe, healthy, and ready to learn. H.R. 2468 will help ensure this is a reality for more children and families managing asthma and food allergies. AAFA is grateful for the subcommittee's consideration of this bill, and stands ready to help in any way.

* * *

Ms. ESHOO. Thank you very much for your testimony to each of the witnesses, and now we will move to—that we have concluded the witnesses' testimony, I will recognize myself for 5 minutes of questions.

I will start with Ms. Zarecky. Again, thank you for being here today. What do you think is the single most important thing Congress can do to address sudden unexplained deaths of infants and children?

Ms. ZARECKY. For me personally, research is very badly needed. Sudden unexplained death in childhood, which is what happened to Scarlett, research is absolutely critical, and we can't do good research unless we have good data, which is what the legislation seeks to accomplish. It is a terrible

[40] American Academy of Allergy, Asthma and Immunology, School-Based Asthma Management Program (SAMPRO). Available at https://www.aaaai.org/conditions-and-treatments/school-tools/SAMPRO; Lemanske, Robert F. et al.
Creation and implementation of SAMPRO™: A school-based asthma management program. *Journal of Allergy and Clinical Immunology*, Volume 138, Issue 3, 711 – 723.

medical tragedy, and we—families need more answers, and research is just so badly needed into why it happens.

Ms. ESHOO. Is there any—I am familiar with what the bill does, but is there any research being conducted today, and if so, where, by whom?

Ms. ZARECKY. Sure. Yes. So we participated in research being done out of New York University. It is the Sudden Unexplained Death and Childhood Registry and Research Collaborative. And my understanding is there is also research being done at Seattle Children's and Boston as well, Boston Children's Hospital, although I am less familiar with that. But there is limited amount of research being conducted already.

Ms. ESHOO. And in the aftermath of Scarlett's death, can you describe to us what was available or what was not available to you given that probably one of the darkest chapters—darkest chapter of your life?

Ms. ZARECKY. Yes. I mean, the Sudden Unexplained Death in Childhood Foundation has been a lifeline to our family. They have provided not only emotional support, they have allowed us to be connected with other families who have experienced this tragedy.

When something like this happens to you, you think you are the only one that it has ever happened to. So being able to be connected with other families has been critical, but also being able to have support in terms of having someone who can make a phone call to the medical examiner's office. I can't tell you how impossible even dialing that phone number is at times.

And even just to ask, you know, after a little while, when is my daughter's autopsy going to be done, having that support not only from an emotional standpoint but also just, you know, logistical things that you never really think of until, you know, you have lost a child, has been—has been really critical.

Ms. ESHOO. And the legislation covers what you just pointed out?

Ms. ZARECKY. It mostly covers data collection and so that we can support research and figure out what happened to these children.

Ms. ESHOO. OK. Dr. Beers—thank you—the United States, you said, is the most dangerous place in the developed world to deliver a baby. I can't believe that that is a statistic next to the two words "United States," but that is our challenge, and we need to meet the challenge.

Each year, 700 American women die and 50,000 women are severely injured due to complications related to child birth. For African-American women in the United States, it is even more dangerous because they are three times more likely to die from childbirth than White women.

In ProPublica's reporting, it found that, quote, "the American medical system is focused more on fetal and infant safety and survival than on the mother's health and well being." Do you agree with that finding?

Dr. BEERS. I don't know that it is focused more on that, but I would say that we need a much greater and more intense focus on maternal health and on access to high-quality, accessible and culturally sensitive——

Ms. ESHOO. We really shouldn't be pitting one against the other.

Dr. BEERS. Correct.

Ms. ESHOO. It is not a race to the bottom.

Dr. BEERS. And healthy mothers and healthy families engender healthy babies.

Ms. ESHOO. Now, do you have recommendations on how the Healthy Start Program—and you gave it very good scores, which I like hearing—how it could improve maternal health while also helping infants?

Dr. BEERS. Yes. Absolutely. I think a couple of the areas where Healthy Start really helps improve maternal health—I think, one, the services are really targeted to areas where there are higher rates of infant mortality, which are often coexistent with higher rates of maternal mortality as well.

The services Healthy Start provides are very individualized and targeted to the individual mother and really do help address some of the social determinants. When we look at maternal mortality rates and infant mortality rates, a significant contributor to those are social influences and social determinants.

Ms. ESHOO. Well, do you think the program is doing enough to address racial disparities in maternal and infant health, and if not, what more should be done?

Dr. BEERS. I think there is always more we can do. When we look at the data and the evidence, we see these tremendous disparities. We see the tremendous disparities in race and ethnicity regardless of socioeconomic status. And if we see those numbers, we know we are not doing enough. And so we need to continue to provide culturally appropriate services. We need to continue to engage communities and families in developing solutions and in addition to addressing bias that exists naturally in healthcare.

Ms. ESHOO. Thank you. Well, I am out of time, so Mr. Mendez, I will submit my questions to you in writing. And I know you will respond in a very timely way.

The Chair now recognizes Dr. Burgess, the ranking member of the subcommittee, for his 5 minutes to ask questions.

Mr. BURGESS. And again I thank the chair, thank our witnesses for being here today. I apologize because some of us have been in and out, but there is another hearing going on downstairs. I don't know why the committee leadership chooses to schedule important hearings on top of each other, but I guess it happened when we were in charge too, so I won't to be too critical.

Ms. ESHOO. We can handle it, that is why.

Mr. BURGESS. Dr. Beers, in your written testimony, you talked about that you get a lot of questions related to the sleep, that they are at the top of any new parent's list when they come to see me, and the guidance I give parents is critical to promoting safe practices.

So here you are in the Subcommittee on Health on the Committee on Energy and Commerce with the vast audience on C– SPAN that tunes in and hangs on every word that we say. So this is your opportunity to give that advice very broadly and recognize it doesn't suffice for advice which you will get from your own doctor, but in general, what are those recommendations that you are giving?

Dr. BEERS. Right, right. So thank you for that opportunity. I appreciate that. There are several very important things for safe sleep. Infants should sleep in their own sleep space—without blankets, pillows, crib bumpers, other things—on their backs. And I think those are very important things, in spaces without exposure to cigarette smoke as well, so——

And I recognize as a pediatrician and as a parent that sometimes that is difficult because sometimes you have babies who don't sleep well, sometimes you have babies who are fussy. You are pretty much always exhausted, and so I recognize that that is difficult, but it is just critically important.

Mr. BURGESS. So that is—is that advice for a newborn, or is that continue—for some time continue in the baby's life?

Dr. BEERS. Well, I think that is a great question. So the evidence and the research that we know shows that infants are at risk for sleep-related death up to a year of age, and so that is relevant up to a year of age. I do think it is important to note, though, that— and particularly with this bill—this really does address other instances of sudden unexplained death in infancy and childhood that may be unrelated to the situation.

So, to Ms. Zarecky's point about more research being needed, I think that is a really important point because there is a lot we don't know, particularly about the older infants and children.

Mr. BURGESS. And that was going to be the point of my question, to widen the focus of what we are examining, not ignoring what perhaps may be the more vulnerable population but not to exclude populations that might also be vulnerable.

I do have to say, Madam Chair, and we, of course, have worked on issues related to maternal mortality in the last Congress, this Congress. Last Congress we passed the first stand-alone bill dealing with maternal mortality that I have seen in my entire time in Congress. And it got signed into law, and that is a good thing. We have continued that work in this Congress, and that is a good thing.

But the hearing we had leading up to the bill that you referenced, we had Dr. Nelson from Parkland Hospital, where I did my residency many, many years ago—many, many, many years ago—and I guess the point for Dr. Nelson's testimony was, here is a hospital that is basically an inner city hospital, serves basically a minority population, a low-income population, and they have very significantly good maternal mortality statistics.

So the point in all of that is, we know that it can be done well, and really I hope at some point, we will have some follow-on discussion where we might identify either the exposition of best practices or even, I dare say, do we need to talk about those institutions that are not doing as well?

But I think we owe it to the patient population to be able to— it is hard to discern, it is hard to know when you are shopping for a hospital in which to deliver your baby. You don't basically go into the deep within the statistical part of it. Maybe that is something that we could look at in the future.

Mr. Mendez, I do want to say, as someone who has lived with asthma my entire life, I appreciate your effort on that.

Mr. MENDEZ. Thank you.

Mr. BURGESS. I know there is always more that we could be doing. I do worry some about things that we might mandate from this committee because then we always—we tend to drive the price up of those products that we mandate, and that has been one of the downsides of some of the work we have done in the past. But I appreciate what your organization does and your work——

Mr. MENDEZ. Thank you.

Mr. BURGESS [continuing]. On that.

And Ms. Zarecky, sorry for your loss. I am glad you are here with us to share your story today. I hope that your presence here will be of benefit to people who might learn something from Dr. Beers' instructions that she so wisely gave us.

Thank you, Madam Chair. I will yield back.

Ms. ESHOO. The gentleman yields back. I would be happy to do follow-through on what you just raised.

Now, on the heels of the hearing that we had on maternal mortality, I raised the issue relative to hospitals, and today the accreditation board now includes what you described, but there is always more to be done.

But I think that that is a positive step, because there has to be internal pressure by those that are in charge of and oversee hospitals so that we can weed out those that—whose rates are deeply troubling from those that are doing well, and learn from those that are doing well. So I will continue to work with you on that.

I now would like to recognize the gentleman from New Jersey, the chair of the full committee, Mr. Pallone, for his 5 minutes of questions.

Mr. PALLONE. Thank you, Madam Chair, and I want to thank all our witnesses, including Ms. Zarecky, for being here today. I can't imagine the pain and grief that you had to endure since losing Scarlett, but I thank you for your courage and for sharing her story with us, really.

This cause has long been something that I support. In 2014, President Obama signed into law the Sudden Unexpected Death Data Enhancement and Awareness Act, a law that I sponsored that required the Secretary to collect info on sudden unexpected infant death and sudden unexplained death in childhood, and educate the public, and collaborate with other agencies and State and local health departments to provide information for medical examiners and other individuals.

And, thanks to this law, we now have a more clear vision of what is known and unknown about sudden unexpected infant death and sudden unexpected death in childhood. And our focus has to turn now, how can we take further action to prevent these tragedies and support families, care providers, and researchers when these tragedies occur.

One of the provisions of the Scarlett's Sunshine Act would provide grants for support services for families who have had a child die, including grief counseling, home visits, and support groups.

So I wanted to ask you, Ms. Zarecky. No amount of support can ever replace what you or your family have lost, but can you tell us how support services can be helpful to families like yours in working through these tragedies?

Ms. ZARECKY. Thank you so much for your question, and thank you for asking because it actually gives me the opportunity to focus on one of the strengths of the House bill, and that, of course, is the support services.

I think, when you have lost a child, there is a before and there is an after, and once you have crossed that line, oftentimes there is no greater gift than being able to connect with another family who really, truly understands. And it is the support services that we have received through national foundations as well as local foundations in Pittsburgh.

It has been absolutely critical in being able to live life after our loss. So, you know, bereavement support for families, of course, is very critical. It is very badly needed, and I truly don't know where I would be today if I didn't have the support of other families who have walked this journey before me.

And I thank you, Congressman, for your leadership on this issue and for working on it for many years.

Mr. PALLONE. Well, thank you. Let me just turn to Dr. Beers from a physician's point of view. In your testimony, Doctor, you discuss the difficulty your team faced when you could not identify timely and accessible grief counseling for a family who just lost a child.

As a physician, can you tell us about the appropriate forms of grief counseling and other support services that should be made available to families, and how these services can help support the mental and emotional health of the family?

Dr. BEERS. Absolutely. And I think, as you and other Members know, access to timely and accessible mental health services is a significant issue across the country, and so—and grief counseling and grief services are particularly important for families. When you need them, you need them immediately. They are not services that you can wait 6, 8, 10 months for.

You need mental health providers who are specifically trained in addressing grief and bereavement issues. And what type of services is going to vary a little bit, depending on the family and their individual desires and needs. For some, individual therapy may be appropriate, and for others, group therapy and support groups may be appropriate as well, but certainly we should make sure that both of those things are available to families.

Mr. PALLONE. I wanted to—thank you. I wanted to ask you one more question in the time remaining. Another important provision of the bill supports grants for infant safe sleep and efforts to decrease risk factors.

You mentioned physicians began recommending positioning babies on their back for sleep starting in the 1990s. I remember that. And after which we saw a decrease in cases of sudden unexpected infant death.

However, as continued tragedies demonstrate, we still have a lot of work to do. So, in your testimony, you suggested that we might need to reframe safe sleep recommendations to address cultural or socioeconomic considerations.

Can you explain what that means and how can we ensure that all families receive the benefit of these recommendations?

Dr. BEERS. Absolutely. And perhaps the best way is to share a short example. I am close colleagues with a pediatrician and researcher who does a lot of research in this area, and we used to work together in Washington, DC, and working with many low-income families who live in neighborhoods with high community violence.

And one of the things they learned through their qualitative research was that many of the families they talked to were not adhering to the safe sleep recommendations because they were fearful of people entering into their house or apartment and wanted their baby very close to them. And they felt like putting their baby in a crib was taking them too far away and was putting them at risk because they were living in unsafe and unstable housing.

And so being able to tailor those recommendations to address those very specific concerns of bringing the crib very close to the bed, making sure that you were set up and your room was set up so that the crib was away from the door, those things made an enormous difference. But the only way that we knew that was by asking those questions and really diving into what a family's specific concerns were.

Mr. PALLONE. Thank you.

Thank you, Madam Chair.

Ms. ESHOO. The gentleman yields back. A pleasure to recognize the gentleman from Michigan, former chairman of the full committee, Mr. Upton.

Mr. UPTON. Well, thank you Madam Chair, and I appreciate the hearing, and I have asked that my name be added as a cosponsor to H.R. 2271, so thank you very much for your testimony.

Dr. Beers, a quick question. Just for new moms, when they deliver, often in a hospital, I mean, is it the standard operating procedure to, in fact, make sure that that new mom is aware of the safe sleep recommendations? I think it is pretty widespread belief about bumpers and stuffed animals, but blankets and—I mean, for the first year?

I mean, is there a checklist? I mean, have you—has it been pretty good in terms of your follow-up with hospitals across the country that, in fact, new moms realize that information is pretty good to receive?

Dr. BEERS. It is, and that is pretty standard education that is given in the hospital. I think one of the important things to remember is that, when you are a brand-new mother having just delivered a baby, you know, maybe 24 to 76 hours previously, you may not remember everything or absorb everything you are being told right in that moment.

So being able to continue that education is also very important.

Mr. UPTON. Dr. Mendez, I was chairman of the committee when we passed and signed into law Leader Steny Hoyer's School Access to Emergency Epinephrine Act. Can you give us an update on how that bill is being implemented as well as the School-Based Allergy and Asthma Management Program Act——

Mr. MENDEZ. Sure. I would say, you know, it is a win-win when you look at the numbers and the results and the outcomes, that, you know, asthma is quite costly, and I think that we reduced by $23 billion the amount of cost to the healthcare system because what that Act has tried to do was provide upstream help in terms of interventions before you end up in the emergency room or the hospital.

I think, for the National Asthma Control Program, $71 is saved for each dollar spent in the program. So, to the extent that we can have forward-facing, more advanced protocols here to prevent asthma attacks or allergy attacks is really helpful. So continuing with this current bill, 2468, will help that by adding the asthma piece as well.

Mr. PALLONE. Well, I look forward to pushing that legislation forward. Appreciate your testimony.

And with that, Madam Chair, I yield back.

Ms. ESHOO. The gentleman yields back.

It is a pleasure to recognize the gentlewoman from California, Ms. Matsui, for her 5 minutes.

Ms. MATSUI. Thank you very much, Madam Chair.

And I want to thank the witnesses for being here today.

You know, I was thinking about the fact that schools play a fundamental part in supporting the health and well-being of children, particularly with asthma and allergies, and given the rapidly growing prevalence of childhood food allergies, we must improve school allergy management programs to ensure the continued safety and inclusion of all students.

Moreover, I am particular on the risk factors for food allergies, and the reasons why these potentially life-threatening diseases are becoming increasingly common among kids are not fully understood at this time.

Further, 1 out of 13 children in the United States is living with food allergies. And my grandson is one of them. And if you have someone in the family, you immediately become sensitized to this. I know too well the serious health, social, and economic impacts that a severe food allergy and related adverse immune responses— like hives, asthma, and shock—can have on children and their families as well as their friends.

So we must do more to recognize and study food allergies, and that is why I have introduced the FASTER Act, legislation that updates labeling laws to include sesame and expands data collection of Americans' exposure to specific food allergens. My bill aims to improve the way we monitor, manage, and treat these complex and multifaceted diseases.

Mr. Mendez, thank you very much for specifically highlighting the growing prevalence and serious concerns related to childhood food allergies in your testimony.

Can you expand on some of the best practices for managing food allergies in schools? I am thinking about the fact that the school seems to be the environment that most children interact in, which means not only the personnel, it is the teachers, it is the parents. There are also fellow students too.

Mr. MENDEZ. Yes.

Ms. MATSUI. So how does this legislation incentivize greater dissemination of these best practices?

Mr. MENDEZ. Yes, sure. Thank you for that. And, you know, things have changed completely in the last 20 years, when 2 of my 3 kids had food allergies, and we have come a long way since then, but there are still a lot of gaps and things that we need to do.

I think having—and they are in the bill—having trained personnel in acknowledgment of food allergies is really important in the school, an explicit anaphylaxis program so you have policy and procedures in knowing how to deal with an asthma attack or an allergy attack in the school, with instructions on administering the medication, having updated school records, having a school nurse involved in things, and then incident reports for usage and medication are really key. And then, again, stock medication and train personnel.

Ms. MATSUI. Well, where do the greatest gaps in understanding food allergies, where do they still exist? And how can we best direct the future direction of food allergy research?

I remember, when my son was going to school, no one ever thought about this at all. We used to bring all kinds of cookies and cakes and things to school. Now it is so prevalent and it is something that everybody is aware of but not knowing quite what to do. And I want to understand where the future direction that you believe we are going in.

Mr. MENDEZ. Yes, sure. I think continuing to increase that awareness level is really important. I mean, there is food allergy bullying that happens—

Ms. MATSUI. Yes.

Mr. MENDEZ [continuing]. In classrooms that we really have to be aware of. And to the extent that this bill, 2468, codifies an approach, then it recognizes that that is not OK, to have food allergy bullying.

I think the other thing is, on the clinical trial side, raising the awareness that they are out there and increasing diversity in clinical trials and recruiting more patients into clinical trials. I think that what we have found is that there is not a high degree of awareness in clinical trials, as well, for future research.

Ms. MATSUI. Do you find that there—in your understanding of schools, are there certain schools that—I mean, I am sure that there are disparities——

Mr. MENDEZ. Yes.

Ms. MATSUI [continuing]. In where the schools are and the economic levels. Do you find that there is more emphasis on certain schools than other schools? And what can we do to ensure that everyone gets covered here?

Mr. MENDEZ. Sure. Well, it is clearly in the health disparities issue where that comes into play. And I think, if you look at the ZIP Codes in some of those schools, those are the ones that are most challenged.

In our State Honor Roll report, we looked at those various school policies. There are 24 that have made that honor roll right now, but we could go a lot further.

This National Asthma Control Program is really important, and if we could expand that as well, in addition to your great work on the FASTER Act, I think it would really go a long way towards helping with asthma and allergies in the school community.

Ms. MATSUI. I want to thank you.

And I am out of time, but, Ms. Zarecky, I think the greatest loss anyone can ever experience is a loss of a child. And thank you so much for being here. And know that we will do everything we possibly can to ensure that we find explanations and to continue our work on these issues. Thank you very much.

And thank you very much.

Ms. ESHOO. The gentlewoman yields back.

I know the gentlewoman has legislation—and I look forward to taking it up—relative to one of the allergies, to sesame seeds. And that is not borne on labels. I did call the FDA, spoke to the person in charge of this issue, of that division of the FDA, trying to make the determination whether they could handle this administratively or we should move ahead legislatively. They said it would take between 5 to 7 years to label. So I think we have to get your bill going, Ms. Matsui.

OK. It is a pleasure to recognize the gentleman from Virginia, Mr. Griffith, for his 5 minutes of questions.

Mr. GRIFFITH. Thank you very much, Madam Chair.

And I, too, support the principles of Ms. Matsui's bill. My family are consummate label readers.

Ms. Zarecky, you know, you talked about—and you got to me because you talked about those moments when you go in to listen to your child breathing, and I did that many times, particularly with my older son, who has lots of food allergies and breathing issues, including asthma. And so I know that feeling, and I am so sorry. That being said, let me switch back to allergies, which is where I had planned on going, but, you know, your testimony is very compelling.

I like the bill. I do have some questions about it.

I will tell you that, you know, this is not something new, as you know. It has been around for a long time. My mother loves to still tell the story of, when I was 5 years old, I got in trouble for a brief period of time because I threw a cookie across the room. They did not understand. I had and still have a wheat allergy. I knew I couldn't eat that cookie. And back in the early 1960s, they didn't have rice cookies readily available or, you know, other flours. Everything had wheat in it. And I knew I couldn't have it, but the aide who had just been hired had no idea and kept handing me the cookie and said, "No, this is for you." And, finally, after having refused it several times, I tossed it across the room. I don't remember it, but my mother loves to tell the story.

Mr. MENDEZ. Uh-huh.

Mr. GRIFFITH. Likewise, and as a part of what I was thinking about when you were testifying, one of the greatest days of my life was when my son, my older son—he is now 14 he will be embarrassed and roll his eyes if he ever sees this—but he was about 21/2. We don't know to this day what he got a hold of, but something that we were eating at a restaurant, he got something he was allergic to. We don't know what it was. We heard the wheezing beginning.

Mr. MENDEZ. Yes. Right.

Mr. GRIFFITH. We had already turned the car around. My wife and I were already going to the hospital. And from the back came this little voice that said, "Mommy, I need to see a doctor." The self-awareness factor is so important.

And so I appreciate the bill that Phil Roe and Steny Hoyer have put in. And Phil has had similar bills in the past.

And they had actually had—and one of my concerns with the bill is that they had actually had some requirements that you have medications in the schools, which I like. This one does not require that. Now, Virginia has epinephrine in the schools now. But, you know, if something were to happen, you know, that is step one, as you know.

But one of the questions that comes up is, the trained individuals, how much training would they need? Because I represent a district that has a—we are 422nd in household income out of 435 in the U.S. House. The school systems don't have the money to necessarily have a school nurse, an R.N., in every building. They have one somewhere in the system most of the time.

Mr. MENDEZ. Sure.

Mr. GRIFFITH. So what kind of training would those folks need? And would it be so extensive that it would be too expensive for poor communities like the ones that I represent to be able to afford?

Mr. MENDEZ. Yes. I don't think so. And that is one of the things that we do with the CDC through their National Asthma Control Program. We publish materials on our website which are completely free for an asthma action plan, for an allergy action plan. So just having those—they are easily downloadable. You could get them on a lot of doctor sites as well.

Then, in terms of training, there are videos that we produce that walk you through what an asthma attack looks like and how to address asthma.

So those——

Mr. GRIFFITH. But somebody——

Mr. MENDEZ [continuing]. Are all free resources.

Mr. GRIFFITH [continuing]. Some health teacher or somebody in the school could do these videos and qualify under the bill?

Mr. MENDEZ. That is absolutely right.

Mr. GRIFFITH. All right. I appreciate that, because that would be a concern. I want those people trained, I want them to be aware, but I also don't want to, you know, price them out of the market or make it so that they can't meet the requirements.

Mr. MENDEZ. Yes. I mean, the legislation is great because it comes full circle. It creates incentives for schools to access some of the free materials that the CDC is working with other partners to address on a public health basis.

Mr. GRIFFITH. Now, let me get this on the record too, because sometimes people will look at the language and then they will get carried away. It says in the bill on page 3 that the schools have to have efforts to reduce the presence of environmental triggers of allergies and asthma.

My son, my 14-year-old, is allergic to every tree in the East. I don't want anybody to interpret it and I don't think you mean to have it interpreted that they have to chop all the trees down around the school. Am I correct in that? Just make sure——

Mr. MENDEZ. Right. No, that is——

Mr. GRIFFITH [continuing]. That they have clean systems inside the school?

Mr. MENDEZ. Yes, that is exactly right. There are some best practices that you could do by looking at your air filtration. I mean, there is indoor air, you know, rugs in the classroom, that kind of stuff, that you can manage. So it is not about cutting down trees.

But there is legislation locally that addresses idling school buses, for example, and idling cars. Those are things that you could do on a local basis to reduce fuel emissions that could trigger an asthma attack.

Mr. GRIFFITH. I appreciate it very much. My time is up, and I yield back.

Mr. MENDEZ. Thank you.

Ms. ESHOO. The gentleman yields back.

It is a pleasure to recognize the gentlewoman from New Hampshire, Ms. Kuster, for her 5 minutes of questions.

Ms. KUSTER. Thank you very much. Great to be with you.

And, Ms. Zarecky, I am so sorry for your loss. And I just want to say that I am here today on behalf of my great-niece, Leah, who passed from SIDS just over a year ago. And as my niece has said, our family will never be the same. So Leah is with me always, every day. And I just—the pain that my niece, Miley, and her husband, Dan, have gone through, and my sister, Debbie, and her husband, Peter, and our entire family. So I am with you every day. I appreciate your courage coming forward.

And I want to thank Dr. Beers and every pediatrician in this country. I find it extraordinary, when I went to do the research after losing Leah to understand the scope of this, it is quite an extraordinary public health success that we cut the number of unexpected infant deaths in half, I believe, from the "Back to Sleep" recommendations.

But I am troubled, having done the research—my staff has given me some statistics. In my home State of New Hampshire, in the period between 2011 to 2018, 62 sleep-related infant deaths in my home State, 15 due to SIDS, 42 undetermined. But, despite the recommendations that all infants be placed on their backs to sleep, the New Hampshire review group found that only 48 percent of cases reviewed had been placed on their backs.

And so I want to support—and I have asked to cosponsor the legislation as well. I want to support the additional research from the truly unexpected, unexplained deaths, but I also want to focus on this issue of education and training.

In our case, my great-niece, Leah, died in a daycare setting. And so one of the questions I have for both of you is, What more can we be doing for training parents? And I think your point was very important about we need to ask why they are not able to comply, what is your fear, what is your worry? But, also, what can we do to be training childcare workers and providers?

Ms. Zarecky?

Ms. ZARECKY. I think Dr. Beers would probably be best suited to answer that question. Scarlett's death was not an incident—it was not related to unsafe sleep practices.

Ms. KUSTER. Right.

Ms. ZARECKY. We followed the same guidelines from the AAP. We followed them until Scarlett was 16 months old, well past the age—so Scarlett's death is truly unexplained——

Ms. KUSTER. Truly unexplained.

Ms. ZARECKY [continuing]. And unknown.

Ms. KUSTER. Yes.

Ms. ZARECKY. So I am really not qualified to answer that and would defer to Dr. Beers.

Ms. KUSTER. And that is true in our case as well.

Ms. ZARECKY. Yes. Yes.

Ms. KUSTER. We followed—my niece followed all of the protocols.

Ms. ZARECKY. Yes.

Ms. KUSTER. So if you could comment, Dr. Beers, both as to the sleep protocols but also as to this unexpected, unexplained, what more we could be doing on research.

Dr. BEERS. Absolutely. Absolutely. I would be happy to.

And I think your point about childcare is absolutely spot on because, as pediatricians, we are providing education to parents and families but don't typically have the opportunity to provide direct education to childcare centers and childcare providers. And so that is a very important place. I think we need to be thinking about providing education to serve larger, licensed-center-based childcares but also smaller, home-based and unlicensed childcare centers, because often that is another group that may slip through the cracks with education.

Certainly, you know, local jurisdictions can think about regulations to sort of require that kind of training, and then, as professionals, we can work to make that training available.

I do——

Ms. KUSTER. Can I ask about, in the research that is happening so far—and my niece and her husband are participating in the protocol at Boston Children's Hospital. And thank God they have had that support and that family support. Do we know from the research, is there an increased risk at the stage when a baby is beginning to roll over, and whether that is an issue to be concerned about?

Dr. BEERS. Yes, I mean, you do see a peak around 3 to 4 months of age, certainly, which is a bit before that period of time. But I do think it really does, then, come back to the point that Ms. Zarecky and others have raised, is that there was a tremendous public health success with the "Back to Sleep" campaign, and it has somewhat plateaued.

And what that tells us is that we really need more information and we need better information and more consistent information when, tragically, infants and children do die inexplicably. And so getting that information so that we can make those decisions is, I think, most important.

Ms. KUSTER. And my time is over. I apologize. But I want to thank you for coming forward.

Ms. ESHOO. The gentlewoman yields back.

It is a pleasure to recognize the gentleman from Indiana, Dr. Bucshon, for his 5 minutes of questions.

Mr. BUCSHON. Thank you, Madam Chairwoman. And thank you for having this hearing today with all of these very important bills. I was a physician before, a surgeon, so a lot of these are near and dear to my heart.

Mr. Mendez, as you highlighted in your testimony, roughly 5.5 million, or 1 in 13, American children currently live with asthma, a disease that is one of the leading causes of school absenteeism.

The Department of Education and the Department of Health and Human Services recommend that schools have comprehensive management plans in place to support children with asthma. However, many schools do not have such programs in place, as we have heard. I am proud that my home State of Indiana is a leader in addressing this growing health challenge and was named to the Asthma and Allergy Foundation of America's 2019 State Honor Roll list.

I know that you just talked with Congressman Griffith about the details of the legislation, but can you elaborate on how H.R. 2468, the School-Based Allergies and Asthma Management Program, would use a proven model to assist all States in experiencing the success we have seen in Indiana by ensuring better outcomes that result from a safe learning environment for every student?

Mr. MENDEZ. Sure. I mean, in Indiana specifically, I think you guys have done, through the National Asthma Control Program, school nurse trainings on asthma management, indoor air quality, and pest management. So what we have seen in many of the States is that, to the extent that you can have this training up front, it reduces asthma attacks, it reduces absenteeism because there is greater awareness among the families that have that and the caregivers.

So this act specifically asks for, you know, in an emergency situation, an asthma action plan or an allergy action plan. And we have seen that, with the asthma action plan implementation over time, it has reduced absenteeism, I think, by 20 percent or so, to the extent that we have increased the number of asthma action plans that have been delivered there.

So this legislation will help do that. There is a direct correlation between awareness and having an asthma action plan and now an allergy action plan to reducing missed school days.

Mr. BUCSHON. Are there certain areas of the country that are more prone to the allergy situation? And it is seasonal, correct?

Mr. MENDEZ. Yes. Yes.

Mr. BUCSHON. So, I mean, Indiana, we have seasonal allergies just like everywhere else, but something like this legislation, which would create some uniformity, would still be applicable to most States, correct, I mean, even though there are obviously differences in the environment?

Mr. MENDEZ. Yes, no, that is correct. I mean, the idea here is to create the incentives for all States to work with the CDC. Because it is a competitive grant program. The CDC works with the public health departments in various States. So to the extent that we could expand that program by having States be more competitive in having these programs is really helpful.

There are belts, you know, that we have looked at. The central part of the U.S.—we do an Asthma Capitals report, and the northeast corridor, I–95, and, kind of, the Midwest are areas that we have seen. And we do that Asthma Capitals report based on prevalence of mortality and emergency room visits. So we clearly see there are pockets of where asthma is more significant.

And we also do an Allergy Capitals report, which looks at some different criteria. And you don't want to be at the top of that list either, because it means that, you know, you are struggling in those areas.

Mr. BUCSHON. Yep. Thank you very much.

Madam Chairwoman, I yield back.

Ms. ESHOO. The gentleman yields back.

It is a pleasure to recognize a California colleague, Mr. Cárdenas, for his 5 minutes of questions.

Mr. CÁRDENAS. Thank you very much, Chairwoman Eshoo and also Ranking Member Burgess, for having this very critical and important hearing on these important matters.

And I would like to thank the panelists for coming forward and giving us your expertise, and especially Ms. Zarecky. Thank you for your bravery and your courage in continuing to make sure that all of us—us on this side of the room and everybody in the room and throughout this country—can benefit from knowledge and investment in efforts so that we can minimize these tragedies.

So thank you all very much.

In particular, I want to focus on the Healthy Start program. This important program addresses the infant mortality rate in America by providing grants to State and local community organizations that are in the greatest need. Now nearing its 30th anniversary, the program has created results—good results. Communities receiving Healthy Start grants have, on average, reduced their infant mortality rate below the national average despite having a history of a higher infant mortality rate.

However, the national infant mortality rate in our great country is still far too high. It is clear that we need to do more to improve the programs and ensure the funds are getting to areas that have the greatest need.

Under current law, the Secretary of Health and Human Services is required to consider several factors that contribute to infant mortality rates when awarding grants, such as low birth weight. H.R. 4801, the Healthy Start Reauthorization Act, would require that the Secretary take other important factors into account, such as social determinants of health, and under consideration when awarding grants.

Dr. Beers, can you give us some examples of social determinants of health that might affect the health outcomes of pregnant women and newborns?

Dr. BEERS. Absolutely. I think there are many examples; I will highlight a couple.

First would be food insecurity. If a family is living in a household where they do not have reliable access to food, that certainly is going to affect the health and nutrition of the mother and the developing baby. So that would be one example.

Housing insecurity is another issue, as we have talked a lot about, environmental toxins, environmental influences on health. And certainly, same for a pregnant mother. If she is living in a housing situation where she is exposed to mold or other unsafe environmental influences, that can have an influence as well.

Transportation is another great example. If your OB–GYN care is across town and you have no way to get there, you are not going come to as many of those appointments. And so access to good, reliable, affordable transportation—I have many patients who have to make a decision between buying diapers and bus fare. And so making sure that families have and mothers have transportation is important.

Mr. CÁRDENAS. So all the top-line determinants that you just outlined—and, as you mentioned, there are many more, but in the interest of time, thank you for sharing those with us—is this exclusively a rural issue or a big city issue, or is it pretty much across the board, the things that you outlined?

Dr. BEERS. It is really across the board. Sometimes, you know— I get asked this question a lot, living here in DC, where we are very close together—but sometimes it is just as long to get to an appointment as it might be in a rural area. So it really is across all jurisdictions.

Mr. CÁRDENAS. Is this a minority issue or is this an American issue across the board?

Dr. BEERS. It is absolutely an American issue across the board. There are significant racial and ethnic disparities that do exist that we need to dive into, but it is an issue for all families.

Mr. CÁRDENAS. OK. Thank you.

Healthy Start grantees also coordinate with other evidence-based programs that serve infants and their families, including the Special Supplemental Nutrition Program for Women, Infants, and Children, or WIC, and the Early Childhood Home Visiting Program.

Dr. Beers, can you explain these programs, how they work together with the Healthy Start program to support newborns, and how coordination with these programs can be streamlined to improve healthy outcomes?

Dr. BEERS. Absolutely. Absolutely.

I think one of the key points of the Healthy Start program is the focus on care coordination and individualized services, and so really, through the program, helping families to access all of those different services that you recommend that they may need. Families have an assessment done when they first enter the program to really target in on what those needs are and then help connect them to existing services to decrease duplication of programming and duplication of services.

Mr. CÁRDENAS. So, again, I would like to clarify—and the reason why I am having this clarification, because far too often, when we see communities in need in America, they tend to show minority communities, poor, inner-city communities, but I just would like you to help clarify, is this an issue that faces all Americans— White, Black, brown, women, men, children? Is it pretty much across the board?

Dr. BEERS. Yes, it is.

Mr. CÁRDENAS. OK. Thank you very much for your clarity and for your expertise.

I yield back.

Ms. ESHOO. The gentleman yields back.

It is a pleasure to recognize the—is he here?

Oh, there you are, leaning back.

Mr. SHIMKUS. I don't have any questions.

Ms. ESHOO. You don't have any questions? Happy New Year to you, John. Lovely to see you.

All right. I will recognize the gentleman from Kentucky, Mr. Guthrie, for his 5 minutes of questions.

Mr. GUTHRIE. Thank you very much.

And I am sorry, there is another hearing of this same committee, a subcommittee, that I have been in this morning. And so I am actually going to kind of follow up with you, Dr. Beers, but Mr. Cárdenas kind of asked some of the questions that I was going to ask.

But first I just want to thank Ms. Zarecky for being here. I have a cousin who has had a similar situation. I know how devastating it can be on families. And as we look at the infant mortality decline, about 14 percent, and we look at numbers, those are important, but it is also important to see faces. Because the ones that are still affected, it is—so your willingness to come here at a difficult, emotional time, present to us, as we deliberate and make decisions. I can tell you, I look at faces I have met when I have to deal with issues like this far more than graphs that people put in front of you, so it is important that you do it. I know it has to be emotionally draining, but it is important and a good honor for your child.

But, Dr. Beers, as Mr. Cárdenas was talking to you, I know that in your testimony you said between 2007 and 2017 infant mortality has dropped by 14 percent, which is good to know because we are actually spending a lot of time in this committee studying mother mortality, which has not has the same decrease, it appears.

So I know you were talking with Mr. Cárdenas about things we need to do about the food insecurity and so forth. So what do you attribute the decrease to? And I think some of the things you mentioned before, can you kind of elaborate more? I know he kind of stepped on my questions, so—but I think it is important to give you more time to elaborate on things we can. But why are we seeing the success? I am always like, let's look at success and see if we can replicate it.

Dr. BEERS. Yes, absolutely. And I do also want to clarify, we have had tremendous success and still have a long way to go.

Mr. GUTHRIE. Right. Exactly.

Dr. BEERS. That is, I think, an important point for us.

So I think there are a couple of things we—there has been tremendous progress in terms of access to care for, you know, pregnant mothers and children. So we have had good progress there.

Families have had some growth in programs that allow them access to services focused on social determinants, such as Healthy Start, to really be able to connect families to those services that they need and those services that really help decrease the barriers to getting the care that they need and deserve.

We have grown quite a bit in our medical knowledge in terms of care of newborn infants and things like sudden infant death syndrome and sleep-related death issues, which contributes to that infant mortality rate.

So it really is a combination of a lot of different things. But some of things that really do remain, as I mentioned in my testimony, there are still tremendous and very troubling racial and ethic disparities in the infant mortality rate. And we need more information, and we need to dive deeper and we need to seek community solutions for how we continue to address those.

Mr. GUTHRIE. OK. Thank you very much.

And then, switching a little bit, Mr. Mendez, there is also—Congress is a snapshot of the American public. And I am a father of a daughter with a nut allergy and an uncle of a nephew who goes here at Georgetown but he was home in Kentucky over Christmas and ended up in the emergency room, eating something that had peanuts in it.

And so, as you are parents and you can—in particular, I am talking about schools now—you can control the environment. You read every label. You become obsessive about anything that might have traces of nuts in it. But then you send them off to school.

So that is why it is important that public policy plays a role in what is happening in schools. And I was in the Kentucky General Assembly, and we took steps. So, I guess, are States—does it take the Federal Government having States do this? Or what are States doing now? I think we have a role, but what are States doing now in terms of allergies? Or what are good examples of States——

Mr. MENDEZ. It really depends on the State, but there are some—for example, Delaware—that have stocked epinephrine, and they encourage that.

I mean, there is always the sensitivity about whether or not you want to have mandatory medication in the classroom. That is kind of some of the issue.

But, to the extent that you have training and an emergency action plan and there are trained personnel within the school to respond to those issues, that is really important.

I mean, anyone who has an allergy or asthma that is life-threatening should have medication and be working with their doctors and should bring it with them to their school and let the school know that they have this. And this legislation helps encourage that and create incentives for that. So that is really important.

Mr. GUTHRIE. OK. Thank you.

And those are my questions, and I will yield back.

Ms. ESHOO. The gentleman yields back.

It is a pleasure to recognize the gentlewoman from California, Ms. Barragán, for her 5 minutes of questioning.

Ms. BARRAGÁN. Thank you.

Dr. Beers, thank you for mentioning the environmental influences. Oftentimes we oversee those or we don't discuss them—don't discuss them enough.

I happen to represent a district, California's 44th. It includes the Port of Los Angeles. It is surrounded by three freeways and the port, and there are high air pollution rates there. These factors, being surrounded by highways, help to contribute to some of the worst air quality in the country.

Unfortunately, because of these factors, back home in Los Angeles asthma is an epidemic. A stunning 1 in 11 children in Los Angeles County have asthma. In my very own district, children walk around with inhalers around their necks. And even the doctor's office, they stock up on boxes and boxes of these asthma inhalers, expecting to see children come in. It is so heartbreaking to see, which is one of the reasons why I am so happy that we are trying to move legislation to address this, although there are a lot of steps that need to be taken.

The rates of asthma in communities of color are even worse. That is my very district. I have a district that is almost 90 percent Latino, African-American. Some of the statistics say that 25 percent of African-American children in L.A. County have asthma, and Hispanic children are 1 1/2 times more likely to die due to asthma when compared with other, non-Hispanic children.

Statistics such as these are one of the reasons that I am a cosponsor of the School-Based Allergies and Asthma Management Program. By incentivizing schools to maintain asthma management programs, students and parents can be assured that the child will be able to have the care they require in case of an emergency.

Mr. Mendez, can you elaborate a little bit on how this bill, H.R. 2468, will help to reduce some of the racial disparities that we see happening with asthma?

Mr. MENDEZ. Yes, sure. I mean, you know, there is going to be a child with asthma or allergies in just about every school in the United States. So, to the extent that this program creates incentives to have an asthma or an allergy action plan in the State will be really helpful to all those communities.

The CDC, which provides grants and works with the public health systems in each State, will favor whatever schools or whatever States have this kind of program. So, to the extent that this becomes legislation and creates incentives for schools and States to do this, then it will improve funding and their likelihood for getting funding to prevent asthma and allergy attacks and have the right systems in place.

Ms. BARRAGÁN. When I was a kid, I remember my father had a home that was right near the freeway. And I didn't know any better. I said, "Well, geez, if you live near the freeway, that must mean it is going to be faster to get to where you want, so it is a great place." And, of course, now knowing what I know and the allergies that I deal with——

Mr. MENDEZ. Yes, definitely.

Ms. BARRAGÁN [continuing]. I know that there is a connection there.

Besides this bill, do you have any ideas on other things that we could be doing to address asthma, you know, in particular on a congressional level?

Mr. MENDEZ. Sure. I mean, you know, there are the outdoor environmental issues as well. I mean, to the extent that there have been rollbacks of some legislation that, you know, have contributed to more dirty air, I mean, that is certainly an area.

You are witnessing it in your district, and I think, in particular, they are trying to come up with specific standards for truck emissions. And, in particular, if you are in that window or that area where—I think it is the port—there is quite a bit of short-haul trucking, and there is quite a bit of pollution that is generated from that.

So there is the outdoor environmental issue, and then, you know, there are indoor environmental issues as well, having, you know, indoor air quality and being aware of that in the schools. I mean, kids spend the majority of their time either at school or at home. Those are areas that we could really be focusing on.

Ms. BARRAGÁN. Great. Thank you.

And, ladies, thank you for being here to talk about the infant mortality rates. Certainly in a community like mine that is majority minority, it is heavily impacted. In L.A. County, they have received over a million dollars and were able to invest in programs such as the MAMA's Neighborhood project, which provides tailored home visits during prenatal, labor, delivery, post partum, and interconception periods up to 18 months following birth. These visits help reduce the rates of infant mortality.

With the last 10 seconds I have, do either one of you—can maybe you comment on how else the Healthy Start program works to reduce the racial disparities in care?

Dr. BEERS. I will give a 2-second answer, which is: I think that engagement with the community and the focus on community impact and collective impact is a really important component of it so that we are codesigning solutions together with families and communities who are most impacted.

Ms. BARRAGÁN. I yield back.

Ms. ESHOO. The gentlewoman yields back.

It is a pleasure to recognize my buddy from Indiana, the gentlewoman, Congresswoman Brooks——

Mrs. BROOKS. Thank you, Chairwoman.

Ms. ESHOO [continuing]. For your 5 minutes.

Mrs. BROOKS. And I want to thank you and the ranking member for holding this critically important hearing, and I am really pleased that we are talking about all of these bills today.

While my colleague Dr. Bucshon talked about the progress that Indiana, our home State, is making on asthma, we are not really doing as well on infant mortality. It has been a huge problem in our State for a very long time. And, in fact, our 2017 statistics, we had 602 Hoosier babies die before their first birthday. So that is about 50 babies a month or 12 a week. I mean, it is a tragic loss.

And so your voice, Ms. Zarecky, on today, of all days, and sharing with us the tragic story of your daughter Scarlett, you are a voice for all of these families across the country. So thank you very much.

And I do want to ask you, though, because you do represent a much larger group of families than we all really appreciate, can you share with us a couple of things. Specifically—and I know you talked about the foundation being such a lifeline, but is that where—and the grief counseling that maybe they provided. How did you get connected to that foundation?

What are the mental health services that are needed? We are hoping that the H.R. 2271—focus on support services for families. But when I heard, you know, 5½ months for you to get the autopsy results, can you—briefly, because I also have a question for Dr. Beers about the review teams. What more do we need to be doing? Mental health. And what were your frustrations?

Ms. ZARECKY. Thank you for your question.

First, I would say that, you know, over 5 months is a very long time to wait, but I am also very grateful that the pathologist took the time to really thoroughly examine what happened to Scarlett. So, while it was excruciating, I am so thankful that they took all measures that they did——

Mrs. BROOKS. Good.

Ms. ZARECKY [continuing]. To try to find out what happened to her.

The main reason that we allowed to have the legislation named after Scarlett is, of course, because we wanted to raise awareness of what happened to her. So many people are aware of children who pass away before, you know, their first birthday, but very few people realize how many of us there are, because children pass long after their first birthday, all the way up to the age of 18 years. So I certainly didn't know it could happen before it happened to me.

So, unfortunately, we—I was lucky. I was connected with services relatively early. But it was through my own efforts and my own research that I was able to be connected to—I actually learned about the foundation that I mentioned through a bereavement group, which is of course why bereavement groups are so important. But it would have been wonderful, you know, if even the term "sudden, unexplained death in childhood," if I had even learned of it earlier, you know, as soon as Scarlett passed away, then I could have found the——

Mrs. BROOKS. And so, even though you dealt with, whether it was law enforcement or coroners or medical professionals, you had to do that on your own.

Ms. ZARECKY. Yes, I found my own bereavement support. And it was just sheer luck that I happened to go to a bereavement group where another mother who lost her 14-month-old was there who told me about it. So, yes, I mean, being able to be connected to those services is critical.

Mrs. BROOKS. Thank you so very much for sharing.

And, Dr. Beers, I think what her story shows and her request for data and more information, I think, shows is that we need more protocols at all different levels, whether it is at the death scene investigations—and I am curious about the child death review teams, which, of course, most of our States all have child death review teams.

How does the CDC's National Fatality Review Case Reporting System work with those review teams? And what more do we need to be doing to institute more protocols that can help make sure the death scene investigations are appropriate, to make sure that families get information they need? Can you share with us a bit more about national standards?

Dr. BEERS. Yes, absolutely.

And I think your point is excellent, because it is very difficult to better understand what is happening with sudden, unexplained infant death and sudden, unexplained death in childhood when the data from across States is very inconsistent, and so it is difficult to get a full picture.

And so your point is very good, in that aligning those reviews with CDC standards, with consistent standards, is very important. I think there is a training piece of it, right, where the review committees need to have clear and consistent training with resources that link into the registry, as well as a resource piece of it. Many of these review committees are underresourced, and so the increased investment in that is also important.

Mrs. BROOKS. Thank you.

And before I yield my time, Madam Chairwoman, I would like to acknowledge all these kids who are in the audience, who are incredibly well-behaved and quiet and so good.

And so kudos to you this far in.

So I yield back.

Ms. ESHOO. The gentlewoman yields back.

The reason they are quiet is because we put them to sleep.

It is a pleasure to recognize the gentlewoman from Illinois, Ms. Kelly, for her 5 minutes of questions.

Ms. KELLY. Thank you, Madam Chair. And I would like to thank you and the ranking member for us discussing this very, very important topic. It is just so astonishing to me when I hear about this, because I have worked 3 years on maternal mortality, and it is so similar, the issues.

And I want to thank all the witnesses, and particularly you and your husband for sharing Scarlett's story. Thank you so much, because that takes bravery and courage. So we really, really appreciate it.

I wanted to know, Dr. Beers, could you speak to why it is not only important to reauthorize the program but why updates to the program are necessary and how that will contribute to the reduction of health disparities, such as the consideration of social determinants of health?

Dr. BEERS. Absolutely. No, I appreciate that. And I think, as we have often talked about the importance of knowledge and research, we have more knowledge and research than when the program was initially authorized, and so incorporating that into the legislation is very important.

I think we have talked about this a bit, but the social determinants of and social influences on health are such key contributors to infant mortality and maternal mortality rates that really incorporating those into the legislation and into the program, I think, is critically important and will help us to continue to bring rates down and continue to move forward.

Ms. KELLY. As the chairwoman said, we were able to pass bipartisan legislation out of this committee on maternal mortality, but one thing we haven't done yet is, after you have the baby and the importance of care not just for 2 months but the whole year, studies have found. So that is something that I am going to continue to pursue and push. In both cases was this so very, very important.

Ms. Zarecky, is there anything that you would like to say that we haven't asked you?

Ms. ZARECKY. That is a tall question.

Ms. KELLY. Just, anything else?

Ms. ZARECKY. Yes. I guess I would just like to, you know, thank you for hearing Scarlett's sorry and recognize that Scarlett is one child but there are thousands of children out there who really need Congress. The families really need Congress's help to figure out what happened to them and stop it from happening in the future.

Ms. KELLY. Thank you so much.

And I yield back.

Ms. ESHOO. The gentlewoman yields back. We are all grateful to her. She is the resident scholar and leader on the issue of maternal mortality.

It is a pleasure to recognize the gentleman from Georgia, the only pharmacist in the Congress, Mr. Carter.

Mr. CARTER. Thank you, Madam Chair. Thank you.

And thank all of you for being here, especially you, Ms. Zarecky. Thank you. I appreciate this very much.

Dr. Beers, I want to start with you. Let me ask you, are you familiar with Dr. John Snow? Did you ever read that book "Ghost Map"?

That is a great read. I hope you will get an opportunity. It is about cholera and how he, back in the mid- or early 1800s, how he finally used data to figure out what was causing that and actually was able to get it down to a single well where people were getting water, and that is how they were getting infected and that is how many people had died.

And that is what I want to concentrate on here, because I am from Georgia, and we are the number-one State in maternal mortality. And I still cannot understand that, for the life of me.

But I just want to ask you, how important is the data collection, and how important is it to make sure you are asking the right questions? And are we asking the right questions?

Dr. BEERS. Thank you for that. And I agree that that story is a wonderful public health story and highlights the importance of data.

The data is very important in this. And we are asking some of the right questions, but I am not sure we are asking all of the right questions. And I am not sure we are always asking the right people the questions.

I think it is important for us to expand our data collection in this area to really be talking to affected families and to mothers who are receiving prenatal care and find what their barriers are, find where they are getting difficulty accessing services and/or what things they are running into.

And when we can match that qualitative data that we get from asking those questions with the, sort of, more number/quantitative data, that is going to give us a more full picture and help us further go down the line.

Mr. CARTER. What kind of challenges are you having now in the way of data collection? What are your obstacles?

Dr. BEERS. Yes. So there are a number of things. I think, you know, we certainly have reasonable, I think, nationwide, reasonable access to, sort of, secondary data, hospital-based data, right? But it is harder to get data on some of the social conditions that families are living in. It is harder to get this more qualitative data. It——

Mr. CARTER. But from what—I don't mean to interrupt you, but from what I understand, with maternal mortality, the economic level doesn't really enter into it.

Dr. BEERS. Correct. And it enters into it, but we see these racial and ethnic disparities despite socioeconomic levels. So it is kind of a "yes, and" situation.

But also recognizing that you can look at an entire neighborhood and every person and family in that neighborhood has a different experience and is living in different circumstances. And understanding those nuances better—

Mr. CARTER. Uh-huh.

Dr. BEERS [continuing]. Will help us then better understand how we address this.

Mr. CARTER. Let me ask you something. Are death certificates uniform all throughout the Nation, or each State has a different one?

Dr. BEERS. No, each State has a different one.

Mr. CARTER. How much of a challenge is that?

I mean, I still question why Georgia is first. I just don't get it. I know we have south Georgia and rural areas, but I still don't understand. I mean—

Dr. BEERS. Right.

Mr. CARTER [continuing]. The death certificates, should they be uniform? I mean, should we be asking the same questions all throughout the Nation?

Dr. BEERS. Right. I think that certainly—I think that would be one thing. I think, often, in these situations—and we certainly see this in Washington, DC, as well. We are not doing very much better than you are in Georgia. And the causes are really multifactorial.

Often you can address certain issues fairly easily, and then when you get to some of these really difficult, complex issues, the causes really are multifactorial. So it has to do with education and access to care and bias in healthcare and social determinants of health and how all those things interrelate. And that is a more difficult thing to tackle, and it requires a deeper investment to tackle it.

Mr. CARTER. But you would agree that most probably not everyone is defining maternal mortality the same throughout the country? In other words, this very well may have been something that is not reported in one State but is reported in another State.

Dr. BEERS. I don't know—I am not 100 percent sure I would say the maternal mortality itself is being defined differently, but some of the, sort of, underlying things may be reported differently and different questions being asked that can help give us a full answer.

Mr. CARTER. And, regardless, we still have to address it. I mean—and this is a challenge. And I thank you for your work.

And I thank all of you for being here. Whether it be maternal mortality or sudden, unexplained death in childhood, God forbid, all of these things are extremely important. We just have to figure it out. And it is like it is right there in front of us, and we just can't figure it out.

So thank you for your efforts, and thank you again for being here.

And I yield back.

Ms. ESHOO. The gentleman yields back.

Our subcommittee is blessed to have more than one physician as a member, and so it is a pleasure to recognize Dr. Ruiz for his 5 minutes of questioning.

Mr. RUIZ. Thank you very much.

As an emergency physician doctor, I have seen some very severe cases of asthma and asthma attacks. In fact, there is one child who I will never forget. He died in the emergency department. He was a young, 6- to 8-year-old, African-American boy, playing games with his stepfather, and then suddenly just went into a dramatic asthma attack. He was brought into the emergency department. After a long and intensive resuscitative effort with multiple doctors, he was pronounced dead.

And I was in the room with the doctors—this was during my training at the time—when they told the parents, and it was so heartbreaking. And I am still haunted by that. And so I really respect the seriousness of asthma, because I have seen the end result of what can happen, especially for kids.

And, many times, it is preventable. It is preventable with the right knowledge, the right training, the right medications, the right follow-up, the right coverage. It is preventable.

So there is actually one area in my district that has a very severe asthma problem. They have 3 times the asthma rate in the State of California. In fact, they have the highest pediatric asthma hospitalization rate in the State of California.

And it is multifactorial. For one, we have a large body of water, the largest in California, called the Salton Sea, and when it recedes, the dust is exposed to the children. Two, it is a very low-income—community, in the setting of very medically uninsured, where there is only 1 doctor per 9,000 residents in that part of my district. To give you perspective, it is recommended to have 1 to 2,000 in this country. One to 3,500 is considered medically underserved. So we are 1 to 9,000.

Then they live in underdeveloped areas, so they have dirt roads. Then they live in overcrowded, substandard housing and trailer parks, like I did in my first few years of life.

So all these point to the conditions that children live under, especially those with asthma. And so those kids are less likely to be able to manage their symptoms, more likely to end up in the emergency department, and more likely to be admitted as the result of an uncontrolled asthma attack, when it could be preventable.

So, Mr. Mendez, can you talk about the importance of the children's asthma treatment grant program for helping ensure that preventable asthma attacks are avoided?

Mr. MENDEZ. Sure. The grant program administered by the CDC, the National Asthma Control Program, takes a public health approach and tries to work with State health agencies in order to provide funding to have upstream remediation to issues like that.

And then, to the extent that this program could be rolled out more and have more States win these grants in the public health systems, then I think we will see on-the-ground improvements. Because we have seen, overall, in the various States that have it right now, reductions in emergency room visits, improvement in adherence to medication, reduction in hospitalizations. So, I mean, those three things are really helpful.

And, you know, with an $82 billion cost of asthma to the healthcare system, there are ways to reduce that through upstream programs like this for the National Asthma Control Program. I think that we increased the budget by a million dollars this year, or you voted for that, but to the extent that we could have even greater funding for it—and I think Representative Engel, through the Elijah Cummings Family Asthma Act, is pushing towards that.

Mr. RUIZ. And can you walk us through how environmental factors and, by extension, the social determinants of health affect the overall public health?

Mr. MENDEZ. Sure. I mean, you know, there is some overlap here, but if you go into housing where there is mold, cockroaches, these are all triggers for asthma attacks. So I have been in housing situations or visited housing where I have gone in with a trained health worker who has basically said, you need to remove the carpeting, you need to work with your landlord in order to have them patch up the rodent holes, and then——

Mr. RUIZ. And how does poverty affect——

Mr. MENDEZ. It is significant.

Mr. RUIZ [continuing]. The asthma?

Mr. MENDEZ. I mean, that is really part of it. So, to the extent that you can control or improve the indoor health environment, then it will have better outcomes for the patient.

Mr. RUIZ. It is also a matter of coverage. It is also a matter of being insured and being able——

Mr. MENDEZ. Yes.

Mr. RUIZ [continuing]. To afford your proper asthma course. You know, most people think it is just the albuterol inhaler when you are having an attack——

Mr. MENDEZ. Right. That is the rescue.

Mr. RUIZ. That is the rescue, but——

Mr. MENDEZ. Yes.

Mr. RUIZ [continuing]. The prevention is the other medications.

Mr. MENDEZ. That is correct.

Mr. RUIZ. Thank you.

Ms. ESHOO. The gentleman yields.

It is a pleasure to recognize the gentleman from Missouri, Mr. Long, for his 5 minutes of questions.

Mr. LONG. Thank you, Madam Chairwoman.

And thank you all very much for being here today on this very important topic.

I think the natural order of things is that, you know, our children are supposed to bury us and we are supposed to bury our parents, and when that doesn't happen, it is just heart-wrenching.

And I have a 30-year-old, now, daughter that was diagnosed with Hodgkin's lymphoma at 25. And when we were at the emergency room over here at G.W. and they said, "Your daughter has a large mass in her chest, and it is malignant," you immediately think that you are going to lose that child. She is 30 now, been through all the chemo. And we are very, very thankful to God and to doctors and the healthcare providers and everybody else that we still have her.

So, Ms. Zarecky, I can't fathom, you know, what you went through, to put a healthy baby down to bed and go in to check on the baby and the baby is deceased. So thank you for being here.

My oldest daughter is 33. She is a pediatrician. And I think I have one of her cards in my pocket. And, unfortunately, I think it is in my left pocket, so I have to figure out how to get it out. But I would like to give it to you, Dr. Beers. And just, if you wouldn't mind, just text her a little note or something and say, "I was with your dad today," because it is great honor to have the president-elect of the American Academy of Pediatrics with us, with my daughter being a pediatrician.

I just wish she didn't have a 6-month-old poodle. Because I was babysitting the poodle, and out under the gate it went, and you see the end result here. But I am advertising for somebody who is this doctor—some sling provider, it looks like. But, anyway, that was my Christmas present to myself, was to break my shoulder on the Friday before Christmas wrangling her poodle. But the poodle did survive, I have to tell you.

Dr. Beers, as a pediatrician with a focus on community pediatrics, what has been your experience with the Healthy Start program, and how it has been able to remove barriers to accessing healthcare?

Dr. BEERS. Thank you very much. And I would be delighted to speak with your daughter. It is wonderful to hear of that connection, so thank you.

So, you know—and we have Healthy Start here in DC, so I have the privilege of having had families and patients who have participated in the program. And I think there are really a couple key pieces that highlight the importance of the program, in my experience.

One is the real patient- and family-centered nature of it. It is very individualized. It really takes the family's preference and needs into account and then really works to help connect the family to the healthcare services, to the other enabling services that can help support them in accessing the care they need to do the best they can for themselves and for their family.

I think it is also—as a program, it is very connected and engaged with the rest of the community and the rest of the community-based services so that you are really utilizing all the resources available to you in your neighborhoods and in your community.

Mr. LONG. OK. How does the Healthy Start program support provider training?

Dr. BEERS. It helps support provider training in a number of different ways. So by giving medical providers the education about how to access these services and about what needs families have and how to connect them to that. It also helps with provider training, nonmedical provider training, as well.

Mr. LONG. OK. And how does the Healthy Start reauthorization address the need for collaboration with these providers?

Dr. BEERS. Yes. Yes. That is great. And I think, you know, one of the most important things that I have learned through my career and through working in the community is that we all work better when we work better as a team. I have my own set of skills and experiences. My colleagues and partners have their set of experiences. Our social workers have their experiences. Our WIC nutritionist has her skills and experiences. And so we do better for families when we all come together and work together as part of a team. And that is what Healthy Start helps promote.

Mr. LONG. OK.

You also mentioned the serious maternal mortality crisis that we are facing. And I am a member of the Black Maternal Mortality Caucus, and we are doing everything we can to figure out what is going on there. Can you discuss the role the Healthy Start program can have in reducing maternal mortality?

Dr. BEERS. Absolutely. And it does, it comes back to some of these tenets of identifying what a family's needs and barriers are to accessing good-quality care and then helping to break down those barriers so that mothers can get there.

And so, you know, one of the first and most important things for a mother when she is pregnant is to be able to get to her OB–GYN care and access those services early and on a regular basis, and Healthy Start can help break down those barriers.

It can help identify what some of the social determinants and what some of the social needs may be that are getting in the way or, as we were speaking earlier, may be contributing to poor maternal health outcomes and start to address those things as well—the food insecurity, the housing insecurity, things like that.

Mr. LONG. Do you hear a tapping, or is it just me?

Dr. BEERS. No, I do hear a little tapping.

Mr. LONG. I yield back.

Ms. ESHOO. Tapping and clapping. How is that?

It is a pleasure to recognize the gentlewoman from Delaware, Ms. Blunt Rochester, for her 5 minutes of questions.

Ms. BLUNT ROCHESTER. Thank you, Madam Chairwoman, for recognizing me and also for this important hearing.

And I would also like to apologize. Some of us may be going in and out because of a competing hearing, but this is a very important hearing.

And I would like to thank the witnesses for joining us as we consider legislation that aims to improve the health coverage of our constituents and also the health outcomes.

Ms. Zarecky, I want to personally thank you so much for taking the time, for sharing your story, and for honoring Scarlett. Having lost a spouse unexpectedly, I understand turning that pain into purpose. And so I thank you, and I thank your family for being here today for something that is vitally important to our country.

Last year, I was proud to support the passage of H.R. 3172, the Safe Sleep for Babies Act. Today, we have an opportunity to continue those efforts by looking at H.R. 2271, Scarlett's Sunshine on Sudden Unexpected Death Act.

We need a strong, multifaceted public health approach in order to understand the causes of sudden, unexpected infant death, SUID, and sudden, unexpected death in childhood, SUDC, and how we can prevent instances of both. I am a cosponsor of H.R. 2271 because I believe this legislation achieves those goals. And I am thankful for my friend and my colleague, Congresswoman Gwen Moore, for introducing this legislation.

As the chairman pointed out, this multifaceted approach includes grant funding for State and local health departments, community-based organizations, and nonprofits so that they can provide support to families who have lost an infant or a child to SUID or SUDC.

And I am pleased to hear that the services had a positive effect on your family as well.

Ms. Zarecky, in your testimony, you shared the important policy priorities that we should be considering. And the strength of H.R. 2271, to me, is that it recognizes those priorities and it puts our money our where our mouth is. The bill authorizes $8 million to improve how we investigate and record the unexpected deaths of infants and children, $1 million to improve case reporting, and $15 million to help States develop and implement prevention strategies.

Ms. Zarecky, do you think that it would be difficult, challenging to make the progress that we need to make without including funding for these critical activities? I think that is an easy question.

Ms. ZARECKY. Absolutely.

Ms. BLUNT ROCHESTER. Absolutely. Are there other sections of the House bill that you think make the House version strong?

Ms. ZARECKY. Of course. One element of the legislation here in the House, of course, is the addition of the family support and the bereavement support. You know, it is a critical piece, I think, to being able to support families after their loss and their unique needs.

Ms. BLUNT ROCHESTER. Yes. Thank you.

Another public health issue facing children across the country and in Delaware is the rate of asthma amongst school-age children. In 2015, the Delaware Survey of Children's Health asked parents if their child had ever been diagnosed with asthma, and, in the responses, 17 percent of parents said that they had had an asthma diagnosis.

For this reason, we must have strong policies in place and equip our schools with the tools they need to support these efforts.

That is why I am proud that Delaware's public schools received an "A" on the Asthma and Allergy Foundation of America's 2019 State Honor Roll for meeting a key number of the 23 core policies laid out to protect students.

Mr. Mendez, how did the AAFA choose the standards used in their State Honor Roll of Asthma and Allergy Policies for Schools?

Mr. MENDEZ. Sure. We have been doing it for a while, but we have a medical and scientific board, and we work with the community, and these really are the best practices that we see as really important to prevent asthma and allergies. A lot of this bill, 2468, picks up on some of those policies that we recommend.

So congratulations to Delaware. I mean, you have some stock epinephrine laws, for example, that are really critical and that have been successful.

So 2468 really tries to include, again, asthma action plans, allergy action plans, how to deal with those kinds of emergency situations, in addition to looking at the environmental controls inside the classroom, where many of the kids spend much of their time.

Ms. BLUNT ROCHESTER. I am almost out of time. I have some additional questions that I will submit to the record.

But I want to thank you all for your work and your commitment to the children and to the families of our country. Thank you so much.

And I yield back.

Ms. ESHOO. The gentlewoman yields back.

It is a pleasure to recognize the gentleman from Montana, Mr. Gianforte, for his 5 minutes.

Mr. GIANFORTE. Thank you, Madam Chair.

Ms. Zarecky, thank you for sharing your testimony today and your story. As a father of four, I can only imagine what you have gone through, and I am so sorry for your loss. And I applaud your bravery for being here to tell your story to honor Scarlett.

In your testimony, you said that we don't know how widespread instances of sudden, unexpected death in childhood are because there is a lack of specific ways to record these deaths. I was hoping you could share with us, from the perspective of a parent, what was the process like for you to determine your daughter qualified as an instance of sudden, unexpected death in childhood?

Ms. ZARECKY. For us in particular, about a little less than 48 hours after Scarlett passed away, we heard the initial results of her autopsy, which is, of course, that it was undetermined, her cause of death. And then we waited a little over 5 months to get the full autopsy and the full gamut of tests back. And then, even then, her cause of death was considered undetermined.

So there are, you know, a lot of different terms that do relate to how these deaths are classified. And so that was—you know, through that process and then being able to speak with other families who experienced similar losses, that is how we found that out.

Mr. GIANFORTE. And at a terrible time, where you wanted answers, there was really just no certainty for you.

Ms. ZARECKY. Yes. And to this day, I mean, it is really, truly terrifying to know that I don't know what happened to my daughter. And you want answers, you know? You want to know what happened, but you also want to know that it is not going to happen again.

Mr. GIANFORTE. Uh-huh.

Ms. ZARECKY. And living with that uncertainty for myself, for my subsequent daughter, for my husband, for my nephews and nieces, it is really—you know, it has been 3 years today, and I am just reliving, you know, all of the triggers. And we just celebrated the second Christmas with my second daughter, and I was reliving Scarlett's second Christmas, which she died shortly after. So it has lasting impacts on me, just the trauma associated with it.

Mr. GIANFORTE. Again, thank you for your bravery and being here today.

Ms. ZARECKY. Thank you.

Mr. GIANFORTE. On a related note, Dr. Beers, in your testimony, you discuss how important death review teams are in understanding how these terrible deaths occur.

Montana is a rural State. Could you talk about the challenges that death review teams have in rural parts of the country?

Dr. BEERS. Yes. It is very difficult, right, because when your populations are smaller and more spread out, your expertise is a bit more spread out as well. It is there, but it is a bit more spread out and perhaps harder to access sometimes.

And so I think it does circle back to the importance of some of the things highlighted in this bill, of training, of standards, of support to be provided to death review teams across all States, regardless of the makeup, regardless of whether they are rural or urban. And so I acknowledge that it is a different challenge, right——

Mr. GIANFORTE. Yes.

Dr. BEERS [continuing]. And, I think, you know, is one of the things that this bill helps to get at.

Mr. GIANFORTE. Yes. Good.

And, also, Dr. Beers, Montana is home to eight federally recognized Native American Tribal governments. And it is incredibly troubling that SUID and SUDC are so common amongst Native American peoples. What can the Indian Health Service do to better prevent these deaths?

Dr. BEERS. Yes. No—and I think it does—and, again, it goes back to some of the services provided through Healthy Start: really taking the time and investing the resources to evaluate families, to do intake assessments, to really get to the heart of what challenges they are facing and what their needs are, and then providing that individualized support to help make sure they get there.

You know, you mentioned living in a rural State. Access to care can be more difficult in a rural State because you have to travel farther and you don't have as easy access to public transportation or other things. And so, really, kind of, diving into what those challenges and barriers are and helping to identify solutions.

Mr. GIANFORTE. OK.

I have a couple seconds left. Also, Native American women, as you noted, face higher rates of maternal mortality. Is maternal mortality and infant mortality linked? And how does fixing one affect the other?

Dr. BEERS. Yes. There certainly are linkages, in that the same influences on maternal mortality are very similar to the influences on infant mortality. And so, if we address those things, it will help both those issues.

Mr. GIANFORTE. OK.

Thank you very much for your testimony.

And I yield back.

Ms. ESHOO. The gentleman yields back.

It is a pleasure to recognize the ever-patient gentleman from Massachusetts, Mr. Kennedy.

Mr. KENNEDY. Thank you, Madam Chair. I am grateful for the opportunity.

Thank you to our witnesses.

And, Ms. Zarecky, thank you for being here as well. I echo the comments of my colleagues. I have a 2-year-old and a 4-year-old. Difficult to listen to your testimony this morning.

And I wanted to start by saying, about a month ago, I was at a coffee shop. I had just finished a meeting, and I was on my way out. And, that evening, it was dark and it was raining. And a gentleman, probably about my own age, maybe a couple years younger, just grabbed me and asked me to read a letter that he had scratched on a napkin as I jumped in the car.

And I got in and I started reading it, and it was a letter about his son, Luke, who was 18 months old—my son at that point was about 22 months old—who told your story. A beautiful, bright, healthy, chaotic baby boy, fully vaccinated, walking, talking, beautiful, who went to bed and didn't wake up.

And I went back inside, and we talked for about a half-hour or so. And listening to that young dad try to make sense out of what happened, wrestle with the stigma associated with the loss of a child and the judgment that came down on him and his wife for the perception of having done something wrong, and not be able to point to anything, and to still, as you articulated, search for answers.

His request was that I cosponsor your bill. And, luckily, I already had. But I think it highlights not just the obvious need to try to ensure that we do everything we can to make sure that this doesn't happen again but to make sure that parents get answers and families get answers.

And one of the things that stuck with me from our conversation was how he said, after searching for answers, they were fortunate to come across a research-based program in Boston that did help eventually diagnose a form of sudden, unexpected death in childhood that was consistent with an epilepsy pathway. But, still, largely unanswered.

What struck me was you had a young dad who was in tears who was talking about how fortunate he was to have come across a program that could help at least point him directionally to some explanation about what happened with his son.

I have a letter from his parents—well, from Garrett and Megan—that I wanted to introduce for the record, Madam Chair, as well.

Ms. ESHOO. So ordered.

Mr. KENNEDY. But I wanted to thank you, Ms. Zarecky, for your courage and the strength that you show for Scarlett. So thank you.

I also wanted to turn briefly, in the time that I have left, to another story of a baby who will be turning a year old next month. He was born far away from Massachusetts, and the baby's esophagus is in two separate segments connected abnormally to the windpipe.

Boston Children's Hospital, Dr. Beers, is one of two places in the country that is capable of the surgery to correct that particularly complex and complicated case. And the family has been forced to reschedule that surgery three separate times since August because of their confusion within the baby's home State Medicaid vendor.

We know the diagnosis. We know we can treat it. We know there are people that can conduct the procedure. And yet the joint Federal-State nature of a Medicaid program prohibits that, oftentimes gets in the way.

Six months ago, the baby could have had surgery to relieve difficulty breathing and the pain that could result in trips to the ER. But confusion over those Medicaid regulations regarding out-of-State treatment for infants and children has prolonged that baby's suffering and that of countless others.

So I know you are aware of similar stories, and I apologize for not giving you a whole lot of time, but do you think it would be beneficial to help simplify Medicaid screening and enrollment for clinicians who are providing the highest quality care, specialist care, to children, enabling them to get access to treatment for rare illnesses that are only available at specialty centers across State lines?

Dr. BEERS. I can be very brief: Yes, we do support that. Anything that can decrease the barriers to care and streamline access to coverage, I would support that. Thank you.

Mr. KENNEDY. Thank you.

Thank you for being here.

Madam Chair, thanks for the hearing.

Ms. ESHOO. The gentleman yields back.

We thought, Mr. Kennedy, that the ACE Kids Act was going to address the very situation that you just pointed out. So I want to work with you to make sure that it is working. We worked so long and so hard to get that legislation over the line, and that was the full intent of it, and it is more than disappointing to me to hear what you just said.

But, at any rate, we need to work on that, because that is an impossible situation for a family to be in. No one can go up against these programs and the Federal Government and the bureaucracy and straighten them out themselves.

Now, the ever-patient, my pal, wonderful Member of Congress, your Representative, Ms. Zarecky. We are fortunate to have him in the Congress. We love Mike Doyle. So we are really pleased to welcome him to our subcommittee. And you have your 5 minutes for questioning.

Mr. DOYLE. I want to thank you, Madam Chair, for your kindness, and the ranking member, for allowing me to waive on to the subcommittee today.

Stephanie, I want to thank you and your husband, Ryan. And I saw Iliana walking down the hallway. She is a very active young lady. But your testimony and your courage to come here today— this is a difficult day, but you are here. What you had to say touched every member of this committee.

This is a start of our regular order hearings. We will move into markups in subcommittee and full committee. I think it is safe to say, based on your testimony and the way you have touched every member of this committee, that this is a bill that will move quickly through the subcommittee and full committee process. And, hopefully, we can get this out to the floor and send this over to our colleagues in the Senate. And this is a great way to honor Scarlett's memory, and I just want to salute you for your courage in being here today.

I know we have spent a lot of time talking about sleep-related deaths, but what happened to Scarlett is different. And maybe Dr. Beers or Stephanie, can you help us understand the difference or the distinction between SUDC or SUID and other sleep-related deaths because of unsafe sleep procedures? Explain the difference, because I think a lot of people see this as some sort of, you know, unsafe practices in sleeping. So if you could take a moment to maybe just explain that.

Dr. BEERS. Absolutely. Yes, absolutely. And I appreciate the question because I think it is an important clarification.

And I should say, I think often the reason that we talk more about sleep-related deaths is because we have more data and information on that, and we are better able to articulate some of the reasons and causes behind it and what to do.

And I think that does, then, highlight one of the challenges for sudden, unexplained infant death that may not be sleep-related and/or sudden, unexplained childhood death, is that we don't have that data to be able to talk about—as much of that data—to be able to talk about how to prevent it.

And so SIDS, or sudden infant death syndrome that is sleep-related is an initially unexplained death in infancy that then is ultimately attributable to sleep positioning or to sleep practices——

Mr. DOYLE. Right.

Dr. BEERS [continuing]. Or sleep related in some way. And that is often determined through the death scene investigation or death fatality review.

But there are many, many children who die unexpectedly in infancy or childhood for whom we don't identify a cause and that it is not sleep-related.

Mr. DOYLE. Yes. And maybe that just leads into my second. You know, what kinds of research are being done into SUID that can be expanded to also older infants and children?

Dr. BEERS. Yes. Yes. No, I think it is a great question. I think Ms. Zarecky spoke, actually, to some of the most important things that are happening and then also highlighting that it is sometimes difficult to do research if you don't have the data.

And so this bill focusing in on making sure that we are starting with good data so that we can then build on that I think is a really important piece of it, and also making sure that we are investing resources to be able to do that research.

Mr. DOYLE. And what kind of data is currently being collected on SUID? And how might that also apply to older children?

Dr. BEERS. Yes. Part of the challenge is that it is inconsistent. So there typically is data collected from autopsy results and/or from death scene investigation, but there is a bit of a lack of consistency in the way that is done across jurisdictions. And so that makes it, then, difficult to bring all those stories and cases together to start to draw some conclusions from them.

Mr. DOYLE. And, Stephanie, I have 48 seconds. I want to give you a chance to add anything you would like to add or say——

Ms. ZARECKY. Thank you.

Mr. DOYLE [continuing]. Since I am the last speaker.

Ms. ZARECKY. Thank you. The party is ours, right?

Thank you so much. And, you know, I thank you so much for being here. It means a lot to see a friendly face. This is very intimidating. And——

Ms. ESHOO. We all have friendly faces here.

Ms. ZARECKY. Well, a face that is a little bit more well-known to me in my little town in Pittsburgh.

Ms. ESHOO. Yes, that is all right. I am teasing you.

Ms. ZARECKY. But I just want to thank everyone for listening to Scarlett's story.

And I do want to also thank you for pointing out the fact that, of course, Scarlett's death is a sleep-related death, but, as far as we know, it is unpreventable. We can't predict it, and we can't prevent it.

So, while we have made great strides in sleep-related deaths as related to potential hazards during sleep, we have barely scratched the surface—barely scratched the surface on what is happening to these other kids. Like, there is a reason the numbers have gone down and then they have kind of stagnated.

So, on the back of my shirt right now, I have the names of hundreds of SUDC children who have been lost, and that is just a small fraction of the children representing the families who have just been shattered, who need answers. And we need systems in place to collect the data so that we can do the good research and we can figure out why this is happening. It really is an area of public health that has just not been addressed.

Mr. DOYLE. Thank you. Well, we will get this done not only for you but for all those families that you have represented here today.

Ms. ZARECKY. Thank you.

Mr. DOYLE. Madam Chair, thank you so much.

Ranking Member, thank you for your indulgence.

Ms. ESHOO. Thank you, Mr. Doyle, for your persistence on the legislation and being so central in the life of Ms. Zarecky and her family.

I think almost all of us are parents here, and it just keeps running through our—that it hasn't happened to us, that it could have, the unimaginable. These little angels, one moment they are breathing, and the next minute they are not.

Well, the first panel, thank you to you. And on behalf of all of my colleagues, I can't thank you enough for the excellent testimony that you have given to us and the expertise that you have shared with us. You can see that the committee was fully engaged, asked excellent questions. And you have now built a very sound foundation for the legislation. So thank you to you.

I want to ask the staff to prepare the witness table for the next panel. And we will get as much done as we can before we have to depart for the classified briefing on Iran and Iraq, which begins at, I believe, 1 o'clock in the Congressional Auditorium. So let's prepare the table as quickly as we can, please.

Thank you, first of all, for being here this morning and waiting and listening, but I am sure you have benefited from it, as did we.

So welcome to the second panel of witnesses.

Dr. Matthew Cooper is the director of kidney and pancreas transplantation at the MedStar Georgetown Transplant Institute.

Thank you for being here.

Mr. Kevin Koser, a patient advocate on behalf of the National Foundation for Ectodermal Dysplasias, thank you to you for being here.

And Mr. Fred Riccardi—welcome to you—president of the Medicare Rights Center.

Dr. Cooper, you are recognized for your 5 minutes of testimony.

Statements of Matthew Cooper, M.D., Director, Kidney and Pancreas Transplantation, Medstar Georgetown Transplant Initiative; Kevin G. Koser, Patient Advocate, on Behalf of the National Foundation for Ectodermal Dysplasias; and Frederic Riccardi, President, Medicare Rights Center

Statement of Matthew Cooper, M.D.

Dr. COOPER. Thank you, Chairwoman Eshoo, Ranking Member Burgess, and members of this committee.

I will attempt to be brief. I know there are pressing issues that are before this committee. I will say, it is an absolute pleasure, a privilege, to be here. I am much more comfortable in a hospital, in an operating room, so this is outside of my boundaries, but I am——

Ms. ESHOO. This is our hospital and operating room.

Dr. COOPER. Yes, I understand.

I am representing hundreds of thousands of successful transplant recipients; several hundred thousands who, actually, are currently waiting for that call for the gift of life; hopefully several million in the future that will receive a lifesaving transplant; living donor families; those that have given the gift of life at the decision of their deceased loved ones; and countless transplant professionals around the country who care tirelessly for these groups of individuals.

My name is Dr. Matthew Cooper. As mentioned, I am a transplant surgeon. I do believe I have the best job in the world in participating in sharing of that gift of life. I actually serve as the director of kidney and pancreas transplantation for the MedStar Georgetown Transplant Institute here in the District.

I am also very much involved in a number of national societies and patient-centered organizations, including the American Society of Transplant Surgeons, the National Kidney Foundation, the American Association of Kidney Patients, whose voices are very important in this and who we have heard very loud and clear, and a spokesperson for Honor the Gift, which is a grassroots organization of professionals and patients who are looking to push this legislation through.

As mentioned in many of the introductory comments, this truly is a no-brainer. We believe that this bipartisan support is very encouraging. And unlike some of the very difficult conversations we had about maternal and fetal death—again, back to some of the comments, almost Dr. Seuss-like, this is nonsensical. And so we really hope that, at the end of this, this is something that becomes very clear.

Organ transplantation is by far a medical success story for the patients that are able to receive an organ transplant. It increases not only their length of life but also their quality of life, not only for they but for their family. Important to recognize that kidney disease, kidney failure is not an individual problem. It is a family problem.

But, unfortunately, everybody who needs a kidney transplant does not receive one. The supply-and-demand problem is real here in the United States. Over 100,000 people waiting for kidney transplants. Unfortunately, about

20,000 a year are transplanted. And, unfortunately, there remains, then, a dramatic shortage of organs.

Unfortunately, the current Medicare policy serves to exacerbate this issue. Under current policy, after that 36 months following a very successful transplant, Medicare coverage for immuno-suppressive medication goes away. That becomes a significant problem for many patients, 80 percent of which are primary Medicare beneficiaries.

And I have witnessed this on a personal basis. I can give many examples. A very simple one that several months ago came through my doors: A young mother of three who was covered by Medicare with a supplemental insurance, who was doing very well following a transplant, unfortunately lost her job and, with that, lost her supplemental insurance. She was, therefore, only covered by Medicare. You can imagine where this story goes.

Three years following a successful transplant, she, unfortunately, was unable to pay for her medications. And while some might say that is her fault for not coming forward and letting us know that this was a problem, recognize that life goes on for these patients. They have families to care for, they have other bills to pay, and, unfortunately, they are a little bit embarrassed that they are unable to care for their own medications.

And so she lost her transplant. She is back on the list, and she is one of the potential only 10 percent of people that will receive a second transplant because of the sheer numbers of supply and demand.

And this is not an only story. Across the country, well over 70 percent of programs can talk about at least one patient who has lost their organ secondary to insufficient coverage.

From a medical standpoint, it makes no sense, and also from a financial standpoint, we have lots of information now that demonstrates that we can save Medicare money. This is an absolute win for all of us. It costs about $86,000 a year for dialysis. Up-front costs for the transplant are around $100,000. But each year of immunosuppressive coverage is about $2,000, $2,300 a year; with generics and patient support programs, perhaps even less. And, again, this own government has recognized the cost savings perhaps being close to $300 million. That is a tremendous win for all of us.

And so, simply put, this legislation can potentially save kidneys, it can save lives, and it certainly saves the Government money.

And I applaud Dr. Burgess not only for this but for all the things that you have done for kidney care. Please know that your efforts have not gone unnoticed.

And I would encourage Chairman Eshoo and the rest of this committee to please help us support this bill. Let's bring this across the finish line. It is time to put the exclamation point on this.

Thank you.

[The prepared statement of Dr. Cooper follows:]

Testimony of Matthew Cooper, M.D., Medstar Georgetown Transplant Institute, Georgetown University, Washington, DC, before the Energy and Commerce Health Subcommittee, U.S. House of Representatives, Support for H.R. 5534, "Comprehensive Immunosuppressive Drug Coverage for Kidney Transplant Patients Act," January 8, 2020

Chairwoman Eshoo, Ranking Member Burgess, and members of the Committee, thank you for the opportunity to testify here today.

My name is Dr. Matthew Cooper, and I am a transplant surgeon serving as the Director of Kidney and Pancreas Transplantation at the Medstar Georgetown Transplant Institute here in the District. I am actively involved with many patient advisory boards and professional societies. I am a member of the National Kidney Foundation's National Board, a council member of American Society of Transplant Surgeons, a member of American Society of Transplantation, a medical advisory board member for American Association of Kidney Patients, and a spokesperson for the Honor the Gift campaign – a national, patient-centered, grassroots movement advocating for the extension of immunosuppression medication coverage for kidney transplant patients.

It is my honor to advocate for the interests of 37 million kidney patients—including the 215,000 Americans living with a functioning kidney transplant, the health of which depends on a lifelong regimen of immunosuppressive drugs to prevent organ rejection.

Thank you for today's discussion about the impact of Medicare's 36-month limit on immunosuppressive drugs for kidney transplant recipients. A special thanks to those Members of Congress who introduced H.R. 5534, including Representatives Burgess, Eshoo and McEachin from this committee. The kidney and transplant communities are especially appreciative of Dr. Burgess and Representative Kind's steadfast leadership on this legislation.

The Medicare program has been at the forefront of quality kidney care for almost 50 years. As many of you know, Medicare created a lifeline for patients with kidney failure when it began covering dialysis for all patients, regardless of their age, in 1973. Similarly, Medicare has covered hundreds of thousands of kidney transplants over the years, allowing countless kidney patients a second chance at life.

Organ transplantation is a medical success story. For the patients who are fortunate enough to receive a donated organ, the quality and length of their lives can be dramatically improved. But not everyone who needs a donated kidney receives one. There are currently more than 103,000 individuals on the kidney transplant waiting list, while just 21,300 transplants were performed in the first eleven months of 2019. There remains a measurable and dramatic shortage of kidneys available for transplant.

Unfortunately, current Medicare policy exacerbates the issue. Under current policy, kidney transplant patients who are neither aged nor disabled – more than 80 percent of the kidney transplant population – lose Medicare coverage of critically important immunosuppressive drugs 36 months after their transplant. Without immunosuppressive drugs to prevent rejection, many patients find themselves back in a risky and frightening place - or worse - in need of a new kidney.

As a transplant surgeon for nearly 20 years, I have witnessed firsthand the impact of this shortsighted policy. Patients struggle to pay for the immunosuppressive drugs needed to maintain the health of their transplant when their Medicare coverage ends, especially lower income patients who lack group health insurance or do not qualify for Medicaid or other assistance. These financial pressures might force a patient into rationing their immunosuppressive drugs or forgoing them altogether, either of which almost absolutely results in graft failure.

I can recall several patients in recent memory who were forced to choose between paying their mortgage or utility bill, <u>or</u> paying for their transplant-saving medication. Many of my colleagues report that they encounter patients in very similar situations. A 2013 *New England Journal of Medicine* article reported that nearly 70 percent of kidney transplant programs reported either a death or organ transplant loss due to patients' inability to pay for their anti-rejection medications.

The 36-month limitation on coverage also has a detrimental effect on live donor organ donations as well. Patients are reluctant to ask a friend or family member to be a living donor if they fear they will be unable to afford their anti-rejection medications long term. As an advocate for increasing organ donation, it is awkward for me to encourage living donors or donor families to give the most amazing "gift of life" knowing that Medicare will cut off immunosuppressive coverage after three years. How does this truly honor the gift?

As a taxpayer, it is doubly frustrating that Medicare will pay for dialysis and for the *first* and *second* transplant but will not pay for the medications needed to maintain and preserve the *first* transplant.

A patient on dialysis costs the federal government almost $86,000 per year. Meanwhile, coverage of immunotherapy under Medicare Part B is approximately, $2,300 per year. Even if you factor in the upfront costs of the transplant surgery - which average over $110,000 – the savings to the government are clear.

In May, the Department of Health and Human Services' (HHS) conducted two analyses which indicated that there was potential significant cost-savings by extending immunosuppressive coverage for kidney transplant patients by averting future dialysis and re-transplantation for these patients. The Centers for Medicare and Medicare's Office of the Actuary concluded that extending coverage could save Medicare up to $300 million over ten years.

By enacting H.R. 5534 – the Comprehensive Immunosuppressive Drug Coverage for Kidney Transplant Patients Act – Congress can provide a lifetime of Medicare coverage of immunosuppressive medications for transplant recipients who lack other coverage. By providing this coverage of last resort, Congress can help reduce the likelihood of graft loss, reduce the demand for another transplant, enable more patients to seek transplant as an option clearly superior to maintenance dialysis, and also protect taxpayers. Importantly, this measure also honors the gift of kidney donation for those who gave selflessly so that others may have their second chance at life.

The 36-month immunosuppressant drug coverage policy is not medically, economically, or ethically justified, and must be fixed by Congress. Thank you for your commitment to advancing H.R. 5534 – for kidney patients, their families, and those who care for them.

* * *

Ms. ESHOO. Thank you, Doctor. This bill is going to move. It has to. And it really needs to be adopted by the Congress, both houses, and sent to the President for his signature. You are absolutely right. It will make all the difference in the world for not only patients but also, you know, the dollars that are attached to this. It is common sense. I never realized that this was the case. So thank you for your testimony and your patience today.

Mr. Koser, welcome. Thank you for your patience in waiting to testify. You have 5 minutes to do so.

Statement of Kevin G. Koser

Mr. KOSER. Wonderful. Good afternoon, Chairwoman Eshoo, Ranking Member Burgess, and distinguished members of this committee. I want to thank you for this opportunity to speak with you about a cause and bill that are very close to my heart.

My name is Kevin Koser, and I am a cochair of the National Foundation for Ectodermal Dysplasias' Family Advocacy Committee. I am here to ask for your support in advancing H.R. 1379, the Ensuring Lasting Smiles Act, on behalf of the estimated 3 to 4 percent of Americans just like my 4-year-old son, Kannon, here in the audience, who are diagnosed with a congenital anomaly.

The bill currently has 266 bipartisan cosponsors, including 21 members of this subcommittee, and the identical Senate bill has 37 bipartisan cosponsors.

This bill will ensure that all private group and individual health plans provide coverages for Americans who are born with congenital anomalies and then require medically necessary treatments to restore function to missing or nonfunctioning body parts.

The intent of this bill might seem like common sense. It is. Health insurance should approve claims for medically necessary treatments of congenital anomalies.

In many cases, that is happening, especially when you think of the more well-known anomalies such as heart defects or spina bifida. The problem is that health insurance systematically denies or delays medically necessary treatments for a host of other congenital anomalies, such as those that affect the mouth, teeth, and the oral cavity.

Insurers call these treatments cosmetic and not medically necessary, despite a medical diagnosis and physician-approved care plan. Or insurers state that these are not covered benefits because they appear to be dental-related, even though they are directly linked to the underlying congenital anomaly. These loopholes must be closed.

My family's story serves as an example of this struggle. There were no signs that anything was wrong when Kannon was born. However, a doctor recognized some of the clinical traits of ectodermal dysplasia when he was 9 months old, and genetic testing at the age of 1 confirmed his diagnosis.

Ectodermal dysplasia is a congenital anomaly that affects development of the hair, skin, sweat and saliva glands, teeth, and sometimes other body parts. But it is specifically issues with the mouth, teeth, and oral cavity that has galvanized support from our families to lead the charge in advocating for this bill. Teeth are missing or completely absent. Their eruption is delayed, their enamel is weak, they are cone-shaped, and the jawbone and gum line recede and decay.

Kannon is now 4 years old and just sprouted his first tooth. X rays indicate that he only has four total teeth. A child without ectodermal dysplasia typically grows about 20, and an adult grows between 28 and 32.

Now, please put yourself in Kannon's shoes and imagine the drastic impact this has on your health and daily life. Your diet is severely restricted. Therefore, you lack proper nutrition and are likely underweight or considered failure to thrive. You will choke even on soft foods, because you cannot chew. Your inability to chew results in gastrointestinal and digestive complications. You struggle to speak properly. Your jawbone and gum line decay and recede from the lack of teeth. You will need a team of physicians across multiple medical disciplines, all of whom tell you that your health is suffering because you don't have a mouth full of functioning teeth.

While there is no cure, there are several common treatments that are medically necessary in order to manage these issues. These treatments are not optional: first, prosthetic teeth or dentures starting between the ages of 2 and 5 and replaced every 1 to 3 years as the mouth grows; second, surgeries to reconstruct and replace the decaying jawbone and gum line; and, third, dental implants that are surgically installed once an individual's mouth stops growing, usually around age 20.

Last Christmas, Kannon asked Santa Claus for teeth so he could, quote, "chomp big bites" of food like other kids in his preschool class. Now, please think about that. Our 3-year-old boy, who loves dinosaurs, dragons, and superheroes, asked for teeth for Christmas.

We started pursuing dentures for him, but imagine the heart-break when our health plan told us that, quote, "any services relating to his teeth or intraoral structure supporting the teeth are not a covered benefit" even though that same policy has mandated coverages for medically necessary treatments of congenital anomalies.

We are not alone. Aidan, a 14-year-old boy from Wisconsin, was first told that his oral treatments only served a cosmetic purpose, and other treatments were denied simply because they addressed issues in his mouth. Alli, a 13-year-old girl from Iowa, was told that her recent surgery to install implants was not a covered benefit due to the inappropriately applied dental exclusion. And Karl, a 47-year-old father from Minnesota, has fought for decades with his health insurance about the medical necessity of a fully functioning mouth, even when that same policy stipulates that accidental injuries to the mouth are covered benefits.

The financial burden of paying for this care 100 percent out of pocket is substantial, especially when our families are already paying for congenital anomaly coverages through our monthly premiums. So why are health insurers bypassing clauses within their own policies, and why are the mouth and teeth being separated from the rest of the body when directly related to a congenital anomaly?

We must close these loopholes that insurers use to bypass State congenital anomaly laws and their contractual obligations to approve claims for medically necessary treatments of congenital anomalies.

Thank you.

[The prepared statement of Mr. Koser follows:]

Testimony of Mr. Kevin G. Koser, Patient Advocate, on Behalf of the National Foundation for Ectodermal Dysplasias, Supporting the Subcommittee on Health of the Committee of Energy & Commerce, Hearing on "Legislation to Improve Americans' Health Care Coverage and Outcomes," Wednesday, January 8, 2020 at 10:00am, 2322 Rayburn House Office Building

Good morning, Chairwoman Eshoo, Ranking Member Burgess, and distinguished Members of this Committee. Thank you for the opportunity to speak with you this morning about a cause and bill that are very close to my heart. My name is Kevin Koser, and I live in central Virginia with my wife, Rachel, and two sons, Kannon (4) and Kage (11-mos). On a volunteer basis, I serve as a Co-Chair of the National Foundation for Ectodermal Dysplasias' Family Advocacy Committee. But my most important title is father and concerned parent. Our son, Kannon, who is sitting in the audience today, was diagnosed with a congenital anomaly called Ectodermal Dysplasia, which requires extensive, medically-necessary treatments so he can live a long, productive, and healthy life.

I am here to ask for your support in advancing H.R.1379, the Ensuring Lasting Smiles Act, on behalf of the estimated 3-4% of Americans just like Kannon who are diagnosed with a congenital anomaly, commonly known as a birth defect. As of Monday, January 6, 2020, the House bill had 261 bipartisan cosponsors (186 Democrats and 75 Republicans), including 21 members of this Subcommittee and 33 members overall from the Energy & Commerce Committee. The identical Senate bill, S.560, had 37 bipartisan cosponsors (19 Republicans and 18 Democrats).

What Is the Ensuring Lasting Smiles Act?

This bipartisan, bicameral bill will ensure that all private group and individual health plans (including self-funded plans regulated by ERISA) provide coverages for Americans who are born with congenital anomalies and then require medically-necessary treatments to restore function to missing, poorly functioning, or non-functioning body parts that resulted directly from the diagnosed anomaly. It further clarifies the inclusion of adjunctive dental, orthodontic, and prosthodontic services for congenital anomalies that impact the mouth, teeth, and oral cavity.

The intent of this bill might seem like commonsense. It is. Health insurance should approve claims for medically-necessary treatments of congenital anomalies. In many cases, that is happening, especially when you think of more well-known anomalies like congenital heart defects, missing or defective limbs, or neural tube defects like Spina Bifida.

However, the problem is that health insurance companies systematically deny or delay medically-necessary treatments for Americans diagnosed with a host of other congenital anomalies, such as those that affect the teeth, mouth, and oral cavity, like Ectodermal Dysplasia. Insurers deny treatments for these congenital anomalies by calling the treatments "cosmetic" and "not medically-necessary," despite an official medical diagnosis and physician-approved care plan. Or insurers state that the requested procedures are "not covered benefits" because they appear to be dental-related, even though they are directly linked to an underlying medical condition.

Why Did I Get Involved in This Effort?

My family's story serves as an example of the struggles that Americans with similar diagnoses face across the country. Kannon was born in September 2015. It was—and still is—one of the happiest days of my wife's and my life. There were no signs that anything was wrong. But it is important to understand that not all congenital anomalies present their symptoms immediately at birth. At a routine dermatology appointment when Kannon was 9-months old, the doctor recognized some of the clinical traits of Ectodermal Dysplasia in our son Kannon: his hair was sparse and platinum white; his skin was prone to rashes; he did not sweat; and there were no signs of teeth. Genetic testing was conducted when Kannon was 1-year old, which confirmed the diagnosis.

Ectodermal Dysplasia is a congenital anomaly that affects the development of the hair, skin, sweat and saliva glands, teeth, and sometimes other body parts, depending on the specific diagnosis. There are at least 180 known variants of Ectodermal Dysplasia—some are more severe and impact limb development, eyesight, or in some cases even lead to death due to infections caused by severe skin erosions. These traits result in a lifetime of medical needs across multiple medical disciplines.

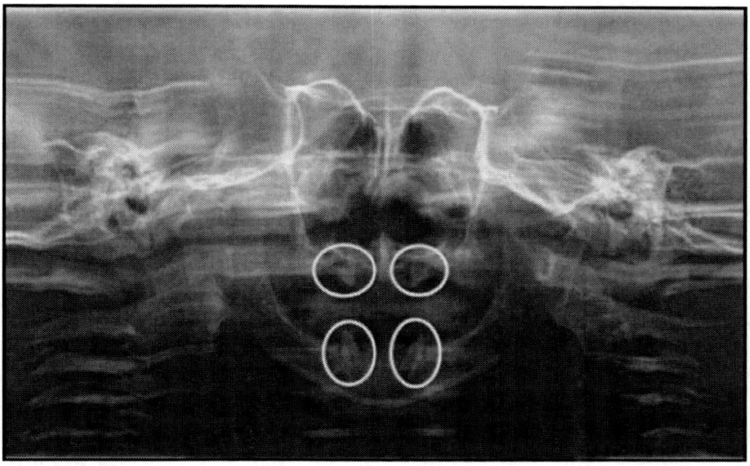

But it is specifically the issues with the teeth, oral cavity, and bone structures supporting the teeth that has galvanized our families to lead the charge in advocating for the Ensuring Lasting Smiles Act. Teeth may be missing or completely absent; their eruption is significantly delayed; the enamel is weak, making the teeth brittle; they will often be conical in shape instead of squared; and the lack of teeth causes the jawbone and gum line to recede and decay.

Kannon is now 4-years old and just recently sprouted his first tooth. X-rays indicate that he only has four (4) total teeth, which are circled in yellow in the image below. A child without Ectodermal Dysplasia typically grows 20 teeth, and an adult grows between 28-32 teeth.

Please put yourself in Kannon's shoes. Imagine the drastic impact this would have on your health and quality of life:

- Your diet is severely restricted—Kannon's diet is limited to soft foods like sliced fruits, hummus with dissolvable crackers, PB&J sandwiches, and pancakes. He is physically unable to eat nutritious foods like fruits or vegetables that are crunchy, and he is unable to eat protein-rich foods like meats or nuts that require teeth to chew.
- Your limited diet results in a lack of proper nutrition, which is the foundation for cognitive and physical development, so you'll likely need daily supplements or meal-replacement products.
- Even with a diet of soft or pureed foods, you'll be prone to choking because you can't chew and have reduced saliva, which is a catalyst for proper digestion.
- Your inability to chew results in gastrointestinal (GI) issues, such as constipation, irritable bowel syndrome; cramping; or ulcers. Otolaryngologists (or ENT) and GI specialists will conduct swallowing studies, and you'll be put under general anesthesia so they can examine your stomach and digestive tract with a scope.
- You struggle to speak properly, requiring speech evaluations and years of speech therapy.
- As your jawbone and gum line decay and recede from the lack of teeth, you require multiple, complex bone grafting surgeries to reconstruct your jaw and facial structures.
- The list of secondary medical issues goes on. You'll need a team of physicians and specialists across multiple disciplines, all of whom tell you that your health is suffering because you don't have a mouth full of functioning teeth.

While there is no cure, and while everyone's medical care plan varies due to differences in how the traits present themselves in the patient, there are several common treatments that are medically-necessary to manage these issues. These treatments are not optional; they must be conducted to restore function to the mouth and for the patient to live a healthy life.

- First, prosthetic teeth (or dentures) starting between the ages of 2-5 and replaced every 1-3 years as the mouth grows.
- Second, surgeries to reconstruct and replace the decaying jawbone and gum line through grafting. The bone is necessary for dentures to rest upon and for our 3rd common treatment, dental implants, to be installed.
- Permanent dental implants are typically installed once an individual's mouth stops growing, usually around age 20. These also help prevent further bone decay through oseointegration.

Last Christmas, Kannon asked Santa Claus for teeth so he could "chomp big bites" of food like other kids in his class. Think about that. Our then 3-year old little boy—who loves dinosaurs, dragons, and superheroes—asked for *teeth* for Christmas. We began pursuing dentures for him, in accordance with a treatment plan established by oral and maxillofacial specialists. Imagine our heartbreak when our health plan told us that "any services relating to his teeth or intra-oral structures supporting the teeth are not a covered benefit," even though the same policy has mandated coverages for medically-necessary treatments of congenital anomalies. This will force us to pay for his medically-necessary treatments 100% out-of-pocket.

We are not alone.

Aidan—a 14-year old boy from Wisconsin—was first told that his oral treatments only served a "cosmetic" purpose and therefore must be paid for 100% out-of-pocket. At a future critical stage in his treatment plan, and after a Medical Review Board agreed that his treatments were medically-necessary, his father's employer, who maintains a self-funded health plan, changed the language of the denial, then stating that the treatments were dental and therefore "not covered benefits."

Alli—a 13-year old girl from Iowa—was told that her recent surgery to install temporary implants is "not a covered benefit." The two implants are absolutely critical in creating anchors for her to receive properly fitted dentures so she can eat and speak properly.

Karl—a 47-year old father from Minnesota—has fought for decades with his health insurance company about the medical necessity of a fully functioning mouth. He has been denied coverage for treatment of his Ectodermal Dysplasia when that same insurance policy stipulates that accidental injuries to the mouth are covered benefits. This is a fight he'll have to continue, not only for himself, but also for his daughter, who has the same condition.

The stories are endless, and they come from all across the country. This is certainly not limited to the Ectodermal Dysplasias community. Dozens of other organizations, representing multiple congenital anomalies and medical professions, have joined this effort too. A full list of supporting organizations is attached to this testimony.

What Are the Physical and Financial Impacts of Claims Denials and Delays on Families?

The patient's health suffers when insurers deny or delay claims for medically-necessary treatments that are meant to restore bodily function as a result of a congenital anomaly. These treatments are not optional. Beyond the physical impact of these denials and delays, the financial burden of paying for this medically-necessary care 100% out-of-pocket is substantial and varies depending on the unique medical care plan that is tailored to fit the individual patient's medical needs. The National Foundation for Ectodermal Dysplasias estimates that some individuals will pay upwards of $150,000 out-of-pocket in their lifetime just for medically-necessary treatments related to the mouth, teeth, and oral cavity.

Coverages for congenital anomalies already exist in an overwhelming majority of private health plans, but insurance companies bypass those clauses by using the aforementioned "cosmetic" loophole or inappropriately applied "dental exclusion." As a result, our families must make tough and often life-altering financial trade-offs by trying to save money for teeth instead of college or retirement, or taking out second mortgages, to pay for these medically-necessary treatments, even though we are already paying for congenital anomaly coverages through our health plan's premiums. So why are health insurers bypassing congenital anomaly clauses within their own policies? Why are health plans separating the mouth and teeth from the rest of the body when directly related to an underlying congenital anomaly?

Moreover, the need for (and costs associated with) secondary treatments—which result directly from the initial denials and delays—would drastically be reduced or even eliminated if health plans appropriately approved claims for medically-necessary treatments such as dentures, reconstructive surgeries, and dental implants. Often, the cumulative cost of these secondary treatments far exceeds the cost of the initial medically-necessary treatment. For example, approving the initial medically-necessary claim for prosthetic teeth would very likely result in an improved ability to chew (reducing or eliminating the need for ENT and GI specialists to conduct swallow studies or endoscopies), improved nutrition (reducing or eliminating the need for appointments with nutritionists who prescribe nutritional supplements, medications, or meal-replacement products), improved speech (reducing the need for speech evaluations and therapy), and improved self-esteem and mental health (reducing the need for psychotherapy appointments with mental health professionals). Approving the claims for medically-necessary treatments would not only improve the health of the patient, but also reduce costs to the patient and insurance company.

What Is the Foundation for This Bill?

The foundation of this federal bill rests on two key points. First, all 50 U.S. states have congenital anomaly statutes, and these are usually written in open-ended ways as if all medically-necessary treatments for all medically-diagnosed congenital anomalies are supposed to be covered health benefits. These state laws apply to all private group and individual health plans issued in that state, otherwise known as "fully-insured" health plans. ("Self-funded" health plans, which are regulated at the federal level, do not have to abide by state laws.) Second, and as previously stated, an overwhelming majority of private health plans—both "fully insured" and "self-funded" plans—include benefits for medically-necessary treatments of congenital anomalies.

Even so, health plans continue to use loopholes and inappropriately applied dental exclusions to bypass the state laws and congenital anomaly clauses that exist in most health plans.

Closing Statement

Our families and children are already dealing with so much due to the diagnosis and physical impact of a congenital anomaly. Fighting health insurance denials and delays—for treatments that are medically-necessary and tied directly to a medically-diagnosed congenital anomaly— causes unnecessary, additional physical suffering for the affected individuals who absolutely require the treatments in order to live a healthy life.

We must close the loopholes and unintended coverage gaps that health insurers use to bypass state congenital anomaly laws and their contractual obligations to approve claims for medically-necessary treatments of congenital anomalies. That is exactly what H.R.1379, the Ensuring Lasting Smiles Act, will do.

On behalf of Kannon and all of our families, thank you for your time and for listening. And thank you to Congressman Peterson, Congressman Riggleman, Senator Baldwin, and Senator Ernst for introducing this bill. It is our hope that you will do everything in your power to pass this important bill for Americans born with congenital anomalies.

Attachments

1. Ectodermal Dysplasia Patient Stories
2. List of Organizations Currently Supporting the "Ensuring Lasting Smiles Act"
3. Support Letter from the National Foundation for Ectodermal Dysplasias, 2 January 2020
4. Support Letter from Members of the "Ensuring Lasting Smiles Act" Coalition, 3 January 2020

Attachment 1. Ectodermal Dysplasia Patient Stories

These stories are representative of the Ectodermal Dysplasias community that has faced significant health setbacks when trying to get medically-necessary treatments to restore function to the mouth and teeth due to a congenital anomaly.

Becky Abbott, M.P.H., on behalf of her son, Aidan Abbott (14-years old), of Wisconsin. My son Aidan was born on January 17, 2005 with health issues and was kept in the hospital for four days. Since birth, he has had chronic health issues and was seen by medical professionals and specialists often. At around the age of 2-3 years old, we noticed that Aidan was missing several of his teeth and we took him to our family dentist for an evaluation. The family dentist referred us to Children's Hospital of Wisconsin, due to the complexity of Aidan's congenital anomaly.

During our first appointment with a pediatric dentist at Children's Dental Center, the dentist mentioned that she believed Aidan had a rare disorder called Ectodermal Dysplasias, due to his missing teeth and health issues, and recommended that he be seen by a geneticist.

Our family made an appointment with the geneticist, and they confirmed the dentist's diagnosis of Ectodermal Dysplasia. Both the pediatric dentist and geneticist noted that Aidan's treatments and procedures to repair his congenital anomaly and replace his missing teeth would be covered under our health insurance. The dentist at Children's recommended that Aidan start out with a lower prosthetic to help with chewing and his speech. That prosthetic was denied on the basis that it served a "cosmetic" purpose. After going through the denial and appeals process, our insurance approved Aidan's first prosthetic and related dental work. However, in the meantime, Aidan developed severe speech, swallowing, and choking issues. Aidan was unable to communicate with family, classmates, or teachers and was referred to a speech therapist and subsequent speech therapy that lasted nearly 3.5 years. He also developed swallowing and choking issues and was referred to specialists at Children's, where he underwent a swallowing study, and endoscopy to determine the underlying issue that was causing him to have issues swallowing. Our family practitioner also prescribed Prilosec, as he believed Aidan had GERD. The endoscopy determined that Aidan did not have GERD and the medication was discontinued. All of his health issues were related to his missing teeth. His diet was altered, and he no longer wanted to eat whole foods for fear that he would choke on his food, as he had done several times in the past. We started supplementing his meals with food pouches and Pediasure to ensure that he was receiving the nutrients he needed. As Aidan refused to eat many of the solid foods that he was recommended at that age, he also developed chronic constipation and severe stomach pain. He was referred to a gastroenterologist who prescribed constipation medication to help relieve his symptoms. These developing issues lasted for several years.

Once his lower denture was placed, he began to develop better speech, and he was able to chew better. He was still hesitant to eat solid foods for quite some time, and it took several years for him to be able to chew slowly enough and feel confident that his food would be digested properly without choking. We believe that most of these issues could have been avoided if the prosthetic was approved in a timely manner.

Over the next several years, Aidan went back to his dental specialist for frequent checkups to determine what the next steps of treatment would involve. At one of his follow-up appointments, the dentist mentioned that, due to Aidan's missing teeth, his two front teeth had erupted too far and were too long. They also noted that the same teeth were at risk for trauma. They recommended that Aidan have orthodontia to move teeth into place to protect those front teeth from risk of trauma. The coverage for that treatment was denied.

On a follow up appointment, his dental specialists believe he should have a frenectomy to remove the tissue that had grown in between the two teeth, as well as four teeth removed to make way for other teeth to be moved into place to protect his two front teeth. The frenectomy was approved, but the subsequent removal of the four teeth were repeatedly denied. The insurance company gave different reasons at different stages of the appeals/denials process and ultimately denied the treatment, saying that the treatment was needed for his upcoming orthodontia, even though the service did not include the use of orthodontia.

Since Aidan's initial prosthetic, we have had to fight insurance for most of his complex treatments. His case has gone to a third-party medical review board. The review board determined that his treatments are medically necessary and that the suggested treatment plan is suitable for the repair of Aidan's congenital anomaly. Even so, our insurance provider used every loophole available to continue to deny his services. One of his initial treatment plans was quoted at approximately $3,080. Since Aidan did not receive that treatment in a timely manner, his treatment plan was forced to change, and the cost of the new treatment has increased to $6,180. Each time his treatment is delayed, he develops new issues and requires additional treatment. His jaw needs to be leveled and aligned, and he has had numerous follow-up appointments, almost weekly, to make adjustments and changes to his dentition.

This is just the start of Aidan's complex treatments, and these treatments will continue for the rest of his life. As Aidan's jaw continues to grow, he will most likely need bone grafting and implants. Our medical insurance policy includes a congenital anomalies clause that includes coverage for the repair of congenital anomalies. The state of Wisconsin also has a state statute that covers the repair of all congenital anomalies from the time of birth. However, our insurance plan is self-funded and federally regulated. Therefore, our plan does not need to adhere to state statutes. Our health insurance company has repeatedly asked for supporting documentation, but no matter how much information we provide from his team of physicians, all of which indicates that his treatments are medically-necessary and required to repair his congenital anomaly, they are still denied.

Jennifer Steele, on behalf of her daughter, Allison Steele (13-years old), and son, Bennett Steele (4-years old), of Iowa. Living with Ectodermal Dysplasia is part of our everyday life. We have two children, Alli (13) and

Bennett (4), who are affected. Alli was diagnosed at age 6, and Bennett was diagnosed at age 4. Two of the largest concerns are their inability to sweat and their missing teeth. We have found ways to adapt and control overheating through various cooling products and methods. Their health and smiles mean everything to us, as we want nothing more than our kids to be healthy and happy. We live everyday with Ectodermal Dysplasia, yet it doesn't stop us from enjoying and loving each day.

Missing teeth makes it very challenging to chew food, and a lack of saliva production makes it easier to choke on food. Nutrition is a major concern and reality that we live with daily. Proper nutrition is directly linked to overall health and growth in children. Lack of teeth also causes the jawbone to deteriorate. As a result of missing teeth, Alli has had several procedures, including swallow studies, an upper endoscopy (or EGD), along with frequent medical appointments and tests by several specialists in an attempt to diagnosis and treat her severe GI symptoms that kept her on the verge of failure to thrive for several years due to her abnormal oral development. These tests and medical appointments could have been avoided with proper treatments, by improving her ability to initiate the digestion process in her mouth, like you experience each time something enters your mouth. She only has one molar, which results in an inability to properly mash or chew food. She is limited on what she can eat, and the foods that are the most difficult are the healthy foods, like vegetables and meat. In the next 9-12 months, she will be ready to be fitted for her first partial denture. Who at the age of 13 wants to wear a denture? Alli does. She wants to have enough teeth in her mouth that she can easily chew her food for the first time in her life. Missing teeth also has had a negative impact on her mental health and self-esteem. She wants to be confident with her smile. This medically necessary process will be a 100% out of pocket cost, even though this is a result of a birth defect.

Alli received her first set of braces at age 7, due to her teeth twisting, turning, and moving into the space that is available in her mouth due to missing teeth. We traveled 260 miles round-trip to the University of Iowa every 3-6 weeks for 4-5 months because there wasn't a local orthodontist that was comfortable with treating her. In December 2016, Alli began the process for her second set of braces, this time requiring only 52 miles round-trip from home to Ankeny, Iowa. Due to the complexity of her dental condition, we make the trip to the orthodontist every 3-4 weeks. She will likely require one more set of braces before she moves on to the more permanent solutions of bone grafting for her jaw and dental implants, which will begin between ages

18-21. Alli currently sees a family dentist in West Des Moines, IA for routine cleaning and care, an orthodontist in Ankeny, prosthodontist at University of Illinois – Chicago, and a pediatric dentist in Iowa City.

On December 10, 2019, Alli had two temporary dental implants surgically placed in her lower anterior jaw to be used as anchors, since she doesn't have posterior teeth to use for anchorage, to correct her deep overbite and to properly make room in her mouth for the partial denture. This will also assist in correcting her crossbite and allow her to improve her ability to chew. Even though we live in the Des Moines metro area, there is not an oral surgeon that is in-network for our medical plan. We had the oral surgeon's office submit a "gap coverage request" to United Health Care in an effort to facilitate Alli's care. We were notified by our UHC Advocate that a prior authorization would be needed. The advocate reached out to the oral surgeon's office and assisted with the gap request and prior authorization. A few days prior to the December 10th surgery, we were notified by the oral surgeon's office that the prior authorization was denied as "not a covered benefit." As this was a medically-necessary surgery for Alli, we went ahead with the surgery as planned, paid $1,200 out-of-pocket, and submitted an appeal on the denied prior authorization. The claim was still submitted to our medical plan, yet it hasn't completed the review process. According to our Advocate, the claim is pending additional information from the provider's office. The outcome at this time is unknown. We plan to utilize our appeal options that our medical plan allows in an effort to obtain coverage.

Without closing the loopholes that insurance companies use to deny claims, such as "not a covered benefit" or "cosmetic," we are paying 100% out-of-pocket for our children's medical needs instead of saving money for their college tuitions or to properly invest in our retirement.

With Bennett's recent diagnosis, we currently don't know what to expect for his treatment plan. We will have frequent appointments with the specialists at the University of Iowa who are familiar with Alli, and monitor his health as he grows, and then develop a plan for his missing teeth that is age- and developmentally-appropriate for him. Our family is fortunate to have dual incomes working for great companies. Despite this, we are facing out-of-pocket expenses that could exceed our annual salaries. We need your help to make sure that families like ours, and others living with congenital anomalies have the coverage they need to live healthy and fulfilling lives. When you have a smile that you can be confident about, you can change the world! We need your help.

Karl Nelsen, PA-C, MS (47-years old), on behalf of himself and his daughter, Samantha Nelsen (9-years old), of Minnesota. My daughter, Samantha (9-years old) and I both have ectodermal dysplasia. I have been fighting for medical insurance coverage for my oral restorations my entire life. I was born with only a few baby teeth and even fewer adult teeth. I received my first set of dentures when I was 5-years old and required a new set every 2-3 years as my body grew. My parents applied for coverage through our health insurance and received denials over and over again to cover my dental prosthetics. As you can imagine, this is a stressful process, both emotionally and financially.

As I reached my 20s, my adult teeth began to fail, my dentures were not well anchored, and I had to make a major decision in my life. I pursued dental implants at the University of Minnesota. I had bone grafting, 10 implants surgically placed into my mandible and maxilla (which can be seen in the image below), and a new set of dental prosthetics made in order to restore my function and appearance. During the 1990s, this cost me approximately $30,000 out-of-pocket as my insurance company denied the restorative treatments on the basis that it was dental and not health-related, even though this work is clearly a restoration for a congenital defect, which was supposed to be a covered benefit.

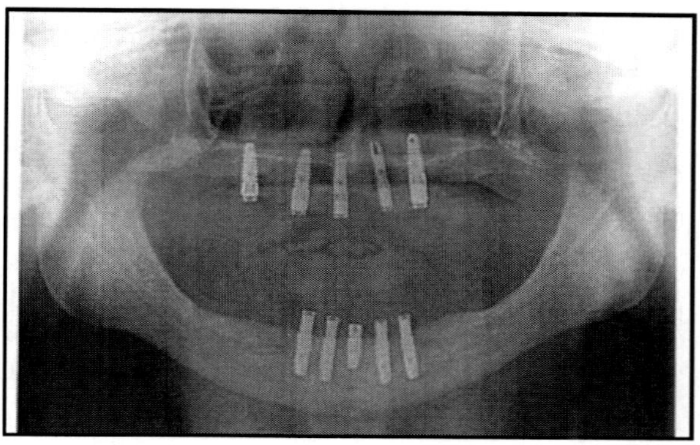

I recently collected estimates for the same work to be done. This same process is now approximately $70,000, which again would be an out-of-pocket expense for a restoration of my congenital changes.

I went approximately 20 years without being active with the National Foundation for Ectodermal Dysplasias until the birth of my daughter, Samantha Grace Nelsen, who is also affected. She is currently 9-years old and will only have a few adult teeth. She will also require dental implants just like her dad. So, the cycle will begin again. Another generation fighting with their insurance companies to get their congenital defects restored.

I believe the success of this bill is entrenched in education. One would think that medical insurance companies provide coverage for congenital defects. For the most part, they do, but our community is caught in the middle since our congenital defect affects oral structures. Thus, they automatically deny claims for our medically-necessary treatments. This is wrong, and we need to close the loopholes that insurers use to deny treatments of congenital anomalies that affect the mouth and teeth.

Julie Claeys, on behalf of her son, Carver Claeys (24-years old), of Michigan. Our son Carver is now 24 years old and completing dental implants after his whole life of wearing dentures starting at age 2 and needing a new set as he grew every two years. In order to obtain implants, Carver had to have bone taken from his hip and implanted into his jaw in order to hold implants in place to prepare for new permanent dentures. An x-ray of his mouth with the implants is included below.

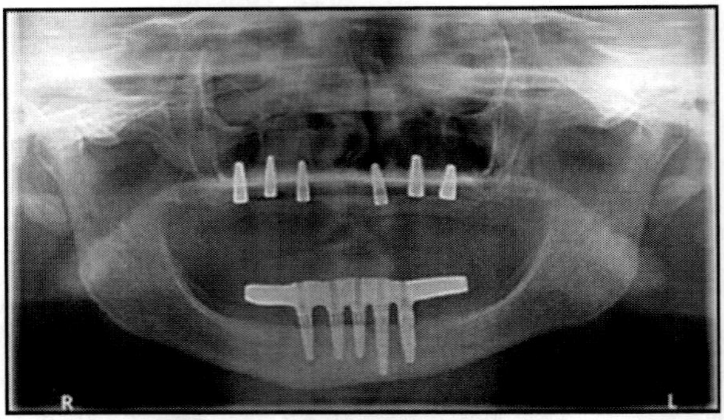

We have paid more than $100,000 out-of-pocket because of denied claims even though our insurance plan stated that they covered medical necessity and birth defects. Congenital anomalies are supposed to be covered by our plan yet our self-funded health plan denied claims. Carver's new set of permanent dentures are billed at a cost of $40,000. He cannot eat or live healthily without these dentures that adhere to his implants. His implants are absolutely medically necessary.

Christine Gottschalk, on behalf of her son, Henry Scott (6-years old), of Washington, D.C. Our son, Henry, has Hypohidrotic Ectodermal Dysplaysia, which is a congenital anomaly. Henry is giggly, tells elaborate tales about fire breathing dragons, and loves to roll down hills with his friends. He also needs teeth. One of Henry's symptoms is anodontia, or the absence of teeth. The lack of teeth impacts his nutrition, speech, and self-esteem. Recently, Henry got his first dentures, and over his lifetime, he will require complex corrective surgeries for normal function. None of the care has been approved by our health insurance. Our claims are automatically denied, and we are forced to cover these expenses out of pocket. My husband is a disabled combat veteran, and our family relies on my income and insurance for Henry's care. This means tough financial trade-offs for our family. We are saving money for teeth and other medically-necessary oral treatments instead of college and retirement, even though our insurance policy has mandated coverages for medically-necessary treatments of congenital anomalies, or when caused by an accident or illness.

Attachment 2. List of Patient and Physician Organizations Supporting the "Ensuring Lasting Smiles Act"

(In Alphabetical Order)

1. Academy of General Dentistry
2. American Academy of Dermatology Association
3. American Academy of Facial Plastic & Reconstructive Surgery
4. American Academy of Neurology
5. American Academy of Oral and Maxillofacial Pathology
6. American Academy of Oral and Maxillofacial Radiology
7. American Academy of Pediatric Dentistry
8. American Association of Oral and Maxillofacial Surgeons
9. American Association of Orthodontists
10. American Association of Women Dentists
11. American College of Prosthodontists
12. American College of Surgeons
13. American Dental Association
14. American Society of Dentist Anesthesiologists
15. American Society of Maxillofacial Surgeons
16. American Society of Plastic Surgeons
17. Bridge the Gap – SYNGAP Education & Research Foundation
18. CCD Smiles
19. Children's Hospital of Wisconsin
20. Colorado Rare

21. Costello Syndrome Family Network
22. Dermatology Nurses' Association
23. Derma Care Access Network
24. EveryLife Foundation for Rare Diseases
25. FACES: The National Craniofacial Association
26. Foundation for Ichthyosis and Related Skin Types, Inc. (FIRST)
27. Genetic Alliance
28. International Pemphigus and Pemphigoid Foundation
29. M-CM Network
30. March of Dimes
31. Moebius Syndrome Foundation
32. National Foundation for Ectodermal Dysplasias
33. National Organization for Rare Disorders
34. Noah's Hope – Hope4Bridget
35. Operation Smile
36. Pathways for Rare and Orphan Studies
37. Project Accessible Oral Health
38. Rare & Undiagnosed Network
39. rareLife Solutions
40. Soft Bones: The US Hypophosphatasia Foundation
41. SunnyStrong
42. The APS Type 1 Foundation Inc.
43. The Marfan Foundation
44. The Sturge-Weber Foundation
45. Usher 1F Collaborative
46. Virginia Council of Nurse Practitioners

Attachment 3. Support Letter from the National Foundation for Ectodermal Dysplasias, January 2, 2020

Dear Members of the Energy and Commerce Committee,

The National Foundation for Ectodermal Dysplasias (NFED) is the only patient advocacy organization in the United States dedicated to individuals who are affected by rare genetic disorders classified as ectodermal dysplasias. The NFED's mission is to empower and connect individuals touched by ectodermal dysplasias through education, support, and research. The NFED has been advocating for individuals affected by ectodermal dysplasias and all rare disorders for almost 40 years.

Ectodermal dysplasias are inheritable conditions that involve defects in the hair, teeth, nails and glands. Individuals may develop only a few teeth; some develop no teeth. As you know, teeth are "medically necessary" to maintain good nutrition, speech, facial symmetry, and normal growth and development. Some affected individuals go a lifetime without teeth. There are significant medical and social implications associated with this. Children who do not develop normal teeth can suffer from failure to thrive, have speech problems, digestive disorders and many other medical problems. As a result, they have to undergo many costly medical procedures and years of costly speech therapy, all that are unnecessary if they just had teeth!

Many individuals call our office on a daily basis seeking help to get teeth for themselves or their children. Insurance companies regularly deny coverage for teeth even though most states have statutes that require such coverage of congenital defects. Insurance companies routinely deny the claims as "cosmetic." When in the world did simply having teeth become cosmetic in this country? Families are denied coverage over and over again after years of fighting. Teeth are not cosmetic and restoration of congenital defects, including congenital dental/oral defects, should be included in all medical insurance policies. It is time for this injustice to stop.

Three years ago, the NFED embarked on a mission to advocate for federal legislation that would mandate coverage for all medically necessary restorations for ALL individuals affected by a congenital disorder. Led by a strong family advocacy committee, we have worked very hard to get legislation introduced. We found great friends and allies, Senators Tammy Baldwin and Joni Ernst and Representatives Colin Peterson and Denver Riggleman. With their dedicated support, the Ensuring Lasting Smiles Act (H.R. 1379, S.560) (ELSA) was introduced as a bill in the U.S Senate and House on February 26, 2019.

Our family advocacy committee has made numerous visits to Capitol Hill and thousands of calls to legislators to garner support for this bill. We are diligent and tenacious in our efforts, and we will not stop until we are successful because this is the #1 issue which most affects our community financially.

People affected by ectodermal dysplasias are expected to have to pay approximately $150,000 out of pocket just for their dental care during their lives.

The NFED and our partners strongly support ELSA. Please hear our voices; listen to our pleas for equal health care for individuals who are affected by rare congenital disorders. Families are counting on you. We urge you to pass this bill in the 2020 year.

Sincerely,

Mary Fete, MSN, RN, CCM
Executive Director

Karl Nelsen, PA-C, MS
Board President

Attachment 4. Support Letter from Members of the "Ensuring Lasting Smiles Act" Coalition, Jan. 3, 2020

The Honorable Anna Eshoo
Chair, Health Subcommittee
House Committee on Energy & Commerce
2125 Rayburn House Office Building
Washington, D.C. 20515

The Honorable Michael Burgess
Ranking Member, Health Subcommittee
House Committee on Energy & Commerce
2125 Rayburn House Office Building
Washington, D.C. 20515

Dear Chairwoman Eshoo and Ranking Member Burgess:

The undersigned organizations write to express our support for HR 1379, the Ensuring Lasting Smiles Act (ELSA). We appreciate your leadership in recognizing the importance of this bill by including it as part of the Health Subcommittee's Jan. 8 hearing entitled, "Legislation to Improve Americans' Health Care Coverage and Outcomes."

This legislation – with more than 260 bipartisan cosponsors – will have a direct impact on patients and will eliminate the existing burdens that prevent access to necessary diagnosis and treatment for those with congenital craniofacial anomalies, such as cleft lip and palate, skeletal and maxillofacial abnormalities, facial paralysis, microtia, hypodontia, and craniosynostosis. Specifically, if enacted, ELSA will ensure all group and individual health plans cover medically necessary services, including needed dental procedures such as orthodontic or prosthodontic support, as a result of a congenital anomaly. It would exclude coverage for cosmetic procedures or surgery on normal structures.

The Centers for Disease Control and Prevention (CDC) classifies birth defects as "common, costly, and critical" and reports that one in 33 newborns in the United States suffers from a congenital anomaly. Craniofacial anomalies, for example, can restrict a patient's ability to breathe, eat, and speak in a normal manner. Therefore, highly personalized surgery to repair an anomaly helps the patient grow and function normally. Early intervention by a team of specialists, including plastic surgeons, oral and maxillofacial surgeons, pediatric dentists, orthodontists, dermatologists and speech therapists, is necessary to assess and oversee the patient's treatment and development, sometimes over the course of several years.

Most private health plans provide coverage for the surgical treatment of congenital anomalies and many states require insurers to provide coverage of any health services related to congenital anomalies or birth defects. Despite this, health plans often deny claims and appeals for oral or dental-related procedures – like orthodontia and dental implants – or other procedures, which are often crucial to the overall success of treatment, claiming these services are cosmetic.

Severe dental anomalies are a common symptom of many craniofacial anomaly conditions requiring serious medical treatment that is outside the scope of procedures covered by dental plans. As a result, patients are forced to incur significant out-of-pocket costs on medically necessary reconstructive dental care related to their disorder during their lifetime. When private insurance denies a child's reconstructive surgery, families many times end up turning to Medicaid, SCHIP, or other state-sponsored programs for coverage.

The Ensuring Lasting Smiles Act would address these coverage denials and ensure that all patients with birth defects or anomalies get the treatment they need.

For these reasons, we support the Ensuring Lasting Smiles Act and urge members of your subcommittee to help advance this bill through the House.

Sincerely,

Academy of General Dentistry
American Academy of Neurology
American Academy of Pediatric Dentistry
American Association of Oral and Maxillofacial Surgeons

American Association of Orthodontists
American College of Surgeons
American Dental Association
American Society of Dentist Anesthesiologists
American Society of Plastic Surgeons
Dermatology Nurses' Association
International Pemphigus and Pemphigoid Foundation
March of Dimes
National Foundation for Ectodermal Dysplasias
National Organization for Rare Disorders
Noah's Hope
Pathways for Rare and Orphan Studies

* * *

Ms. ESHOO. Thank you for your testimony. Powerful testimony.

Mr. Riccardi, it is a pleasure to welcome you, and you have 5 minutes for your testimony.

Statement of Frederic Riccardi

Mr. RICCARDI. Good afternoon. I am Fred Riccardi, president of the Medicare Rights Center. Medicare Rights is a national, non-profit organization that works to ensure access to affordable healthcare for older adults and people with disabilities through counseling and advocacy, educational programs, and public policy initiatives.

Thank you for the opportunity to speak with you today about two bipartisan bills that can help improve healthcare coverage and outcomes for people with Medicare.

One such bill, the BENES Act, introduced by Representatives Ruiz, Bilirakis, Walorski, and Schneider, would update Medicare enrollment rules for the first time in over 50 years to better empower beneficiaries to make informed coverage choices. These modernizations are needed due to major changes in how people experience their initial Medicare eligibility.

Today, as in 1965 when the program was created, most people are automatically enrolled in Medicare Part A, the hospital coverage benefit, and Part B, outpatient coverage, when they turn 65 because they are receiving Social Security benefits. However, as an increasing number of Americans are working longer and delaying Social Security benefits, in 2016 only 60 percent of Medicare-eligible 65-year-olds were taking Social Security, compared to 92 percent in 2002. That is a big difference.

Unlike those who are automatically enrolled, this growing cohort of employed older Americans must actively do so. Most can sign up for Part A at any time without a penalty, but enrolling in Part B is much more complicated. Enrolling requires that individuals understand when to sign up during Medicare's time-limited enrollment windows, how their current insurance might work with Medicare, and what penalties may result if they delay enrollment, even by honest mistake.

And the stakes are, indeed, very high. The consequences of any missteps can be significant and may include a lifetime Part B late-enrollment penalty. This penalty accrues at 10 percent for every year the individual should have been enrolled but wasn't. Currently, there are approximately 760,000 people who are paying a Part B late-enrollment penalty, and the average amount represents a 30 percent increase in the monthly premium.

They may also face harmful gaps in coverage and exposure to high out-of-pocket costs. Because Part B enrollment periods do not align, coverage starts later, and beneficiaries may have to wait several months before coverage begins. This is true for the initial enrollment period—this is the window around someone's 65th birthday—and then also for the general enrollment period, the period that we are in right now, where there is a larger gap in coverage of up to 7 months.

Americans who have other insurance when they become eligible for Medicare have even more to wade through, like whether Medicare will pay primary or secondary and whether they can delay Part B without a penalty.

The rules are so confusing that HR experts in employer benefits departments struggle to understand them. And clear advice from the Federal Government to those approaching Medicare eligibility would help, but no such notice is required at this point. As a result of this information vacuum, among the most frequent calls to our national consumer help line are those from people or on behalf of people with Medicare who are struggling to enroll into Part B and experiencing severe gaps in coverage.

Without immediate action, a growing number of Americans are going to experience these pitfalls in the current system. People are working longer and also delaying Social Security to collect their full retirement benefit, and more and more beneficiaries are going to face these critical Part B enrollment decisions.

Eight former CMS Administrators who served in both Democratic and Republican administrations endorse the BENES Act's commonsense solutions, which are needed now more than ever.

In part, the bill, for the first time, would require the Federal Government to notify individuals about eligibility, update enrollment timelines to eliminate unnecessary and harmful breaks in coverage, and inform future alignment strategies.

I would also like to take some time and speak to H.R. 3935, the Protecting Patients Transportation to Care Act. Led by Representatives Carter, Cárdenas, Graves, and Bishop, this bill would strengthen healthcare access for people with Medicaid, including some of the 12 million enrollees who are also eligible for Medicare.

And so, for these people with Medicaid, dual enrollees who also have Medicare, they tend to have very complex healthcare needs that require regular visits to medical appointments. And reliable transportation to and from these visits is absolutely crucial but not always readily available. In these instances, Medicaid's NEMT benefit can be a lifeline, facilitating access to needed care for those who have no other way to get to medical visits.

And in some States, like Georgia, there are innovative things happening where people are able to access prescription drugs. Codifying this benefit into Medicaid statute would ensure that enrollees have meaningful health coverage going forward.

Thank you.

[The prepared statement of Mr. Riccardi follows:]

Testimony of Frederic Riccardi, President, Medicare Rights Center, "Legislation to Improve Americans' Health Care Coverage and Outcomes," United States House of Representatives, Committee on Energy & Commerce, Subcommittee on Health, January 8, 2020

Introduction

Chairwoman Eshoo, Dr. Burgess, and members of the House Committee on Energy & Commerce, Subcommittee on Health: I am Fred Riccardi, president of the Medicare Rights Center (Medicare Rights). Medicare Rights is a national, non-profit organization that works to ensure access to affordable health care for older adults and people with disabilities through counseling and advocacy, educational programs, and public policy initiatives. We provide services and resources to nearly three million people with Medicare, family caregivers, and health care professionals each year.

Thank you for the opportunity to speak with you today about two bipartisan bills that would help older adults and people with disabilities access and afford needed care, the Beneficiary Enrollment Notification and Eligibility Simplification (BENES) Act (H.R. 2477) and the Protecting Patients Transportation to Care Act (H.R. 3935).

The Beneficiary Enrollment Notification and Eligibility Simplification (BENES) Act (H.R. 2477)

Medicare Part B Enrollment Challenges and Consequences

Medicare is the federal government program that provides health care coverage if you are over 65, under 65 and receiving Social Security Disability Insurance (SSDI) for a certain amount of time, or under 65 and living with End-Stage Renal Disease (ESRD). As you know, there are four parts of Medicare: Part A, Part B, Part C, and Part D:

- Part A provides inpatient/hospital coverage.
- Part B provides outpatient/medical coverage.
- Part C offers an alternate way to receive your Medicare benefits.
- Part D provides prescription drug coverage.

People with Medicare can choose to receive their Parts A and B benefits from Original Medicare, the traditional fee-for-service program offered directly through the federal government that was enacted in 1965, or from a Medicare Advantage Plan, a type of private insurance offered by companies that contract with the federal government. This option was added in 1996. Regardless of how a beneficiary ultimately chooses to receive coverage, the transition to Medicare can be a daunting task for people who are not yet collecting their Social Security benefits.

The BENES Act would help. It would update the Part B enrollment process for the first time in 50 years, making it easier for beneficiaries to understand and navigate. These modernizations are needed due to significant changes in how people experience their initial Medicare eligibility.

While most beneficiaries are still automatically enrolled in Medicare Parts A and B at age 65 because they are receiving Social Security benefits, a growing number of Americans are not. In 2016, only 60% of Medicare-eligible 65-year-olds were taking Social Security, compared to 92% in 2002.[41] Several factors are responsible for this shift, including the decoupling of the Medicare and Social Security eligibility ages, changing demographics, and evolving employment patterns. More older adults are working later in life and deferring Social Security, though they may not realize that doing so impacts their Medicare coverage.[42] Others may choose—appropriately or not—to delay signing up for Medicare because they have another source of coverage, such as an employer-based plan.

Unlike those who are auto-enrolled, individuals who defer Social Security until after age 65 must take steps to enroll in Parts A and B. To sign up for Part A, the decision is relatively straightforward: people who qualify for premium-free Part A—the majority of Medicare beneficiaries—are not bound by any enrollment periods; they can sign up any time after they are eligible, without penalty.

Delaying and then enrolling in Part B without penalty is a much more complicated and high-stakes endeavor. It requires beneficiaries to understand and consider specific enrollment periods, existing coverage, and the penalties associated with delayed enrollment. If this process is mismanaged, the consequences can be significant—including lifetime financial penalties, high out-of-pocket costs, and periods of non-coverage.

Unfortunately, many people do make mistakes. Year after year, among the most frequent calls to our National Consumer Helpline are those from or on behalf of people eligible for Medicare who inadvertently and through no fault of their own failed to enroll in Part B on time and are experiencing severe repercussions.[43]

The rules are so confusing that even sophisticated Human Resources (HR) experts can struggle to follow them, and many employers' benefits departments lack the Medicare knowledge to effectively guide their employees and retirees on Medicare enrollment. Further, the federal

---

[41] Medicare Payment Advisory Commission, "Report to the Congress: Medicare and the Health Care Delivery System" (June 2019) available at: http://www.medpac.gov/docs/default-source/reports/jun19_medpac_reporttocongress_sec.pdf?sfvrsn=0.

[42] Johnson, R.W., Urban Institute, "Older Workers: Opportunities and Challenges" (July 2010) available at: http://www.urban.org/UploadedPDF/412166-older-workers.pdf.

[43] Medicare Rights Center, "Medicare Trends and Recommendations: An Analysis of 2017 Call Data from the Medicare Rights Center's National Helpline" (April 2019) available at: https://www.medicarerights.org/pdf/2017-helpline-trends-report.pdf.

government provides virtually no notification to people who are nearing Medicare eligibility about their responsibilities, including if they must actively enroll. Instead, only people who already receive or have applied for Social Security benefits before turning 65 are notified by the federal government when they first become eligible for Medicare.

This notification process is chiefly managed by the Social Security Administration (SSA), the federal agency responsible for Medicare enrollment. SSA identifies individuals collecting retirement benefits and sends their records to the Centers for Medicare & Medicaid Services (CMS)—the federal agency that manages the Medicare program—four months before they turn 65.[44] CMS then sends them a "Welcome to Medicare" packet three months before their 65th birthday that includes their new Medicare card, a letter confirming their enrollment and explaining how Medicare works, and information about how to decline automatic enrollment.[45]

Because this Medicare notification process is tied to the collection of Social Security benefits, it is reaching a shrinking subset of beneficiaries.[46] In part, this is due to the gradual two-year increase in the Social Security eligibility age, from 65 to 67.[47]

Historically, the eligibility age for both Medicare and Social Security was 65. This made the linkage between the programs' beneficiary notification systems less problematic than it is now that the ages are no longer aligned. Today, Medicare-eligible individuals who do not begin taking Social Security until they reach the age for full retirement benefits (currently 66) receive nothing from the federal government about their initial Medicare eligibility at age 65. And existing law offers no remedy: there is no requirement that either SSA or CMS notify people if they have not yet applied for Social Security.

As a result, many people bear the full burden of navigating Medicare's complex enrollment process alone, to disastrous effect. We frequently hear

---

44 Medicare Payment Advisory Commission, "Report to the Congress: Medicare and the Health Care Delivery System" (June 2019) available at: http://www.medpac.gov/docs/default-source/reports/jun19_medpac_reporttocongress_sec.pdf?sfvrsn=0.

45 Centers for Medicare & Medicaid Services, "Welcome to Medicare booklet and letter" available at: https://www.medicare.gov/forms-help-resources/mail-you-get-about-medicare/welcome-to-medicare-booklet-and-letter.

46 Medicare Payment Advisory Commission, "Report to the Congress: Medicare and the Health Care Delivery System" (June 2019) available at: http://www.medpac.gov/docs/default-source/reports/jun19_medpac_reporttocongress_sec.pdf?sfvrsn=0.

47 The Social Security Amendments of 1983 gradually raised the full retirement age for Social Security benefits, also known as the Old-Age, Survivors, and Disability Insurance (OASDI) Program, from 65 to 67. The increase in the full retirement age began in 2003 and will be complete in 2027.See: *Ibid.*

from beneficiaries who, in this information vacuum, have made enrollment missteps that have left them functionally uninsured and on the hook for sizable costs.

All too often, there is no easy solution. Under Medicare enrollment rules, these individuals may be unable to get coverage quickly. Absent access to a Special Enrollment Period (SEP) based on qualifying job-based insurance,[48] people who do not enroll in Part B during their Initial Enrollment Period (IEP)—a seven-month around their 65th birthday—must wait until the next General Enrollment Period (GEP) to sign up. This can mean gaps in coverage, as the GEP runs from January 1 to March 31 each year but coverage does not begin until July 1.

Consider Medicare Rights' client, Mr. A. He was laid off at age 65. As part of his termination, he was provided two years, through September 2018, of continued enrollment in the company's large employer group health plan. Before the group coverage was due to terminate, Mr. A went to his local Social Security office to enroll in Medicare. There, for the first time, he was told that when he lost his job, it triggered a change in how his group health coverage was treated under Medicare rules. He learned that he was ineligible to enroll in Part B through a SEP and would have to wait until the next GEP in January 2019 to sign up, and until July of that year for coverage to begin—leaving him without adequate health coverage for nearly a year. Mr. A also learned that he would be required to pay a Part B Late Enrollment Penalty (LEP), which can be a lifelong burden.[49]

The Part B LEP accrues at 10% of the current Part B premium for every year a person should have been—but was not—enrolled in Part B.[50] Because Mr. A delayed enrollment for two years, he must pay 20% more every month, amounting to a lifetime penalty.[51] The Part B LEP is intended to encourage individuals newly eligible for Medicare to enroll in the program and ultimately

---

[48] The Part B Special Enrollment Period (SEP) is an eight-month period during which an individual can enroll in Medicare Part B after they no longer have coverage from current work (job-based insurance). *See*: Medicare Rights Center, "Job-based Insurance and Medicare" (2019) available at: https://www.medicareinteractive.org/get-answers/coordinating-medicare-with-other-types-of-insurance/job-based-insurance-and-medicare.

[49] Those who are eligible for Medicare as a result of disability and who are not yet 65 have an IEP when they turn 65. During this IEP, a previously assigned late enrollment period for wrongfully delayed enrollment upon becoming eligible for Medicare due to disability may be removed. *See*: POMS at HI 00805.015.

[50] 42 C.F.R. § 407.15; POMS at HI 00805.025.

[51] 10% multiplied by the number of years delayed. *See*: Medicare Rights Center, "Medicare Part B Late Enrollment Penalties" (2018) available at: http://www.medicareinteractive.org/page2.php?topic=counselor&page=script&script_id=316.

to ensure that a younger, healthier population balances the Medicare risk pool.[52] But because the rules concerning Medicare enrollment are often unknown or misunderstood, many people end up paying LEPs due solely to honest error. In 2018, roughly 760,000 Medicare beneficiaries were paying a Part B LEP, with the average penalty representing nearly a 30% increase in a beneficiary's monthly premium.[53]

The prevalence, amount, and efficacy of the LEP is concerning, especially given the financial status of many Medicare beneficiaries. Currently, half of all people with Medicare—nearly 30 million seniors and people with disabilities—have annual incomes below $26,200 and one quarter have less than $14,550 in savings.[54] At the same time, high and rising health care costs are taking up an increasing share of beneficiaries' limited budgets. In 2016, nearly 30% of Medicare households spent 20% or more of their income on health care, while only 6% of non-Medicare households did so.[55] Most people with Medicare simply cannot afford to pay more for their care.

Another complication is that people like Mr. A, who have other insurance when they become eligible for Medicare, must try to make sense of Medicare's intricate coordination of benefits requirements. These rules govern how other types of insurance works with Medicare, which pays first, or primary, and which pays secondary. This is important because when Medicare is primary, the other insurance may not pay until Medicare does, whether the individual is enrolled in Part B or not. Accordingly, if an individual has secondary insurance—such as COBRA or retiree coverage—and does not enroll in Medicare, it is as if they have no coverage at all.

The rules are different for each type of insurance and are not easily understood, if a beneficiary even knows they exist. Like others not yet collecting Social Security, individuals with other coverage do not get a notice from the federal government explaining these interactions and other considerations when they turn 65. Some employers may know the rules, but

---

[52] Davis, P.A., Congressional Research Service, "Medicare: Part B Premiums" (August 4, 2016) available at: https://fas.org/sgp/crs/misc/R40082.pdf.

[53] Congressional Research Service, "Medicare: Part B Premiums" (April 4, 2019) available at: https://fas.org/sgp/crs/misc/R40082.pdf.

[54] Jacobson, Gretchen; et al., Kaiser Family Foundation, "Income and Assets of Medicare Beneficiaries, 2016-2035" (April 21, 2017) available at: https://www.kff.org/medicare/issue-brief/income-and-assets-of-medicare-beneficiaries-2016-2035/.

[55] Cubanski, Juliette; et al., Kaiser Family Foundation, "The Financial Burden on Health Care Spending: Larger for Medicare Households than for Non-Medicare Households" (March 1, 2018) available at: https://www.kff.org/medicare/issue-brief/the-financial-burden-of-health-care-spending-larger-for-medicare-households-than-for-non-medicare-households/.

many may not, which can result in well-intentioned but incorrect guidance on which employees rely, often to their detriment.

This was the case for Medicare Rights' client Ms. R. She was covered by COBRA and undergoing cancer treatment.[56] She declined to enroll in Part B because her employer told her that COBRA pays primary to Medicare. Unfortunately for Ms. R, it's the other way around—Medicare pays primary to COBRA. While she was receiving needed treatment, the COBRA plan realized she was not enrolled in Part B and should have been. As is allowed in these circumstances, the plan then stopped paying for her care and recouped several months' worth of payments. Because losing COBRA coverage does not trigger a SEP, Ms. R had to wait until the next GEP to enroll in Part B. Consequently, she was left without health insurance for nearly a year, charged thousands of dollars in medical bills, and put at risk of losing needed care, as her providers threatened to cut off her cancer treatment because she lacked outpatient coverage.

Demographic and Employment Trends

Without immediate solutions, more and more Americans will have experiences like Mr. A and Ms. R. The population is aging rapidly[57] and more older adults are working later in life.[58] At the same time, the gap between Medicare and retirement benefit eligibility continues to grow. As a result, an increasing number of individuals will face critical Part B enrollment decisions, lending an urgency to the need for improvements to the current system.

From 2006 to 2016, the number of Americans age 65 and over rose by 33%—from 37 to 49 million. Over that same time period, the number of Americans aged 45-64 (who will reach age 65 over the next two decades) increased by 12%, and the number of Americans age 60 and over increased by

---

[56] The Consolidated Omnibus Budget Reconciliation Act (COBRA) is a federal law passed in 1986 that lets certain employees, their spouses, and their dependents keep group health plan (GHP) coverage for 18 to 36 months after they leave their job or lose coverage for certain other reasons, as long as they pay the full cost of the premium. *See*: Medicare Rights Center, "COBRA Basics" (2019) available at: https://www.medicareinteractive.org/get-answers/coordinating-medicare-with-other-types-of-insurance/cobra-and-medicare/cobra-basics.

[57] Administration for Community Living, "A Profile of Older Americans: 2018" (April 2018) available at: https://www.acl.gov/aging-and-disability-in-america/data-and-research/profile-older-americans.

[58] Mitra Toossi and Elka Torpey, Bureau of Labor Statistics, "Older Workers: Labor Force Trends and Career Options" (May 2017) available at: https://www.bls.gov/careeroutlook/2017/article/older-workers.htm.

36%. By 2040, estimates suggest that the U.S. will be home to 82 million older adults, over twice their number in 2000.[59]

Aside from this sheer increase in volume, a growing share of this population is likely to delay taking Social Security benefits at age 65, while the full retirement age raises to 67.[60] Recent data show this shift, illustrating that an increasing number of older adults are working later in life: between 1999 and 2009, the share of workers ages 55 and older increased from 12 to 19%, the largest proportion on record.[61]

Further, the number of employed older Americans rose by nearly 35% just between 2011 and 2016, and this demographic is projected to be the fastest-growing segment of the workforce in the coming years.[62] Over the 2014 to 2024 decade, the labor force growth rate of 65- to 74-year-olds is expected to be about 55%. This number climbs to 86% for those 75-and-older, compared with a 5% increase for the labor force as a whole.[63]

These realities demand that policymakers act now to improve Medicare Part B enrollment. Otherwise, a growing number of newly eligible beneficiaries will struggle to access and afford meaningful health care and coverage.

The BENES Act

As discussed throughout, Medicare's rules are complex. The resulting beneficiary confusion is compounded by the lack of federal government outreach and notification to people as they approach Medicare eligibility. Exacerbating these systemic issues is the growing disconnect between the eligibility ages for Medicare and full Social Security benefits, along with changing demographics and employment patterns. As these trends show no sign of abating, the BENES Act's commonsense solutions are needed now more than ever.

---

[59] Administration for Community Living (ACL), "A Profile of Older Americans: 2017" (2017) available at: https://www.acl.gov/aging-and-disability-in-america/data-and-research/profile-older-americans.

[60] Favreault, M.M., Urban Institute, "Raising Social Security's Retirement Age" (July 2010), available at: http://www.urban.org/UploadedPDF/412167-Raising-Social-Security.pdf.

[61] Johnson, R.W., Urban Institute, "Older Workers: Opportunities and Challenges" (July 2010), available at: http://www.urban.org/UploadedPDF/412166-older-workers.pdf.

[62] SeniorLiving, "Elderly Employment: Analyzing Rates of Employment for Older Americans" (December 2017) available at: https://www.seniorliving.org/research/elderly-employment/.

[63] Mitra Toossi and Elka Torpey, Bureau of Labor Statistics, "Older Workers: Labor Force Trends and Career Options" (May 2017) available at: https://www.bls.gov/careeroutlook/2017/article/older-workers.htm.

Championed by Reps. Ruiz (D-CA) and Bilirakis (R-FL), as well as Reps. Schneider (D-IL), and Walorski (R-IN), the bipartisan and bicameral BENES Act (H.R. 2477) would take major steps to (I) Strengthen Education for the Soon-to-Be Eligible; (II) Eliminate Harmful Gaps in Coverage; and (III) Inform Future Policymaking on Enrollment Period Alignment.[64]

Strengthen Education for the Soon-to-Be Eligible

Today, no federal entity is responsible for notifying people about their Medicare eligibility if they are not already collecting Social Security when they first become eligible. As a result, many Americans do not receive the enrollment information they need, when they need it. This is a rapidly intensifying problem. In 2002, 8% of those who were eligible for Medicare at age 65 were not auto-enrolled in the program and did not receive government notification until after their IEP—past the point in time that an individual can always enroll in Medicare without facing any late enrollment penalties. By 2016, this number had risen to 40%.[65]

As noted by MedPAC in its June 2019 report, "the Medicare program should not rely on alternative sources to properly inform potential beneficiaries to sign up for Medicare during their IEP."[66] We agree with the commissioners that this should be addressed, and that "[i]mprovement in the timeliness of notification to eligible individuals about Medicare enrollment and potential late enrollment penalties is essential."[67]

The BENES Act offers a logical solution. It would require the federal government to notify people nearing Medicare eligibility about their rights and responsibilities. The notification would be sent to individuals attaining ages 63, 64, and 65 as part of their annual Social Security statement and to people with disabilities who are in the 24-month Medicare waiting period. It would, in part, clearly explain the individual's Medicare eligibility, the potential effects of delayed Part B enrollment, and the need for coordination of benefits.

---

[64] The legislation has also been included as Title I of the Beneficiary Education Tools Telehealth & Extenders (BETTER) Act of 2019 (H.R. 3417) and has been introduced in the Senate as S. 1280 by Senators Casey (D-PA) and Young (R-IN). The Senate bill has eight other bipartisan cosponsors.

[65] Medicare Payment Advisory Commission, "Report to the Congress: Medicare and the Health Care Delivery System" (June 2019) available at: http://www.medpac.gov/docs/default-source/reports/jun19_medpac_reporttocongress_sec.pdf?sfvrsn=0.

[66] Medicare Payment Advisory Commission, "Report to the Congress: Medicare and the Health Care Delivery System" (June 2019) available at: http://www.medpac.gov/docs/default-source/reports/jun19_medpac_reporttocongress_sec.pdf?sfvrsn=0.

[67] *Ibid.*

With this important reform in place, people approaching Medicare eligibility—including those who are not already receiving Social Security—would, for the first time, get trusted, understandable information from the federal government about how, whether, and when to enroll in Medicare.

This consumer-friendly notice would be developed by the federal government in consultation with relevant stakeholders, including older adults, people with disabilities, low-income individuals, HR professionals, private health plans, and others. The notice would also be posted online in a prominent location on both the SSA and CMS websites.

Eliminate Harmful Gaps in Coverage

The BENES Act would also modernize the Medicare IEP and GEP to allow coverage to begin more quickly post-enrollment. This significant update would eliminate gaps in coverage that can leave people exposed to high costs and inadequate care.

Currently, if a newly eligible beneficiary enrolls in the fourth through seventh month of their IEP, the initiation of Medicare coverage is needlessly delayed. The BENES Act would restructure the IEP so that Medicare coverage begins on the first of the month or the first of the following month when a person enrolls. Similarly, the annual GEP includes a significant gap between enrollment and the start of an individual's coverage—up to a seven-month delay. The BENES Act would also restructure the GEP to start coverage as soon as possible.

Inform Future Policymaking on Enrollment Period Alignment

Medicare's annual GEP does not coincide with the program's annual open enrollment periods for private Medicare plans, including Medicare Advantage and Part D. Nor does it align with commercial insurance open enrollment periods, which traditionally take place between October and December of each year. This fragmentation is inconsistent with the goals of maximizing coverage continuity and informed beneficiary choice and easing beneficiary transitions to Medicare. The BENES Act would take steps to correct this, by directing the U.S. Department of Health and Human Services to make recommendations to Congress regarding opportunities to better align Medicare's enrollment periods.

Taken together, the BENES Act's long overdue, commonsense changes would better empower people who are approaching Medicare eligibility to make optimal, timely coverage decisions that build their health and economic security.

These reforms have been endorsed by eight past CMS Administrators who served in both Democratic and Republican administrations. In an August 2016 letter supporting the BENES Act when it was first introduced, they wrote "…we frequently disagree among ourselves about any number of issues. But we all agree on the importance of treating Medicare beneficiaries fairly, efficiently, and as helpfully as possible. That's why we have come together in support of the bipartisan [BENES Act]."[68] The bill is also strongly supported by the Medicare Rights Center and a diverse array of nearly 100 stakeholder organizations, including consumer advocates, health plans, unions, service providers, and faith-based groups.[69] We reiterate this long-standing support again here, and urge you to pass the BENES Act without delay.

The Protecting Patients Transportation to Care Act (H.R. 3935)

Medicaid is an important source of health care for 12 million people with Medicare, covering needed services that Medicare does not, such as long-term services and supports (LTSS) and some types of nonemergency medical transportation (NEMT) to medically necessary health services. Medicaid also makes Medicare more affordable by helping low-income beneficiaries pay their premiums and cost-sharing amounts.[70]

Individuals who are eligible for both programs, known as dual eligibles, tend to have complex health care needs which can require recurring doctor appointments, strict adherence to prescription medication, and frequent medical tests: 41% of dually eligible individuals have at least one mental health diagnosis, 49% receive LTSS, and 60% have multiple chronic conditions, such as ESRD, diabetes, or heart disease.[71]

---

[68] Letter from eight former CMS Administrators to leaders of the House Committee on Energy & Commerce, the House Committee on Ways & Means, and the Senate Committee on Finance (August 22, 2016) available at: https://www.medicarerights.org/pdf/CMS-Admin-Support-Ltr-BENES-Act-S3236-HR5772-082216.pdf.

[69] Letter from 85 stakeholder organizations to Chairman Richard Neal and Ranking Member Kevin Brady of the House Committee on Ways & Means (June 25, 2019) available at: https://www.medicarerights.org/pdf/062619-benes-act-support-letter.pdf. *See also:* List of 95 supporting organizations submitted for the hearing record.

[70] Centers for Medicare & Medicaid Services, "People Enrolled in Medicare and Medicaid" (March 2019) available at: https://www.cms.gov/Medicare-Medicaid-Coordination/Medicare-and-Medicaid-Coordination/Medicare-Medicaid-Coordination-Office/Downloads/MMCO_Factsheet.pdf.

[71] *Ibid.*

For these and other high-need Medicaid enrollees, consistent, reliable transportation to and from their medical appointments is crucial but may not always be readily available. Health and affordability issues may make it impossible for them to drive a car, use public transit, or pay for a ride. Others, such as those who live in rural areas, may have limited public transportation options and face long travel times. In these instances, Medicaid NEMT can be a lifeline. It facilitates access to medical services for low-income beneficiaries who have no other means of transportation—helping them receive the care they need to manage their conditions and improve their outcomes.

Consider Ms. V, a Medicare Rights client who is a dual eligible and lives independently in an apartment building. She has several health challenges and is unable to walk without assistance, much less drive a car or navigate public transportation. Through her Medicaid NEMT benefit, she is able to safely attend her medical appointments. Another client, Ms. L, has ESRD and multiple chronic conditions. She doesn't qualify for a kidney transplant and needs dialysis regularly to stay healthy and independent. Without Medicaid NEMT, she wouldn't be able to access this life-sustaining care while living at home and participating in her community.

Of the less than 10% of Medicaid enrollees who qualify for and use NEMT,[72] many, like Ms. V and Ms. L, rely on the benefit to access services that help them stay healthy—such as dialysis, substance use disorder/behavioral health care, adult day health care, preventive care, specialist visits, and physical therapy/rehabilitation.[73] Assisting individuals in getting to their routine medical appointments allows them to receive preventive care and stick to treatment regimens that help them build and maintain their health—as well as avoid costly medical emergencies, hospitalizations, and institutionalizations.

Multiple studies agree the benefit is cost-effective.[74] One such review found that for the estimated 3.6 million people who miss or delay medical care each year due to lack of transportation, NEMT was a cost-effective or cost-

---

[72] Letter from the Congressional Black Caucus to Chairwoman Rosa L. DeLauro and Ranking Member Tom Cole of the House Committee on Appropriations, February 15, 2019.

[73] MaryBeth Musumeci and Robin Rudowitz, Kaiser Family Foundation, "Medicaid Non-Emergency Medical Transportation: Overview of Key Issues in Medicaid Expansion Waivers" (February 2016) available at: https://www.kff.org/medicaid/issue-brief/medicaid-non-emergency-medical-transportation-overview-and-key-issues-in-medicaid-expansion-waivers/.

[74] Justice in Aging, "Medicaid Non-Emergency Medical Transportation for Older Adults: A Critical Benefit at Risk" (May 1, 2019) available at: https://www.justiceinaging.org/fact-sheet-medicaid-non-emergency-medical-transportation-for-older-adults-a-critical-benefit-at-risk/.

saving way to help them manage their conditions.[75] Another concluded that NEMT yielded impressive returns on investment for dialysis and wound care.[76] And still another found that adults who lack transportation to medical care are more likely to have chronic health conditions that can escalate to require more expensive care if not properly managed.[77]

NEMT can also help people travel to their pharmacies to pick up their prescriptions and medical supplies. In some states, such as Georgia, the benefit covers rides to pharmacies whether or not they are part of a trip to a medically necessary health service. This function—and its potential to improve prescription drug access and adherence—is especially critical for dual eligibles. In part this is due to utilization. Older adults take an average of four to five prescriptions per month, and over two-thirds have multiple chronic conditions that require ongoing medical treatment.[78] At the same time, many live on fixed or limited incomes, which can make paying for medications or transportation to the pharmacy difficult.[79] Those who cannot purchase or collect their prescriptions may be forced to go without care—leading to worse health outcomes and quality of life. The Medicare and Medicaid programs are also impacted by barriers to enrollee prescription drug access and affordability, as those who forgo medication and experience declining health as a result may need more extreme interventions later.[80]

NEMT has been a mandatory Medicaid benefit by regulation since the Medicaid program's inception in 1966,[81] based on the Department of Health

[75] P. Hughes-Cromwick and R. Wallace, et al., Transit Cooperative Research Program, "Cost-Benefit Analysis of Providing Non-Emergency Medical Transportation" (October 2005) available at: http://onlinepubs.trb.org/onlinepubs/tcrp/tcrp_webdoc_29.pdf.

[76] Adelberg, Michael; et al., "Non-Emergency Medical Transportation: Findings from a Return on Investment Study" (July 2018) available at: https://mtaccoalition.org/medical-transportation-101/health-economic-benefits/.

[77] Richard Wallace, et al., "Access to Health Care and Nonemergency Medical Transportation: Two Missing Links" (2005) available at: http://www.researchgate.net/publication/39967547_ Access_to_Health_Care_and_Nonemergency_Medical_Transportation_Two_Missing_Links.

[78] Purvis, Leigh; et al., AARP Public Policy Institute, "Trends in Retail Prices of Prescription Drugs Widely Used by Older Americans: 2017 Year-End Update" (September 2019) available at: https://www.aarp.org/content/dam/aarp/ppi/2019/09/trends-in-retail-prices-of-prescription-drugs-widely-used-by-older-americans.doi.10.26419-2Fppi.00073.003.pdf.

[79] Jacobson, Gretchen; et al., Kaiser Family Foundation, "Income and Assets of Medicare Beneficiaries, 2016-2035" (April 21, 2017) available at: https://www.kff.org/medicare/issue-brief/income-and-assets-of-medicare-beneficiaries-2016-2035/.

[80] Lee, Shinduk et al., "Attitudes, Beliefs, and Cost-Related Medication Nonadherence Among Adults Aged 65 or Older With Chronic Diseases" (December 6, 2018) available at: https://www.ncbi.nlm.nih.gov/pmc/articles/PMC6292137/#.

[81] 42 C.F.R. § 431.53.

and Human Services' statutory authority to require state Medicaid plans to provide for methods of administration necessary for their proper and efficient operation.[82] Additionally, as part of the Early and Periodic Screening, Diagnostic, and Treatment (EPSDT) benefit, states are required to offer children from birth to age 21 and their families "necessary assistance with transportation" to and from providers.[83]

As all 53 members of the Congressional Black Caucus noted in a February 15, 2019 letter, "over half of Medicaid transportation services are utilized by patients with the highest burden of chronic diseases, including those diagnosed with cancer, HIV, mental illness, substance abuse, and end-stage renal disease....without this help, they could not access the chemotherapy, dialysis, and other services that allow them to remain at home and out of the hospital."[84] In 2017, members of the Blue Dog Coalition also weighed in to support the benefit, writing "NEMT is an essential component of our nation's health care system, especially in rural areas."[85]

The Protecting Patients Transportation to Care Act (H.R. 3935), introduced by Reps. Carter (R-GA) and Cardenas (D-CA), along with Reps. Graves (R-GA) and Bishop (D-GA), would formally codify this long-standing requirement, ensuring that beneficiaries have meaningful health care coverage. The Medicare Rights Center and nearly 60 other NEMT stakeholders strongly support H.R. 3935 and urge its swift enactment.[86]

Conclusion

Based on our work with people with Medicare and their families, we know that health care access and affordability are ongoing challenges. Every day on our National Consumer Helpline, we hear from older adults and people with disabilities who are struggling to cover these costs and obtain services for which they are eligible.

---

[82] 42 U.S.C. § 1396a(a)(4)(A).

[83] 42 C.F.R. § 441.62; *see also* 42 U.S.C. § 1396a(a)(43).

[84] Letter from the Congressional Black Caucus to Chairwoman Rosa L. DeLauro and Ranking Member Tom Cole of the House Committee on Appropriations, February 15, 2019.

[85] Letter from Reps. Sanford Bishop, Charlie Crist, Jim Cooper, Henry Cuellar, Vincente Gonzalez, Josh Gottheimer, Daniel Lipinski, Tom O'Halleran, Collin Peterson, David Scott, and Kyrsten Sinema to Chairman Greg Walden and Ranking Member Frank Pallone of the House Committee on Energy & Commerce, October 17, 2017.

[86] *See:* List of 58 supporting organizations submitted for the hearing record.

To improve the health and financial well-being of current and future Medicare beneficiaries, I urge you to pass the BENES Act and the Protecting Patients Transportation to Care Act this year. These urgently needed legislative solutions would help an ever-growing number of Americans make informed Medicare enrollment choices and stay healthy in their homes and communities.

Additionally, as you work to strengthen the Medicare and Medicaid programs this year through an extenders package or otherwise, I respectfully ask you to address several programs and policies that require prompt action due to looming expirations or other circumstances. Recently championed by the Medicare Rights Center and 71 other national organizations representing older adults, people with disabilities, consumers, and providers, these time-sensitive matters include relief for Medicare beneficiaries who will face even higher prescription drug out-of-pocket costs this year due to the January 1 increase in Medicare Part D catastrophic coverage eligibility thresholds from $5,100 to $6,350; at least five-year extensions of the Medicaid Home and Community-Based Services (HCBS) Money Follows the Person Program (MFP), and Spousal Impoverishment Protections; and permanent, increased funding for Medicare low-income outreach and enrollment efforts.[87]

Again, thank you again for the opportunity to be here today. I look forward to continuing to work together to improve Americans' health care coverage and outcomes.

* * *

Ms. ESHOO. Thank you, Mr. Riccardi, for your testimony.

To each one of you, thank you.

And we are going to ask you for some patience. You can have a somewhat leisurely lunch. We are going to break now and attend the classified briefing. And I would say we will return—the House is going to go back into session at 2:15, so I think that is a safe time for us to come back into session and give us time to get back from at least an hour of the classified briefing.

So we will see you in a bit. Have a nice lunch. Thank you. [Recess.]

Ms. ESHOO. OK. Good afternoon again. Thank you to or second panel of witnesses for your patience in staying with us. We have now concluded the

---

[87] Letter from 72 stakeholder organizations to Speaker Nancy Pelosi, Minority Leader Kevin McCarthy, Majority Leader Mitch McConnell, and Minority Leader Chuck Schumer (December 16, 2019) available at: https://d2mkcg26uvg1cz.cloudfront.net/wp-content/uploads/Medicare-Medicaid-Extenders-Group-Letter-12-16-19.pdf.

opening statements, your opening statements, and we will move to Member questions. And I will recognize myself for 5 minutes to get the ball rolling on that.

Dr. Cooper, thank you again. You gave excellent testimony today. Eleven thousand Americans—and you already know this, but I think it is important to state for the record that 11,000 Americans will die waiting for transplants this year. In the meantime, the Medicare program is putting people who are lucky enough to have a kidney transplant at risk by cutting off their coverage for immno—immunosuppressive drugs. Why is that such a tongue twister?

Why do you think this has gone on for 50 years? I can't help but ask that question.

Dr. COOPER. Yes. I knew you were going to ask me that question, and I wish I had answers for it.

Ms. ESHOO. I mean, because there are advocates. There have been transplants, people waiting, people knowing that they were going to die because of the way this thing is set up. Why has it taken 50 years?

Dr. COOPER. Well, I think the easy answer, Madam Chairwoman, is that, when you look at Medicare, I am not sure the A's, the B's, and the D's sort of all communicate with each other all the time, and what is potentially a loss in one area is a gain in the other. And, unfortunately, it probably took your examples and probably the voices of those many patient organizations that I talked about to continually bring this up, for folks to sit down and finally put all the numbers together in one place and recognize, again, overall this is a cost savings. But, again, beyond that, you know, this really is an ethical and moral obligation now.

Ms. ESHOO. It is. It certainly is.

Let me ask you this, because you are a transplant—you do transplants. Do you think that—the only hearing I ever remember since I came to Congress and have served on this committee was a hearing when I was in my second term. So that would have been 1995, 1996, and it was an examination of what are—of the system that we have that allocates——

Dr. COOPER. Organs.

Ms. ESHOO [continuing]. Organs. Are you satisfied with how that works in our country?

Dr. COOPER. That is a great and very timely question, Madam Chairwoman. So the problem that we started this conversation with, the supply and the demand that has sort of led to some——

Ms. ESHOO. Because there are very few that get one, get a part, get an organ.

Dr. COOPER. Yes, ma'am. And so I think we as a transplant community, we as the public, you know, continue to seek for better ways to make sure that that valued and cherished resource gets to the people that need them the most. There is currently afoot an effort to try and change the allocation system so that we remove geographic boundaries, which is currently the primary way in which organs are allocated, so that we, in fact, are getting the organs to where they need to get to.

We hope to eventually get to a point where we don't have that supply-and-demand problem, but until we get there, there is a need to continue to look at more ingenious ways to be able to assure that the organs are getting to the people that need them.

Ms. ESHOO. Do you think there should be an reexamination of the system that we have?

Dr. COOPER. Well, I think there—it continually is a reexamination, Madam Chairwoman.

Ms. ESHOO. No, but—at Congress.

Dr. COOPER. Oh, I actually think that the groups that have been contracted to oversee organ transplants through HRSA, UNOS, the SRTR actually recognize, again, that there is, you know, an opportunity for us to do better. We certainly would like to continue to have the support, things like the Executive order, things like Congress to continue to move those initiatives forward, but I truly believe the passion that exists within the transplant community is fairly capable of moving things forward and looking at other ways to do things better, particularly the allocation.

Ms. ESHOO. Thank you.

Mr. Riccardi, one of the—a problem you identified is that CMS doesn't notify soon-to-be-eligible Medicare beneficiaries about enrolling in Medicare if they don't receive Social Security benefits. Seems to me that this could be fixed administratively. Why doesn't CMS do this notification now?

Mr. RICCARDI. The practical, you know, solution to providing the notice involves not only CMS but also Social Security and the IRS.

Ms. ESHOO. Why can't they do it? Is there something that—does there have to be a statute?

Mr. RICCARDI. There has to be—yes.

Ms. ESHOO. There has to be a statute?

Mr. RICCARDI. There has to a statutory change to provide this notice. And what we have observed over time, now that people are working longer and delaying their Social Security, people are——

Ms. ESHOO. They run into this.

Mr. RICCARDI [continuing]. Missing their Medicare enrollment.

Ms. ESHOO. Yes. Another issue identified is that Medicare coverage is delayed until after the enrollment period ends. Why doesn't CMS begin Medicare coverage on the first of the month after a person enrolls, similar to how private business enrollment works?

Mr. RICCARDI. Exactly. That is the most commonsense solution, and I think this is the point where the enrollment periods just need to be modernized. Most Americans are now used to enrolling in coverage and having it start the following month, and that is what this bill would do.

Ms. ESHOO. Right. Thank you very much.

The Chair now recognizes Dr. Burgess, the ranking member of our subcommittee, for his 5 minutes of questions.

Mr. BURGESS. I thank our witnesses for staying with us today, and these are important topics that we are talking about.

Dr. Cooper, you have referenced the passion in the transplant community. I just have to tell you, when I went to the President's executive order on kidney care, I didn't figure there would be many people that showed up for that. Who is going to be there? That place was packed, and it was packed with very passionate advocates and it was—it really brought home to me, and although this has been a long-term fight that we have done on this immunosuppressive bill, it is important work and it needs to be done. It needs to get across the finish line.

Just in general, take us back to 1972 or when the End Stage Renal Disease Program started. Why was this—why was this incorporated into the program this way?

Dr. COOPER. Again, I want to take the opportunity to thank you for everything you have done, Dr. Burgess. It has been, I understand, a very difficult and challenging battle for you, and I am hoping, again, together we can see this through to the finish line.

I think the answer to your question is that perhaps there wasn't the appreciated unintended consequences that would come about through this. Like I said, the way that Medicare was set up, the charges for the actual procedure and, you know, everything that came soon thereafter was not fully appreciated, you know, by another part of Medicare that paid for the long-term care of the post-transplant patient.

And like I said, you know, in the responses to Madam Chairwoman, I think we didn't really take time to sit down together and say how do we make this whole and recognize it as—bring it all together will ultimately result in a cost savings for all this. So I think it was just we kept speeding forward with transplants, we kept demonstrating the successes. And perhaps even the numbers that were shared earlier of the grafts that were lost from lack of immunosuppressive coverage did not fully appreciate the significance of the problem. There were several hundred. There is probably more like several thousand. And it really is now coming, I think, full circle, particularly with the voices, the patient organizations that said, you know, we have to recognize really the unintended consequences in how we are losing too many grafts from something that is absolutely preventable.

Mr. BURGESS. And it is almost as if we were sugarcoating the issue when we talk about, you know, loss of a graft. I mean, this is a bad deal when it happens to someone. I mean, they have been lucky enough to get a transplant either from a living donor—good news is God gave us each two kidneys, and you can give one to someone else if you choose—or somebody got a cadaveric donor, and they were on a waiting list, they waited a long time to get a match, got a tissue match. They were able to go.

And now for want of—I mean, cyclosporine now is, what, $250 a month? I mean, it is not a big expense. It is not like some of the other things we talk about in this committee where it is $65,000 a month to be on your medicine. This is relatively manageable, and yet for that small investment, the agency is letting these patients go into something for which they cannot recover without another surgery.

Dr. COOPER. I understand. We I think, unfortunately, look at the expression of gifts of life and don't really recognize that that is exactly what it is. This is a gift. It does provide new life for individuals, and the fact that we are unable to protect that gift with, like you said, something that is truly manageable and truly affordable and recognize, again, that with each graft lost, that potentially puts someone else on an already list that is overwhelming and prevents other people from potentially receiving a graft.

And so, again, if we just figure out that we can get out of our own way and protect a lot of the kidneys that are currently successful, being transplanted, we are going to make, I think, a potential effort towards the same thing that the President put forward on Executive order of trying to increase the numbers of transplants by 2023.

Mr. BURGESS. Now, you are a transplant surgeon. Do you do other transplants besides renal transplants?

Dr. COOPER. I do pancreas transplants also and combinations of the two, particularly those that have end-stage renal disease from type 1 or type 2 diabetes, another remarkable operation that changes people's lives.

Mr. BURGESS. So somebody gets a transplant remote from the ESRD Program, somebody gets a heart transplant, what happens to them? Do they get—I mean, I presume their regular health insurance will cover their antirejection drugs?

Dr. COOPER. Yes. The majority of that, like I said, for kidney transplants, you know, far over 80 percent of our patients are Medicare primary. It is a little bit different for the other organs. Their private insurance is probably much better set up to take care of those organs. I think there is effort afoot after this gets approved to potentially make certain that we are not losing other organ systems through the cracks also. But primarily, number one, because of the volume of kidney transplants and the primary payer being Medicare do we see this as such a significant problem in the kidney population.

Mr. BURGESS. OK. So ironically we may have disadvantaged people by setting up the ESRD Program who were covered by commercial insurance. Perhaps their immunosuppressant would be covered.

Dr. COOPER. That is certainly one way of looking at it, sir, yes.

Mr. BURGESS. OK. Mr. Riccardi, I just have to ask you, because it came to my attention in a constituent meeting last week, about the COBRA not being credible coverage and the gap that some people can fall into. You have kind of alluded to that. Can you speak to that a little bit?

Mr. RICCARDI. Yes. Yes, I can. And this is another aspect of where the eligibility periods for Medicare haven't been modernized now that there is the existence of COBRA. Currently, if somebody has Medicare part A and they enroll in COBRA, they will be continuing to pay their COBRA premiums, and then typically they will learn from either the health insurance plan or from a physician that the COBRA plan is no longer active or refuses to pay, and then they are locked out of coverage.

And it reminds me—every day we are hearing from people who are calling our helpline, but it reminds me of one individual that I had worked with many years ago. She happened to be from Texas, and she had been paying her COBRA premium. And then, when she was ready to enroll in Medicare, she realized that she couldn't. And she hadn't received any information about needing to enroll and was essentially misinformed by her employer, and this was a large company.

And typically we hear from people after they have already spoken to Social Security, Medicare, they have reached out to their elected officials, and they are desperate for needed assistance. And so we do increasingly over the last several years have more and more calls from people who are on COBRA. Either they have been paying these premiums, which is, if anybody has seen a

COBRA premium, it is much more costly than a Medicare part B premium. And so most people are scrambling to get into Medicare, but then they are locked out of this punitive gap in coverage.

Mr. BURGESS. OK. I don't think we addressed that in this bill, but that is something we do need to take on at some point. I thank you.

I will yield back.

Ms. ESHOO. The gentleman yields back.

I am just stunned that no administration that I know of has ever come forward in these areas saying we need a statute to fix this. I think that is what is jaw-dropping to me. I have never had a constituent, in terms of organs and what we are trying to correct with the legislation, ever point this out to me. But what stands out is we are in Washington, DC, is that no Secretary of Health and Human Services has ever come forward and said this needs to change and we need you to write a new statute.

I now would like to recognize the gentlewoman from California, Ms. Matsui, for her 5 minutes of questioning.

Ms. MATSUI. Thank you. My microphone seems to be very powerful.

Older adults today face a challenging healthcare landscape with rising medical costs and fixed financial resources. It is unacceptable that Medicare's complex enrollment process often further exacerbates these challenges.

Mr. Riccardi, in your testimony, you note that modernizations to the part B enrollment process are needed due to a shift in how people are experiencing their initial Medicare eligibility. Can you elaborate on some of the factors responsible for this shift?

Mr. RICCARDI. Sure. As people are working longer and the Social Security eligibility age for full retirement benefits is now separate—the Medicare eligibility, someone is eligible at age 65, and currently for someone who is retiring, they have to wait till age 66 to collect full retirement benefits, and that age will increase to 67. So increasingly there are fewer people who are taking their Social Security right now, and these people are going without an individual notice.

And what the BENES Act will do are three key things. First, they just will simply provide a notice about somebody's upcoming Medicare eligibility prior to age 65. They will—it will inform people about the basic rules related to Medicare, including this late enrollment penalty. So it will prevent people from incurring a late enrollment penalty. And, lastly, it is going to eliminate this disastrous gap in coverage that I was just speaking about by ensuring that people who do enroll into Medicare can have their coverage start the following month or the current month.

Ms. MATSUI. Right. Absolutely. And it is important to me that, as we recognize the modern realities of how Americans are aging and transitioning through life stages, that we need to streamline part B to reflect these realities, and I think it is time to do that certainly.

Mr. Koser, thank you for your testimony today. I appreciate it very much. I am grateful you are here today. It is so admirable you are advocating for many of the patients and children across the country.

Mr. Koser, can you tell us a little more about your journey and how you came to be involved in advocacy?

Mr. KOSER. Thank you, Congresswoman. I appreciate that. So Kannon is 4 years old. We had no family history of ectodermal dysplasia. We had never heard of it until the doctor at University of Virginia mentioned it to us. It was at that point obviously I got heavily involved with the National Foundation for Ectodermal Dysplasias.

What I found there was that there was a systematic issue across this entire country where people affected not only by ectodermal dysplasia but other congenital anomalies were running into these issues, despite maintaining a full comprehensive health insurance plan.

For Kannon specifically we are very early in his treatment plan right now. We have started trying to pursue these dentures for him. Got rejected in the initial denial from insurance. We plan to pursue them further. We are going to end up having to pay 100 percent out of pocket for him probably in the next several months. We are waiting for his first tooth to fully erupt. That will cost thousands.

But I just wanted to not only represent Kannon and ectodermal dysplasia, but within the written testimony you will see there is about 46 other organizations representing different disorders and congenital anomalies that are facing these same issues.

Ms. MATSUI. And the health plans often deny these claims, right?

Mr. KOSER. Correct.

Ms. MATSUI. OK. You know, although all 50 States already have some sort of congenital anomaly law, it is really clear from your testimony that State regulation alone is not enough to ensure coverage for treatment. Can you expand on how some of these short-comings occur and how Federal policy will help reenforce State protections for congenital anomalies?

Mr. KOSER. Certainly. And thank you for that. I think it is important to understand the foundation of this bill. As you mentioned, all 50 States have statutes that already exist, many of them existing for decades, regarding that any insurance plan issued and regulated by the State must include medically necessary treatments of congenital anomalies.

Those laws are written in open-ended ways as if all congenital anomalies are to be treated equally. Those plans, otherwise known as fully insured plans, the State-regulated plans, there is only approximately 50 million Americans with such plans. The flip side and the other important piece here is to note that self-funded or self-insured plans, which are regulated at the Federal level through ERISA of 1974, there are 110 million Americans with such plans. These are private, employer-sponsored health plans, regulated at the Federal level. Beyond that, both types of plans, fully insured and self-funded, are both overwhelmingly telling us that within their policies we have mandates for coverage of medically necessary treatments related to congenital anomalies. It is just these loopholes. That is the only way that the insurers can bypass those things.

Ms. MATSUI. OK. Fine. Thank you very much, and I know how we must come forward to address these loopholes. And thank you very much for being here today. Thank you.

Ms. ESHOO. The gentlewoman yields.

It is a pleasure to recognize the gentleman from Florida who is sitting in the ranking member's chair, my friend Mr. Bilirakis, for his 5 minutes.

Mr. BILIRAKIS. Thank you. Thank you, Madam Chair. It is an honor to sit in this chair next to you as ranking member, even though it is probably for only 2 minutes. I will take it.

Again, Mr. Riccardi, complex Medicare enrollment rules and lacking notification costs tens of thousands of older adults and people with disabilities that face lifetime fines—which I think is ridiculous—coverage gaps and other harmful consequences. With fewer people automatically enrolled in Medicare and 10,000 baby boomers aging into Medicare each day, more people new to the Medicare must actively enroll in the program.

In your estimate, what percentage of seniors today have a proper understanding of their current Medicare eligibility and the enrollment process?

Mr. RICCARDI. So thank you for your question. And, you know, currently as more and more people are working longer, you know, there are millions of people who are not well informed about their Medicare coverage because they are not receiving any notification about that. They are relying on information from HR departments, from benefit administrators, from commercial insurance brokers.

And so, currently, there are, you know—approximately only 60 percent of people are automatically enrolled into Medicare. So that is millions of people who are going uninformed about these basic enrollment rules and the penalties, as you had mentioned, these lifetime penalties associated with them. And this problem is only going to snowball, as you mentioned, with, you know, 10,000 people every day turning 65.

Mr. BILIRAKIS. Yes. So it looks like we have an easy solution here with this bill.

Mr. RICCARDI. Yes, very straightforward.

Mr. BILIRAKIS. Again, can you explain how seniors might confuse the merits of delayed enrollment into Social Security with late enrollment into Medicare? I mean, it is complicated.

Mr. RICCARDI. It is very complicated.

Mr. BILIRAKIS. Yes.

Mr. RICCARDI. And so, you know, the people who are receiving their Social Security benefits, enrollment is automatic and it is streamlined. People are automatically enrolled in part A and part B, and they can choose a drug plan or Medicare Advantage. For older adults who are continuing to work or who are waiting to collect their full retirement benefit, they have much more to consider, whether Medicare is going to be primary or secondary. And then they are juggling multiple enrollment periods—an initial enrollment period, a special enrollment period, a general enrollment period—and none of these periods are aligned.

So what the BENES Act will do, it will prevent many of these errors from occurring by providing a simple notification a few years out before someone turns 65 versus individuals kind of scrambling after they have turned 65 and realize that they have been working their entire life, they have had insurance, and then once they are eligible for Medicare, they are locked out of the program for several months. It is very unfair.

Mr. BILIRAKIS. As far as—so, again, you know, obviously people have to have a sense of responsibility. But how are they going to be informed? We are talking about emails. We are talking about letters, hopefully with big letters, big font because I have a hard time, I need big font, and I will be a senior pretty soon.

Mr. RICCARDI. Well, one thing that I have observed over the years and what we have heard from our helpline clients is that, when Social Security or Medicare sends a mailing, people open it and they read it. And what the BENES Act will do, will provide notification as part of somebody's Social Security annual award statements. And for many of you, if you have spoken to someone who is near retirement or thinking about retirement, they are starting to wonder, well, how much can I collect at 62 and 65 and 67 and 70.

And so providing this information as part of that notice will ensure that people are obtaining it, and then they can make more informed decisions around whether they should enroll into Medicare part B.

Mr. BILIRAKIS. Thank you very much.

Madam Chair, the BENES Act is important to help individuals who are approaching Medicare eligibility, but as we all are aware, there are many issues that beneficiaries face once they are enrolled in Medicare—and I am sure you will agree—and begin accessing services and filing claims. Once those have to do with the—one of those things that has to do with Medicare is reimburse in its secondary payer status. That is confusing too.

I cosponsored a bill with Congressman Kind, and it is called the—well, it's H.R. 1375, the Provide Accurate Information Directly, or the PAID Act, that would help achieve efficiencies for beneficiaries, build better information sharing, again, through better information sharing. I would ask members of the committee to consider that particular bill and maybe cosponsor the bill.

And I will yield back, Madam Chair. Thank you.

Ms. ESHOO. The gentleman yields back.

I now would like to recognize the gentleman from Oregon, Mr. Schrader, for his 5 minutes of questions.

Mr. SCHRADER. Thank you very much, Madam Chair. I appreciate it.

Mr. Riccardi, thank you very much for taking the time to be here today and speaking with us on these important problems in Medicare. The BENES Act is a great piece of legislation. We are a big supporter of the BENES Act, and your testimony speaks to the reasons that we need to do legislative solutions.

I also have introduced a bill, bipartisan bill, with some of the colleagues here on the Energy and Commerce Committee, as well as others, dealing with the Medicare Enrollment Protection Act. It is much along the lines of what you and Chairman Burgess just discussed. I became personally aware of these types of situations shortly after I first got elected back in 2009. A constituent of mine, Bill Bergman, came to me, and like many Americans we have just talked about, he worked past the age of 65. He got COBRA coverage, a voluntary retirement package and COBRA through his employer. Felt he was in pretty good shape. Then, you know, fast forward, he assumed—he actually asked, "Could I switch to Medicare after getting off of COBRA?" Was given inaccurate information, and he was really surprised when he faced lack of coverage when his COBRA terminated. And he tried to get Medicare, because there was no enrollment period for him to get Medicare.

And that is a huge problem, one of the many problems that we have talked about here today. And he was subject to the late enrollment penalty as a result of that.

The bill I have introduced, H.R. 2565, with Mr. Bilirakis, Mike Thompson, and Vern Buchanan, provides a permanent remedy to folks who face barriers to enrolling in part D and penalties due to electing to utilize COBRA coverage after they are Medicaid eligible. Basically, what it does is, at the conclusion of Medicare—excuse me—of COBRA coverage, that would be considered a qualifying event for a new enrollment period. So they would be able to enroll and get coverage within a month of, like we just talked about is common in a lot of other plans.

I would hope that, while the BENES Act goes forward, this would be a nice complement. And I wonder if you would agree that this is probably a nice complement to the BENES Act and perhaps could be a great amendment to work into this legislation to further deal with some of the Medicare enrollment problems that we are seeing.

Mr. RICCARDI. Yes. I agree that I think it is important to look for strategies and solutions to individuals who have other types of employer coverage, extensions of that coverage, like retiree insurance or COBRA coverage, to allow for a special enrollment period.

Again, these are many people who have done everything right. You know, they have worked a long time. They have had coverage through their employer. They have kept continual coverage, because as we age, you know, people do not want to have gaps in coverage or periods of time where they are uninsured, and then it is a surprise when they can't enroll.

It reminds me of a client that Medicare Rights had worked with many years ago who had worked for a very large company, and he was enrolled into a retiree insurance and was informed that he did not need to have Medicare part B because he was going to be taken care of. And so many of us can kind of look back and remember the time where, if you did have insurance, you know, a company could guarantee it to you for life. Well, you know, for this individual, you know, eventually he developed stage IV cancer, and then the COBRA coverage began to deny payment and he was forced to, you know, personally take out a reverse mortgage to pay for his care to cover himself during that gap in coverage.

And I remember speaking to him and his daughter and how the family really struggled, and for him, he was less concerned about himself but more about the financial impact that it was going have on his wife.

Mr. SCHRADER. Very good. Very good story also.

So I would hope the leaders of the committee would take into consideration our legislation, along with the BENES Act, is one of many solutions that, when this bill gets marked up, be brought to the floor and hopefully pass and help our seniors get the coverage they deserve and think they have earned and especially after they have done all the right things.

And I yield back.

Ms. ESHOO. The gentleman yields back.

If I might make a suggestion, it seems to me, Mr. Schrader, that you need to get into a huddle with Dr. Ruiz. How is that? Friendly suggestion. Sounds like an amendment to a bill to me, but it is nice when everybody agrees.

I now would like to recognize the gentleman from Virginia, Mr. Griffith.

Mr. GRIFFITH. Thank you, Madam Chair. I appreciate it.

I appreciate you all being here today. I know it has been a long day. As you know, we had a significant briefing that I think just about every Member attended. It is the first time I have been to one of those where there was not enough seats, but it was important. It was good for all us to do that.

Mr. Koser, I am with you in principle. I am looking for ways we can tighten up that language to make sure that we are doing exactly what you want to do and not getting too carried away. And I think we are going to be able to work that out.

Mr. KOSER. Thank you, Congressman.

Mr. GRIFFITH. And I think we get that done, we can move forward on this.

Everybody else has had great testimony. I was here for the testimony. So I heard that and appreciate you all being here.

And with that, because I know it is late, I yield back.

Ms. ESHOO. Well, I called him a gentleman. Now he is a really timely one.

A pleasure to recognize the gentleman from California, Mr. Cárdenas, for his 5 minutes of questions.

Mr. CÁRDENAS. Thank you very much, Madam Chair, and Ranking Member as well. And I don't know how timely I am going to be, but hopefully I can be a gentleman.

I would also like to thank my colleague on the other side of the aisle, Congressman Carter, for working on the issue that I would like to bring up today, and also not to mention, we have a colleague who is not on this committee who is a champion on this issue, and it is Congressman Bishop from Georgia.

And I would also like to give a personal thanks to Mr. and Ms. Koser for coming and tirelessly advocating on behalf of not only your family but thousands and thousands of children and families across this country. And hopefully we can do some good work as a result of that, and so thank you for bringing your beautiful family with you.

I would like to talk about the importance of access to reliable transportation for Medicaid beneficiaries. As you said in your testimony, Mr. Riccardi, this benefit can be a lifeline for Medicaid beneficiaries who may not be able to afford other means of transportation. I think it is just common sense. If you can't get to your doctor, it doesn't matter if you have health insurance or not.

Mr. Riccardi, I would like to ask you a few questions about the folks who rely on this benefit and what sort of treatments they are using it for and what they are trying to get to with this transportation.

First, Mr. Riccardi, just to clarify, when we talk about non-emergency medical transportation, otherwise known as NEMT, we are talking about rides to healthcare providers, pharmacies and that sort of thing, not trips in and ambulance or to the ER. And so can you clarify what kind of access these people are getting when they utilize this transportation?

Mr. RICCARDI. Yes. The NEMT benefit is a key Medicaid benefit that helps the most vulnerable Medicaid enrollees access medical services. This is not emergency care, say, ambulance rides to a hospital, but for medical visits. And these people are any combination of elderly, have a disability, and very low income and have no other means of transportation.

And so this benefit allows people to receive both preventive care and a number of type of services. Many of our clients who are receiving this benefit are using it for dialysis treatments and also for behavioral health and substance abuse disorder treatment and medical services.

I can think of one client who, you know, is unable to leave her home and, without this benefit, she would not be able to receive her medical treatment. And, you know, she needs some assistance in leaving the home, and this benefit is crucial for her to get to her medical appointments.

And in many cases, people who are using this benefit are women, and they are elderly and unable to, you know, drive or transport themselves, and this is why this benefit is so important.

Mr. CÁRDENAS. Thank you.

And to clarify, and this is a benefit that benefits people in rural and inner city communities pretty much equally, right?

Mr. RICCARDI. Equally.

Mr. CÁRDENAS. It doesn't discriminate.

Mr. RICCARDI. Yes. So individuals in rural communities can access this benefit. And what is unique about this transportation benefit is our helpline is available for people with Medicare and Medicaid to call us up with questions and issues. And so many of the people that we speak to who are accessing this benefit are not calling us with complaints about NEMT. They are calling us with other Medicare-related questions, but we hear about the chronic conditions they have and how this transportation benefit allows them to receive the services that they need.

And the majority of our clients are receiving dialysis. What is great about this benefit—and I know this—States have flexibility with this benefit—they are able to access this service, you know, 24 hours a day, and it really is a lifeline for them. Otherwise, if this benefit did not exist, people would not be able to stay and live independently and in the community.

Mr. CÁRDENAS. And also I would venture to say—and I will go on to my next question—that without this benefit, the cost expense would exacerbate for the individual and for our system.

Mr. Riccardi, according to the Medicaid and CHIP Payment and Access Commission, about 42 percent of the people who use the NEMT benefit are dual eligibles, meaning they are eligible for both Medicare and Medicaid. In your testimony, you said that these dual-eligible individuals often have complex medical needs, that 60 percent have multiple chronic conditions, and 41 percent have at least one mental health diagnosis.

Is it fair to say that these individuals likely need a significant amount of Medicaid—excuse me—Medicare throughout the year?

Mr. RICCARDI. So, yes, on average, someone who is dually eligible for Medicare and Medicaid can have anywhere from four to five chronic conditions and, additionally, at least one behavioral health issue. And increasingly more and more older adults are suffering from anxiety and depression, and so this benefit truly is crucial for people who are either elderly or disabled and low income where they are unable to afford transportation. So this really enables for them to receive their services and then also prevent either relapses or a worsening of a chronic condition.

Mr. CÁRDENAS. Thank you very much. And I yield back the balance of my time.

Ms. ESHOO. The gentleman yields back.

It is a pleasure to recognize the gentleman from Oklahoma, Mr. Mullin, for 5 minutes of questions.

Mr. MULLIN. Thank you, Madam Chair.

Dr. Cooper, the Medicare ESRD Program has saved lives but has also impact on overall medical expenses. What are the easiest ways to reduce expenses connected with this program?

Dr. COOPER. Thank you, Congressman. So certainly, on the one side, which is obviously transplant, and we spent a lot of time today talking about the value of a transplant and how it saves lives. The other part is identifying chronic kidney disease early and preventing people from ever needing the point where transplant is necessary.

And so—and some of your efforts have certainly, I think, garnished a lot of interest in the kidney community of early identification and getting people the care they need for problems such as high blood pressure and diabetes so that they can receive the appropriate treatment for those and avoid kidney disease. But, unfortunately, a lot of people without access to primary care eventually get to the need of a transplant. And I think that is why we are here today, is to recognize transplant is the best treatment for end-stage organ disease. Dialysis is in many ways, we think, a stop-over.

And, unfortunately, there is a lot of misperceptions about whether or not, number one, people can avoid dialysis altogether. They can and receive a transplant immediately, rather than go on dialysis. And also, who are the appropriate candidates for transplant? We are finding more and more myths exist about who is not a candidate for transplant, and we should spend more time recognizing that most people who have end-stage renal disease should be referred to a transplant program because it is the best treatment for end-stage renal disease.

Mr. MULLIN. All right. Unfortunately, I have had my wife's grandfather and two good friends of mine who have passed away while they were on dialysis, awaiting a transplant, because in Indian Country it is disproportionately high, roughly 50 percent more likely to find themselves on dialysis, needing a transplant, than any other groups. And so it is vitally important, and it is something that we take to heart.

I can't simply drive any direction outside of our house, going to the big city of Tulsa, without passing a dialysis center. There are 2 within 30 miles of each other, and we are pretty rural for that to happen.

When you compare a transplant to dialysis, is a return on investment a short period of time? Is it noticed?

Dr. COOPER. Yes. So there has been lots of studies that have demonstrated that people who undergo a transplant versus remaining on dialysis, at approximately 90 to 100 days after they receive their transplant, that they have a decreased risk of death versus remaining on dialysis. And so the return on the investment, to use your term, is actually very quick following transplant.

Now, that appreciates the fact that we do have some absolute contraindications and relative contraindications to being listed for transplant, albeit, like I said, those are getting shorter and shorter. But recognize again that the data has clearly shown that people should be transplanted who meet the criteria for transplantation because, again, their return on investment, not only from a length of life but from a quality of life, both for them and for their family, as I mentioned, it is an important consideration that end-stage renal disease not only affects the individual but affects their family and support system who often have to plan around three-times-a-week dialysis and all of the rigors that are associated with suffering through end-stage renal disease.

Mr. MULLIN. All right. And this is just more of a statement. This isn't a question, because I am supporter of H.R. 5334, but I am concerned to see that under section 2, individuals eligible for services in this, which is Indian Health Services, would be barred from this coverage under Medicare.

As I have stated before, American Indians and Alaska Natives are 50 percent more likely to have kidney failure compared to others. I know the bill sponsors are friends of Indian Country, and I look forward to continuing to work with them to ensure American Indians have the access to the medical services they need.

And with that, I will yield back.

Ms. ESHOO. The gentleman yields back.

I don't understand the reason why that is the case, but——

Mr. BURGESS. May I address that?

Ms. ESHOO. Sure.

Mr. BURGESS. Well, the bill was introduced by another Member of Congress. We did not have absolute editorial authority before it was introduced.

Mr. MULLIN. Yes.

Mr. BURGESS. I think that is something that can be remedied.

Mr. MULLIN. And we understand that the sponsor is looking into it. We have clarification, but they have made us assured they are going to do what they can to——

Ms. ESHOO. Good. I would——

Mr. MULLIN [continuing]. Amendment under the rule.

Ms. ESHOO. You obviously are already working with the authors of the legislation. And, if anything, we want the tremendous benefits that the legislation brings about to have, I would say, you know, first and foremost in the Native American community to be——

Mr. MULLIN. And I understand that this is last payer anyways, but it still has to be written in. That is the way I——

Ms. ESHOO. Exactly. Well, it can't be prohibited.

Mr. MULLIN. Right.

Ms. ESHOO. That is where—that is kind of chilling to me, to draw a line and say, oh, you who need this desperately are definitely out. Mr. BURGESS. If I may offer, when this was an Energy and Commerce product, that did not happen. We will fix it.

Ms. ESHOO. Good. OK.

Dr. Ruiz of California.

Mr. RUIZ. Thank you, Madam Chair, and thank you for considering my bill, H.R. 2477, the Beneficiary Enrollment Notification and Eligibility Simplification Act of 2019, otherwise known as the BENES Act.

I would also like to thank my friend and colleague, Mr. Bilirakis, on this committee for introducing this important piece of legislation with me.

I grew up in the Coachella Valley, and oftentimes people think of Palm Springs, Indian Wells, Rancho Mirage with lush country clubs and that is a place where you go to retire and spend a lot of money playing golf and enjoying life, and that is definitely an option. However, the vast majority of seniors in my district are not so well off, and they still struggle and they still have bills, and their Social Security doesn't cut it, and they still take care of their grandchildren, and they still have other bills that they need to pay, and so they have to work. And when they work, they don't get the notification of automatic enrollment into Medicare part A, part B. Therefore, they miss out and they are late, and that has consequences, multiple consequences.

One is, for every year that they are late, they incur a 10 percent lifetime penalty on their premiums. So let's say they work for 3, 4, 5 years. That is a 50 percent increase in premiums for the rest of their lives.

Second, when they don't enroll, they just don't have coverage. Simple as that. And some of these jobs don't offer that kind of insurance, and they just think that they are automatically going to get Medicare, and they don't.

And then, finally, there are some innate enrollment coverage gaps that are unacceptable, up to 6 months at times. And, because they don't have insurance during that time, even after they enroll, then they have to pay those expensive bills. They have to get private health insurance, which has higher premiums than the Medicare. And we have seen how that can be detrimental, especially for those who have to decide between paying their bills, working, food, those that have to take reverse mortgages, those that simply go into extreme financial hardship, which adds to their sickness and ailments with anxiety.

And so this bill wants to prevent those—not only prevent seniors from not having insurance once they turn 65, it also wants to prevent them from incurring the penalty for late enrollment, per se, after 65, but even closes those loopholes within the enrollment coverage gap that currently exist simply because it is outdated, it is complex, and people are really losing out.

So this bill really protects seniors, and it is aimed for seniors by making sure they get notification, starting as early as the age of 60, every year when they are anticipating what they may be able to get in terms of their Social Security years later, even if they have to work. And it also aligns the enrollment period for part B with the other private insurance enrollment period so it is not as confusing. So it is just what they would normally—when they would normally enroll, they would enroll.

So those two provisions will prevent them from making the mistake of not enrolling in a proper fashion.

And then, finally, the third thing is that it closes that nuanced systematic flaw, which has a loophole of an enrollment coverage gap by ensuring that, once they enroll, even those 3 months after they turn 65, but also when they do their first enrollment, their first late enrollment, that they don't have to wait up to 6 months, that it can happen in the same month or soon after.

So let me ask you some questions. In your written testimony, you state that in 2018, approximately 760,000 Medicare beneficiaries were paying the late enrollment penalty. And many of the seniors I know can't afford their medicines or their Medicare premiums in the first place. They certainly cannot shoulder the additional burden of a penalty, and this is not to mention the potentially devastating effect of having a potential gap in coverage, especially when you are at most risk of getting sick. So these laws are over 50 years old, and healthcare has changed in the last 50 years.

Have the enrollment laws been amended since they were initially enacted, and how is the enrollment environment different today than it was back then?

Mr. RICCARDI. So the——

Ms. ESHOO. We will allow Mr. Riccardi to respond, but your time is up. Yes.

Mr. RICCARDI. Thank you.

Ms. ESHOO. Please proceed.

Mr. RICCARDI. The enrollment rules for the initial enrollment period and the general enrollment period have not changed in over 50 years.

And to speak to your point about the struggles that older Americans have with finances is that approximately 50 percent of older adults are living on $26,000 a year or less, and a quarter of them have less than $13,000 in savings and they simply cannot bear the burden of these late enrollment penalties and these gaps in coverage.

Our helpline hears, you know, approximately a quarter of our calls around these issues, and the worst call that we receive happens to be every year during the month of April after somebody misses the general enrollment period, because they would not be able to enroll for another approximately 18 months for coverage.

And so what is so important about the BENES Act is it will eliminate this punitive gap in coverage for people, as you have mentioned, who have had other types of insurance, in many cases have been paying more than what it costs—what it would cost to be in the Medicare program.

And so this bill will prevent these errors from happening. It is very commonsense and practical that they would receive a notice from the Federal Government about the best decision for them to make.

Mr. RUIZ. Thank you. I yield back my time.

Ms. ESHOO. Wonderful. The gentleman yields back.

And I recognize the gentleman from Georgia, Mr. Carter.

Mr. CARTER. Thank you, Madam Chair.

And thank all of you for being here. We appreciate this very much.

Madam Chair, I want to start by thanking you and thanking Chairman Pallone for including my bill, H.R.—and Representative Cárdenas' bill—H.R. 3935, the Protecting Patients Transportation to Care Act, in today's hearing.

H.R. 3935 is pretty simple. It just codifies what is already in rule, and that is important, and it codifies something that is beneficial and is helping us.

You know, I have been in the State legislature. I was in the State legislature for 10 years. I have been in Congress now for 5 years. One of the most difficult tasks I have had as a healthcare professional is explaining to some of my colleagues the value of and benefit of healthcare and well care, of making sure we are getting patients the care that they need and how it can actually save us money, and save us a lot of money. But all this does is to just codify current regulations that the States have to offer nonemergency medical transportation for medically necessary services to patients who don't have access to transportation on their own.

Now, I represent a lot of south Georgia, a very rural area, and that is very important. However, it is important to note also that this could have an impact on people in urban areas just as well. There are certainly people who need this service in the urban areas just as we obviously need it in the rural areas.

Now, to tell you the truth, generally speaking, I am not in favor of mandating things and of codifying these type of things; however, the benefit outweighs the risk here. There is no question about it. The benefit of this far outweighs any risk.

And, having said that, I will say that there are a number of my colleagues who have expressed some concern about fraud, waste, and abuse, and I get that, and I understand that. This bill actually addresses that as well and actually puts some areas in place, some programs in place, to make sure that we are checking on that. And we are going to continue to work on that. It is extremely important.

But the lack of access to transportation can be a barrier across the country, and as I say, patients who use the nonemergency medical transportation benefit do it for a number of reasons, for a variety of reasons. Dialysis would be one. And that is a perfect example. Substance abuse, and let's talk about that for one second. This committee, in a bipartisan effort—as I have always said, I think this is the most bipartisan committee in Congress, and I do believe that sincerely—but what we have done for substance abuse and for addressing that situation, this is an extension of that. We need to make sure that people have access to those programs. So that is vitally important as well.

Mental health treatment, day support for patients with intellectual and developmental disabilities, physician services, pharmacy services, physical therapy, the list goes on and on. All of these are extremely important to making sure that we have a healthy citizenship, and that is very important.

So it is no surprise—and just to give you one example—it is no surprise that people who miss medical appointments due to a lack of reliable transportation experience worse health outcomes and are more likely to end up in the emergency room. You talk to any doctor, you talk to any hospital administrator, and they will tell you, where is the main cost? Emergency rooms. We got to keep people out of the emergency rooms. We have got to get them in the habit of primary care, getting them in the habit of making sure that they are not using the emergency room as their primary care physicians.

There is a study from Florida State University that found that, if just 1 percent—1 percent—of nonemergency medical transportation trips prevented an emergency room visit, the State of Florida would receive a 1,108 percent return on investment. Now, who wouldn't take that? So I am just trying to show you the value of this, because I believe there is a great value here.

So, as I said, we are going to be working on this as far as the fraud, waste, and abuse goes. Think about the future. Now we have got Uber. Now we have got Lyft. We have got other things, and this requires the States to use prior authorization or some other form of utilization management to help cut down on bad actors, and we have bad actors in everything, including this. We need to do that. So we have got stipulations in here for that.

Have I missed anything?

Mr. RICCARDI. No, you haven't missed anything. But what was— what I was thinking about was an individual, say, somebody who is frail and elderly. And as people are living longer and diagnosed with dementia and Alzheimer's, this benefit is cost effective and ultimately a cost saver, helping people stay in the home, reducing hospital visits, reducing ER visits, and allowing people to live in the community. And it is difficult to quantify what that would mean for someone's life, but this benefit, although it is not highly utilized, it is very important and vital to keeping people healthy and at home. So——

Mr. CARTER. Great. Well, thank you. And I know I am out of time, but before I yield back, I would like to submit the following letters for the record—these are in support of this bill—from Generate Health, Access Living, Greater Hartford Legal Aid, Connecticut Legal Services, New Haven Legal Assistance Association, Together Colorado, Center for Health Progress, American Network of Community Options & Resources, Community Catalyst, and Georgians for a Healthy Future.

Ms. ESHOO. Thank you. Wonderful. So ordered.

[The information appears at the conclusion of the hearing.]

Mr. CARTER. Thank you. And I yield back, Madam Chair.

Ms. ESHOO. So ordered.

I would just like to say this about Mr. Carter's bill. I think it would be a godsend to people, in plain English, just a godsend.

I would like to submit the following statements for the record and request unanimous consent to enter them into the record: a statement from the National Kidney Foundation in support of H.R. 5534; a letter from the American Dental Association in support of H.R. 1379; a letter from the American Society of Plastic Surgeons in support of H.R. 1379; a letter from the Healthcare Leadership Council in support of H.R. 2477 and H.R. 3935; a letter from the American Network of Community Options and Resources in support of H.R. 3935; a letter from the March of Dimes in support of H.R. 4801; testimony of John Kahan, president of Aaron Matthews SIDS Research Guild of Seattle Children's, in support of H.R. 2271; a letter from Food Allergy Research and Education in support of H.R. 2466.

This is really an honor roll of organizations, and kudos to all the authors and cosponsors of the seven bills that we heard today. This is quite something.

Testimony of the American Academy of Allergy, Asthma and Immunology in support of H.R. 2468; a letter from former CMS Administrators—well, that is nice—in support of H.R. 5772; a list of 95 organizational supporters of H.R. 2477; a letter from 72 stakeholder organizations in support of H.R. 2477; a one-page summary of H.R. 2477 developed by the Medicare Rights Center. Thank you. An October 2018 New York Times article entitled, "Why You Shouldn't Wait to Sign Up for Medicare, Part B." Well, I don't think very many people read it. So that is why we are here today. A December 2019 Wall Street Journal article entitled, "Medicare Enrollment Can Be Confusing and Lead to Unexpected Costs"; a joint statement of Representatives Ryan, Underwood, and Stivers in support of H.R. 4801; a letter from Generate Health in support of H.R. 3935; a letter from Access Living in support of 3935; a letter from the Blue Dog Coalition in support of the NEMT benefit; a letter from the Congressional Black Caucus in support of the NEMT benefit; a list of 59 organizational supporters of 3935; a study on NEMT's return on investment prepared by the Medicare Rights Center. Thank you again. A statement from CVS Health in support of 5534.

Without objection, so ordered.

[The information appears at the conclusion of the hearing.]

Ms. ESHOO. So to each of you at the witness table, on behalf of all of the members of this subcommittee, I want to thank you for your tremendous patience. You have been here since early this morning, and even though you weren't at the witness table, you stuck with it, and we sincerely appreciate it.

Hearings—legislative hearings are foundational to strengthen bills, and so the expert testimony, the testimony of a parent describing what takes place in their day-to-day lives and informing us of what we need to do, is always very powerful. You operate on people. We are listening. Your family experience strengthens our hand in terms of producing good legislation.

And, Mr. Riccardi, thank you for your work and the work of your organization. It really is superb, and I have confidence that—someone said the Magnificent Seven—that we move these bills. I have every intention of doing so, and because the American people will be bettered by them.

So thank you to all of you. I want to thank your families that are here, the little ones, these angels. We should have brought them up here and had them sitting with me, but one of them actually gave me a big hug. Isn't that something? That looks good. I feel like crawling in there with him.

With that, we thank all of you. And the subcommittee is now adjourned.

[Whereupon, at 3:25 p.m., the subcommittee was adjourned.]
[Material submitted for inclusion in the record follows:]

Representative Kennedy,

My wife and I are writing in support of Scarlett's Sunshine Act. We request that you submit the following to the Subcommittee on Health of the Committee on Energy and Commerce hearing on "Legislation to Improve Americans' Health Care Coverage and Outcomes" on January 8, 2020. We are grateful to you for co-sponsoring Scarlett's Sunshine Act and for elevating this bi-partisan, bi-cameral bill.

Our son Luke was a healthy, fully-vaccinated, walking, playful, and carefree 18-month-old toddler. Luke stood out for his serenity and joy; he was an old soul who loved to smile, eat berries, and laugh. In March 2019, we put our apparently healthy son to bed. We never thought that our son would not wake up, yet our worst nightmare unfolded the next morning. Tragically, we are not alone: hundreds of healthy children over the age of one die suddenly and unexpectedly every year.

Scarlett's Sunshine Act will work to improve investigations into and statistical reporting of unexplained death in children under 5 years. Unexplained death is the 5th leading category of toddler (age 1-5) death in the U.S.. However, medical examiners are ill-prepared to handle these cases, resulting in the full scope of the problem being unclear. Our own son's cause of death was not classified as Sudden Unexpected or Unexplained Death in Childhood (SUDC), even though he is a classic case, because of local medical examiner autopsy reporting norms. Many parents have waited many months or even years for autopsy results all the while living with the anxiety and guilt provoked by the sudden and unexplained nature of their loss.

We are exceptionally fortunate to have stumbled into the Robert's Program at Boston Children's Hospital, a Boston-based research program conducting leading-edge research in SIDS and SUDC. Having a clearer sense of our son's cause of death—and that there was no way we could have predicted or prevented it—ameliorated the considerable guilt we feel as bereaved parents. The guilt and stigma that follows these deaths is a burden no parent should bear. Guilt and stigma are especially acute for parents of SIDS (age <1) victims, who face the public misconception that sleep position causes SIDS when unsafe sleeping efforts is only a risk factor, not a cause. Low-income bereaved parents face even greater legal suspicion and are much less likely to find community resources.

More than anything, we hope that greater attention and research in sudden and unexplained death in children will one day help us identify and treat children who are at risk. We hope future parents will be spared the greatest pain they can know.

Best regards,

Garrett Johnson
Assistant Professor
Questrom School of Business
Boston University

Megan Greenfield
Partner
McKinsey & Company

More information
SUDC Foundation: https://sudc.org/
Robert's Program at Boston Children's Hospital: http://www.childrenshospital.org/robertsprogram

January 8, 2020

The Honorable Earl L. "Buddy" Carter
2432 Rayburn House Office Building
Washington, DC 20515

Re: January 8, 2020 hearing on H.R. 3935 by the Subcommittee on Health of the House Committee on Energy and Commerce

Dear Representative Carter:

Generate Health would like to thank you for sponsoring H.R. 3935, the "Protecting Patients Transportation to Care Act" and express our support. As an organization whose mission is to eliminate racial disparities in infant and maternal health, we are acutely aware of how important non-emergency medical transportation (NEMT) is to helping patients access the care they need. We primarily serve/represent Black moms and babies in the St. Louis region, and our constituents have identified transportation as a top issue impacting the racial disparities in infant and maternal health outcomes.Without NEMT, Black moms and babies would not be able to access critical health services, like prenatal care, primary care, preventive care and care for substance use disorders. Therefore, we strongly support making NEMT a statutorily mandated Medicaid benefit.

Non-emergency medical transportation is both a critical and cost-effective benefit. In a recent survey of NEMT recipients, 58 percent reported that they would not be able to make any medical appointments without NEMT.[1] By helping patients access routine and preventive care, NEMT helps prevent avoidable medical emergencies and costly hospitalizations. More specifically, while NEMT provides transportation to 10 percent of, or about 7 million, Medicaid enrollees, it only constitutes 1 percent of Medicaid's total budget.[2] Recent data has also shown that NEMT has resulted in a return on investment for both wound care for diabetics and dialysis.[3]Additionally, one Florida study estimated that if just 1 percent of all medical transportation trips prevent a one-day stay in a hospital, the resulting return on investment would be 11:1.[4]

In recent years, both the benefits of NEMT as well as the consequences of not providing NEMT have been demonstrated across states. While providing NEMT has been shown to help patients stay healthy and states save money, as explained above, forgoing NEMT has been shown to be a barrier to receiving care and maintaining overall health.[5]

---

[1] Medical Transportation Access Coalition, *The Value of Medicaid's Transportation Benefit – Results of a Return on Investment Study*, https://mtaccoalition.org/wp-content/uploads/2018/08/NEMT-ROI-Study-Results-One-Pager.pdf and https://mtaccoalition.org/wp-content/uploads/2018/07/NEMT-ROI-Methodology-Paper.pdf

[2] Letter from the Congressional Black Caucus to Chairwoman Rosa L. DeLauro and Ranking Member Tom Cole of the House Committee on Appropriations, February 15, 2019

[3] Medical Transportation Access Coalition, *The Value of Medicaid's Transportation Benefit – Results of a Return on Investment Study*, https://mtaccoalition.org/wp-content/uploads/2018/08/NEMT-ROI-Study-Results-One-Pager.pdf and https://mtaccoalition.org/wp-content/uploads/2018/07/NEMT-ROI-Methodology-Paper.pdf

[4] The Stephen Group, *Volume II: Recommendations to the Arkansas Health Reform Task Force Re: Health Care Reform/Medicaid Consulting Services*, October 2015, https://www.stephengroupinc.com/images/engagements/Final-Report-Volume-II.pdf

[5] The Lewin Group, *Indiana HIP 2.0: Evaluation of Non-Emergency Medical Transportation (NEMT) Waiver*, March 11, 2016, https://www.in.gov/fssa/hip/files/Indiana%20HIP%202.0%20NEMT%20Report%20Updated%203-11-16.pdf

For all of these reasons, we support H.R. 3935 and thank you for your leadership on this issue. By codifying NEMT as a required Medicaid benefit, all Medicaid enrollees, including those that we serve, will be able to access this critical health care service that will help them lead healthy, productive lives.

Sincerely,

Kendra Copanas
Executive Director
Generate Health

Cc: The Honorable Frank Pallone, Chair, House Committee on Energy and Commerce
The Honorable Greg Walden, Ranking Member, House Committee on Energy and Commerce
The Honorable Anna G. Eshoo, Chair, House Subcommittee on Health
The Honorable Michael C. Burgess, Ranking Member, House Subcommittee on Health
[SUBCOMMITTEE MEMBER FROM YOUR STATE, IF RELEVANT]
The Honorable Tony Cárdenas
The Honorable Tom Graves
The Honorable Sanford D. Bishop Jr.

January 7, 2020

The Honorable Earl L. "Buddy" Carter
2432 Rayburn House Office Building
Washington, DC 20515

Re: January 8, 2020 Hearing on H.R. 3935 by the Subcommittee on Health of the House Committee on Energy and Commerce

Dear Representative Carter:

Established in 1980, Access Living is the Center for Independent Living for Metropolitan Chicago. We are a cross disability rights and services organization providing individualized, peer-based independent living supports, legal and advocacy services. As a provider representing thousands of Chicagoans with disabilities, we would like to thank you for sponsoring H.R. 3935, the "Protecting Patients Transportation to Care Act" and express our support.

As an organization whose mission is to ensure that Chicagoans with disabilities live fully-engaged and self-directed lives in their homes and communities, we are acutely aware of how important non-emergency medical transportation (NEMT) is to helping patients access the care they need. The overwhelming majority of the consumers we serve are low-income racial and ethnic minorities with a wide range of disabilities across the Chicago region. Without NEMT, these Chicagoans with disabilities would not be able to access critical health services, like dialysis, primary care, preventive care and care for substance use disorders. Therefore, we strongly support making NEMT a statutorily mandated Medicaid benefit.

Transportation options in general for people with disabilities are limited, inefficient, and often expensive, especially in suburban and rural areas. Even in urban centers like the city of Chicago, more options may exist, but they still fail to provide service that is on par with what is available to non-disabled people. Additionally, there exists a state of flux for mass transit, ADA paratransit, and other travel options in urban areas across the US due to the rapid growth of, and attendant instability created by, Transportation Network Companies (TNCs) and the on-demand services they provide. Since TNC service is almost always inaccessible to wheelchair users who cannot transfer from their mobility devices, and since explosive expansion in the TNC sector has begun to threaten the viability of lower ridership transit routes and the ADA paratransit coverage connected to those routes, options for people with disabilities are receding rather than expanding. For these reasons, NEMT is a crucial lifeline to improved health outcomes and quality of life for disabled people everywhere.

Non-emergency medical transportation is both a critical and cost-effective benefit. In a recent survey of NEMT recipients, 58 percent reported that they would not be able to make any medical appointments without NEMT.[1] By helping patients access routine and preventive care, NEMT helps prevent avoidable medical emergencies and costly hospitalizations. More specifically, while NEMT provides transportation to 10 percent of, or about 7 million, Medicaid enrollees, it only constitutes 1 percent of Medicaid's total budget.[2] Recent data has also shown that NEMT has resulted in a return on investment for both wound care for diabetics and dialysis.[3]Additionally, one Florida study estimated that if just 1 percent of all medical transportation trips prevent a one-day stay in a hospital, the resulting return on investment would be 11:1.[4]

In recent years, both the benefits of NEMT as well as the consequences of not providing NEMT have been demonstrated across states. While providing NEMT has been shown to help patients stay healthy and states save money, as explained above, forgoing NEMT has been shown to be a barrier to receiving care and maintaining overall health.[5]

For all of these reasons, we support H.R. 3935 and thank you for your leadership on this issue. By codifying NEMT as a required Medicaid benefit, all Medicaid enrollees, including those that we serve, will be able to access this critical health care service that will help them lead healthy, productive lives.

Sincerely,

Angel Love Miles, PhD
Healthcare/Home and Community Based Services Policy Analyst
Access Living of Metropolitan Chicago

Adam Ballard
Housing and Transportation Policy Analyst
Access Living of Metropolitan Chicago

Cc: The Honorable Frank Pallone, Chair, House Committee on Energy and Commerce
The Honorable Greg Walden, Ranking Member, House Committee on Energy and Commerce
The Honorable Anna G. Eshoo, Chair, House Subcommittee on Health
The Honorable Michael C. Burgess, Ranking Member, House Subcommittee on Health
The Honorable Bobby Rush
The Honorable Robin Kelly
The Honorable John Shimkus

---

[1] Medical Transportation Access Coalition, *The Value of Medicaid's Transportation Benefit – Results of a Return on Investment Study*, https://mtaccoalition.org/wp-content/uploads/2018/08/NEMT-ROI-Study-Results-One-Pager.pdf and https://mtaccoalition.org/wp-content/uploads/2018/07/NEMT-ROI-Methodology-Paper.pdf
[2] Letter from the Congressional Black Caucus to Chairwoman Rosa L. DeLauro and Ranking Member Tom Cole of the House Committee on Appropriations, February 15, 2019
[3] Medical Transportation Access Coalition, *The Value of Medicaid's Transportation Benefit – Results of a Return on Investment Study*, https://mtaccoalition.org/wp-content/uploads/2018/08/NEMT-ROI-Study-Results-One-Pager.pdf and https://mtaccoalition.org/wp-content/uploads/2018/07/NEMT-ROI-Methodology-Paper.pdf
[4] The Stephen Group, *Volume II: Recommendations to the Arkansas Health Reform Task Force Re: Health Care Reform/Medicaid Consulting Services*, October 2015, https://www.stephengroupinc.com/images/engagements/Final-Report-Volume-II.pdf
[5] The Lewin Group, *Indiana HIP 2.0: Evaluation of Non-Emergency Medical Transportation (NEMT) Waiver*, March 11, 2016, https://www.in.gov/fssa/hip/files/Indiana%20HIP%202.0%20NEMT%20Report%20Updated%203-11-16.pdf

ghla Greater Hartford Legal Aid | Connecticut Legal Services | LAA NEW HAVEN LEGAL ASSISTANCE ASSOCIATION, INC.

January 8, 2020

The Honorable Earl L. "Buddy" Carter
2432 Rayburn House Office Building
Washington, DC 20515

Re: January 8, 2020 hearing on H.R. 3935 by the Subcommittee on Health of the House Committee on Energy and Commerce

Dear Representative Carter:

Greater Hartford Legal Aid, Connecticut Legal Services, and New Haven Legal Assistance Association would like to thank you for sponsoring H.R. 3935, the "Protecting Patients Transportation to Care Act," and express our support. Through our mission "to achieve equal justice for poor people, to work with clients to promote social justice, and to address the effects and root causes of poverty," we are acutely aware of how important non-emergency medical transportation (NEMT) is to connecting patients to the care they need. We primarily serve low-income residents of the greater Hartford, Connecticut region. Without NEMT, many of our clients would not be able to access critical health services, like dialysis, primary care, preventive care and care for substance use disorders. It is critical that Connecticut continue to provide federally-mandated NEMT services under the state's Medicaid program. Although we currently have significant challenges in our state regarding the delivery of these services, there is no question that it is a critical service for our clients. Connecticut's NEMT program provides an average of 387,000 trips each month statewide. In a small state like Connecticut, that's a significant number and has a noticeable effect in ensuring our clients access to timely medical services. We strongly support making NEMT a statutorily mandated Medicaid benefit for all states.

The need for this to be a statutorily-mandated service arises from the fact that currently it is mandated only by federal regulations, which have been held to be unenforceable by private parties, and states have therefore attempted to evade their responsibilities to provide it. Indeed, several states have sought and even obtained a waiver from the federal Medicaid agency, CMS, to avoid providing this service to certain groups of Medicaid enrollees. Without a statutory mandate, this trend will continue and such a waiver could be obtained for our state as well.

Non-emergency medical transportation is both a critical and cost-effective benefit. In a recent survey of NEMT recipients, 58 percent reported that they would not be able to make any medical appointments without NEMT.[1] By connecting patients to routine and preventive care, NEMT helps prevent avoidable hospitalizations. More specifically, while NEMT provides transportation to 10 percent of, or about 7 million, Medicaid enrollees, it only constitutes 1 percent of Medicaid's total budget.[2] Recent data also show that NEMT has a positive return on investment for both wound care for diabetics and dialysis.[3] Moreover, one Florida study estimated that if just 1 percent of all medical transportation trips prevent a one-day stay in a hospital, the resulting return on investment would be 11:1.[4]

Providing NEMT has more benefits than not. NEMT has proven effective in helping patients stay healthy and states save money. Forgoing NEMT has been shown to be a barrier to receiving care and maintaining overall health.[5]

For all of these reasons, we support H.R. 3935 and thank you for your leadership on this issue.

Sincerely,

Alison Weir
Policy Advocate
Greater Hartford Legal Aid

Kristen Noelle Hatcher
Managing Attorney
Connecticut Legal Services

Sheldon Toubman
Benefits Attorney
New Haven Legal Assistance Association

Cc: The Honorable Frank Pallone, Chair, House Committee on Energy and Commerce
The Honorable Greg Walden, Ranking Member, House Committee on Energy and Commerce
The Honorable Anna G. Eshoo, Chair, House Subcommittee on Health
The Honorable Michael C. Burgess, Ranking Member, House Subcommittee on Health
The Honorable Tony Cárdenas
The Honorable Tom Graves
The Honorable Sanford D. Bishop Jr.

---

[1] Medical Transportation Access Coalition, *The Value of Medicaid's Transportation Benefit – Results of a Return on Investment Study*, https://mtaccoalition.org/wp-content/uploads/2018/08/NEMT-ROI-Study-Results-One-Pager.pdf and https://mtaccoalition.org/wp-content/uploads/2018/07/NEMT-ROI-Methodology-Paper.pdf

[2] Letter from the Congressional Black Caucus to Chairwoman Rosa L. DeLauro and Ranking Member Tom Cole of the House Committee on Appropriations, February 15, 2019

[3] Medical Transportation Access Coalition, *The Value of Medicaid's Transportation Benefit – Results of a Return on Investment Study*, https://mtaccoalition.org/wp-content/uploads/2018/08/NEMT-ROI-Study-Results-One-Pager.pdf and https://mtaccoalition.org/wp-content/uploads/2018/07/NEMT-ROI-Methodology-Paper.pdf

[4] The Stephen Group, *Volume II: Recommendations to the Arkansas Health Reform Task Force Re: Health Care Reform/Medicaid Consulting Services*, October 2015, https://www.stephengroupinc.com/images/engagements/Final-Report-Volume-II.pdf

[5] The Lewin Group, *Indiana HIP 2.0: Evaluation of Non-Emergency Medical Transportation (NEMT) Waiver*, March 11, 2016, https://www.in.gov/fssa/hip/files/Indiana%20HIP%202.0%20NEMT%20Report%20Updated%203-11-16.pdf

1.

January 7, 2020

The Honorable Earl L. "Buddy" Carter
2432 Rayburn House Office Building
Washington, DC 20515

Re: January 8, 2020 hearing on H.R. 3935 by the Subcommittee on Health of the House Committee on Energy and Commerce

Dear Representative Carter:

Together Colorado would like to thank you for sponsoring H.R. 3935, the "Protecting Patients Transportation to Care Act" and express our support. As an organization whose mission is to put human dignity at the center of public life, we are acutely aware of how important non-emergency medical transportation (NEMT) is to helping patients access the care they need. We primarily serve/represent people in schools and congregations throughout Colorado. Without NEMT, those most vulnerable in our community would not be able to access critical health services, like dialysis, primary care, preventive care and care for substance use disorders. Therefore, we strongly support making NEMT a statutorily mandated Medicaid benefit.

Non-emergency medical transportation is both a critical and cost-effective benefit. In a recent survey of NEMT recipients, 58 percent reported that they would not be able to make any medical appointments without NEMT.[1] By helping patients access routine and preventive care, NEMT helps prevent avoidable medical emergencies and costly hospitalizations. More specifically, while NEMT provides transportation to 10 percent of, or about 7 million, Medicaid enrollees, it only constitutes 1 percent of Medicaid's total budget.[2] Recent data has also shown that NEMT has resulted in a return on investment for both wound care for diabetics and dialysis.[3]Additionally, one Florida study estimated that if just 1 percent of all medical transportation trips prevent a one-day stay in a hospital, the resulting return on investment would be 11:1.[4]

In recent years, both the benefits of NEMT as well as the consequences of not providing NEMT have been demonstrated across states. While providing NEMT has been shown to help patients stay healthy and states save money, as explained above, forgoing NEMT has been shown to be a barrier to receiving

---

1

Medical Transportation Access Coalition, *The Value of Medicaid's Transportation Benefit – Results of a Return on Investment Study*, https://mtaccoalition.org/wp-content/uploads/2018/08/NEMT-ROI-Study-Results-One-Pager.pdf and https://mtaccoalition.org/wp-content/uploads/2018/07/NEMT-ROI-Methodology-Paper.pdf

2

Letter from the Congressional Black Caucus to Chairwoman Rosa L. DeLauro and Ranking Member Tom Cole of the House Committee on Appropriations, February 15, 2019

3

Medical Transportation Access Coalition, *The Value of Medicaid's Transportation Benefit – Results of a Return on Investment Study*, https://mtaccoalition.org/wp-content/uploads/2018/08/NEMT-ROI-Study-Results-One-Pager.pdf and https://mtaccoalition.org/wp-content/uploads/2018/07/NEMT-ROI-Methodology-Paper.pdf

4

The Stephen Group, *Volume II: Recommendations to the Arkansas Health Reform Task Force Re: Health Care Reform/Medicaid Consulting Services*, October 2015, https://www.stephengroupinc.com/images/engagements/Final-Report-Volume-II.pdf

1.

care and maintaining overall health.[5]

For all of these reasons, we support H.R. 3935 and thank you for your leadership on this issue. By codifying NEMT as a required Medicaid benefit, all Medicaid enrollees, including those that we serve, will be able to access this critical health care service that will help them lead healthy, productive lives.

Sincerely,

Judy Danielson
Community Leader
Together Colorado

Cc: The Honorable Frank Pallone, Chair, House Committee on Energy and Commerce
The Honorable Greg Walden, Ranking Member, House Committee on Energy and Commerce
The Honorable Anna G. Eshoo, Chair, House Subcommittee on Health
The Honorable Michael C. Burgess, Ranking Member, House Subcommittee on Health
[The Honorable Tony Cárdenas
The Honorable Tom Graves
The Honorable Sanford D. Bishop Jr.

5

The Lewin Group, *Indiana HIP 2.0: Evaluation of Non-Emergency Medical Transportation (NEMT) Waiver*, March 11, 2016, https://www.in.gov/fssa/hip/files/Indiana%20HIP%202.0%20NEMT%20Report%20Updated%203-11-16.pdf

CENTER FOR
HEALTH PROGRESS

January 8, 2020

The Honorable Earl L. "Buddy" Carter
2432 Rayburn House Office Building
Washington, DC 20515

Re: January 8, 2020 hearing on H.R. 3935 by the Subcommittee on Health of the House Committee on Energy and Commerce

Dear Representative Carter:

Center for Health Progress thanks you for sponsoring H.R. 3935, the "Protecting Patients Transportation to Care Act" and would like to express our support. We believe our health care system should work for everyone, so we work across the state of Colorado to create opportunities and eliminate barriers to health equity. We are acutely aware of how important non-emergency medical transportation (NEMT) is to helping patients access the care they need. According to a rigorous state survey, 14 percent of Colorado's Medicaid enrollees had to skip a medical appointment because they couldn't get transportation to their doctor's office,[1] and patients who are elderly, disabled, or live in rural areas are disproportionately affected by transportation challenges. Without NEMT, these patients would not be able to access critical health services, like dialysis, primary care, preventive care, and care for substance use disorders. Therefore, we strongly support making NEMT a statutorily mandated Medicaid benefit.

Non-emergency medical transportation is both a critical and cost-effective benefit. In a recent survey of NEMT recipients, 58 percent reported that they would not be able to make any medical appointments without NEMT.[2] By helping patients access routine and preventive care, NEMT helps prevent avoidable medical emergencies and costly hospitalizations. More specifically, while NEMT provides transportation to 10 percent of, or about 7 million, Medicaid enrollees nationally, it only constitutes 1 percent of Medicaid's total budget.[3] Recent data has also shown that NEMT has resulted in a return on investment for both wound care for diabetics and dialysis.[4] Additionally, one Florida study estimated that if just 1 percent of all medical transportation trips prevent a one-day stay in a hospital, the resulting return on investment would be 11:1.[5]

---

[1] Colorado Health Institute, *2019 Medicaid and Commercial Access to Care Index*, July 2019, https://www.coloradohealthinstitute.org/research/2019-medicaid-and-commercial-access-care-index

[2] Medical Transportation Access Coalition, *The Value of Medicaid's Transportation Benefit – Results of a Return on Investment Study*, https://mtaccoalition.org/wp-content/uploads/2018/08/NEMT-ROI-Study-Results-One-Pager.pdfhttps://mtaccoalition.org/wp-content/uploads/2018/08/NEMT-ROI-Study-Results-One-Pager.pdf and https://mtaccoalition.org/wp-content/uploads/2018/07/NEMT-ROI-Methodology-Paper.pdf

[3] Letter from the Congressional Black Caucus to Chairwoman Rosa L. DeLauro and Ranking Member Tom Cole of the House Committee on Appropriations, February 15, 2019

[4] Medical Transportation Access Coalition, *The Value of Medicaid's Transportation Benefit – Results of a Return on Investment Study*, https://mtaccoalition.org/wp-content/uploads/2018/08/NEMT-ROI-Study-Results-One-Pager.pdf and https://mtaccoalition.org/wp-content/uploads/2018/07/NEMT-ROI-Methodology-Paper.pdf

[5] The Stephen Group, *Volume II: Recommendations to the Arkansas Health Reform Task Force Re: Health Care Reform/Medicaid Consulting Services*, October 2015, https://www.stephengroupinc.com/images/engagements/Final-Report-Volume-II.pdf

PO Box 18877 | Denver, Colorado 80218 | TELE 720.583.1760 | www.centerforhealthprogress.org

In recent years, both the benefits of NEMT as well as the consequences of not providing NEMT have been demonstrated across states. While providing NEMT has been shown to help patients stay healthy and states save money, as explained above, forgoing NEMT has been shown to be a barrier to receiving care and maintaining overall health.[6]

For all of these reasons, we support H.R. 3935 and thank you for your leadership on this issue. By codifying NEMT as a required Medicaid benefit, all Medicaid enrollees, including those that we serve, will be able to access this critical health care service that will help them lead healthy, productive lives.

Sincerely,

Maggie Gómez
Deputy Director
Center for Health Progress

Cc: The Honorable Frank Pallone, Chair, House Committee on Energy and Commerce
The Honorable Greg Walden, Ranking Member, House Committee on Energy and Commerce
The Honorable Anna G. Eshoo, Chair, House Subcommittee on Health
The Honorable Michael C. Burgess, Ranking Member, House Subcommittee on Health
The Honorable Tony Cárdenas
The Honorable Tom Graves
The Honorable Sanford D. Bishop Jr.

[6] The Lewin Group, Indiana HIP 2.0: Evaluation of Non-Emergency Medical Transportation (NEMT) Waiver, March 11, 2016, https://www.in.gov/fssa/hip/files/Indiana%20HIP%202.0%20NEMT%20Report%20Updated%203-11-16.pdf

ANCOR

January 7, 2020

The Honorable Earl L. "Buddy" Carter
2432 Rayburn House Office Building
Washington, DC 20515

Re: January 8, 2020 hearing on H.R. 3935 by the Subcommittee on Health of the House Committee on Energy and Commerce

Dear Representative Carter:

The American Network of Community Options & Resources (ANCOR) would like to thank you for sponsoring H.R. 3935, the "Protecting Patients Transportation to Care Act" and express our support. As an organization that represents community-based disability service providers, we are acutely aware of how important non-emergency medical transportation (NEMT) is to helping the people our members support to access the care they need. Without NEMT, people with disabilities would not be able to access critical health services, like dialysis, primary care, preventive care and care for substance use disorders. Therefore, we strongly support making NEMT a statutorily mandated Medicaid benefit.

ANCOR is a is a national, nonprofit trade association representing more than 1,600 private community providers of services to people with disabilities. Combined, we support over one million individuals with disabilities, and work to shape policy, share solutions and strengthen the community.

Non-emergency medical transportation is both a critical and cost-effective benefit. In a recent survey of NEMT recipients, 58 percent reported that they would not be able to make any medical appointments without NEMT.[1] By helping patients access routine and preventive care, NEMT helps prevent avoidable medical emergencies and costly hospitalizations. More specifically, while NEMT provides transportation to 10 percent of, or about 7 million, Medicaid enrollees, it only constitutes 1 percent of Medicaid's total budget.[2] Recent data has also shown that NEMT has resulted in a return on investment for both wound care for diabetics and dialysis.[3]Additionally, one Florida study estimated that if just 1 percent of all medical transportation trips prevent a one-day stay in a hospital, the resulting return on investment would be 11:1.[4]

In recent years, both the benefits of NEMT as well as the consequences of not providing NEMT have been demonstrated across states. While providing NEMT has been shown to help patients stay

[1] Medical Transportation Access Coalition, *The Value of Medicaid's Transportation Benefit – Results of a Return on Investment Study*, https://mtaccoalition.org/wp-content/uploads/2018/08/NEMT-ROI-Study-Results-One-Pager.pdf and https://mtaccoalition.org/wp-content/uploads/2018/07/NEMT-ROI-Methodology-Paper.pdf

[2] Letter from the Congressional Black Caucus to Chairwoman Rosa L. DeLauro and Ranking Member Tom Cole of the House Committee on Appropriations, February 15, 2019

[3] Medical Transportation Access Coalition, *The Value of Medicaid's Transportation Benefit – Results of a Return on Investment Study*, https://mtaccoalition.org/wp-content/uploads/2018/08/NEMT-ROI-Study-Results-One-Pager.pdf and https://mtaccoalition.org/wp-content/uploads/2018/07/NEMT-ROI-Methodology-Paper.pdf

[4] The Stephen Group, *Volume II: Recommendations to the Arkansas Health Reform Task Force Re: Health Care Reform/Medicaid Consulting Services*, October 2015, https://www.stephengroupinc.com/images/engagements/Final-Report-Volume-II.pdf

1101 King Street, Suite 380, Alexandria, VA 22314-2944 P: 703.535.7850 F: 703.535.7860 E: ancor@ancor.org www.ancor.org

healthy and states save money, as explained above, forgoing NEMT has been shown to be a barrier to receiving care and maintaining overall health.[5]

For all of these reasons, we support H.R. 3935 and thank you for your leadership on this issue. By codifying NEMT as a required Medicaid benefit, all Medicaid enrollees, including those that we serve, will be able to access this critical health care service that will help them lead healthy, productive lives.

Sincerely,

Sarah Meek
Senior Director of Legislative Affairs

Cc: The Honorable Frank Pallone, Chair, House Committee on Energy and Commerce
The Honorable Greg Walden, Ranking Member, House Committee on Energy and Commerce
The Honorable Anna G. Eshoo, Chair, House Subcommittee on Health
The Honorable Michael C. Burgess, Ranking Member, House Subcommittee on Health
The Honorable Tony Cárdenas
The Honorable Tom Graves
The Honorable Sanford D. Bishop Jr.

[5] The Lewin Group, *Indiana HIP 2.0: Evaluation of Non-Emergency Medical Transportation (NEMT) Waiver*, March 11, 2016,
https://www.in.gov/fssa/hip/files/Indiana%20HIP%202.0%20NEMT%20Report%20Updated%203-11-16.pdf

COMMUNITY CATALYST

January 7, 2020

The Honorable Earl L. "Buddy" Carter
2432 Rayburn House Office Building
Washington, DC 20515

Re: January 8, 2020 hearing on H.R. 3935 by the Subcommittee on Health of the House Committee on Energy and Commerce

Dear Representative Carter:

Community Catalyst would like to thank you for sponsoring H.R. 3935, the "Protecting Patients Transportation to Care Act" and express our support. As an organization whose mission is to ensure everyone has access to quality, affordable health care, we are acutely aware of how important non-emergency medical transportation (NEMT) is to helping patients access the care they need. Without NEMT, Medicaid enrollees would not be able to access critical health services, like dialysis, primary care, preventive care and care for substance use disorders. Therefore, we strongly support making NEMT a statutorily mandated Medicaid benefit.

Non-emergency medical transportation is both a critical and cost-effective benefit. In a recent survey of NEMT recipients, 58 percent reported that they would not be able to make any medical appointments without NEMT.[1] By helping patients access routine and preventive care, NEMT helps prevent avoidable medical emergencies and costly hospitalizations. More specifically, while NEMT provides transportation to 10 percent of, or about 7 million, Medicaid enrollees, it only constitutes 1 percent of Medicaid's total budget.[2] Recent data has also shown that NEMT has resulted in a return on investment for both wound care for diabetics and dialysis.[3]Additionally, one Florida study estimated that if just 1 percent of all medical transportation trips prevent a one-day stay in a hospital, the resulting return on investment would be 11:1.[4]

In recent years, both the benefits of NEMT as well as the consequences of not providing NEMT have been demonstrated across states. While providing NEMT has been shown to help patients stay healthy

---

[1] Medical Transportation Access Coalition, *The Value of Medicaid's Transportation Benefit – Results of a Return on Investment Study*, https://mtaccoalition.org/wp-content/uploads/2018/08/NEMT-ROI-Study-Results-One-Pager.pdf and https://mtaccoalition.org/wp-content/uploads/2018/07/NEMT-ROI-Methodology-Paper.pdf

[2] Letter from the Congressional Black Caucus to Chairwoman Rosa L. DeLauro and Ranking Member Tom Cole of the House Committee on Appropriations, February 15, 2019

[3] Medical Transportation Access Coalition, *The Value of Medicaid's Transportation Benefit – Results of a Return on Investment Study*, https://mtaccoalition.org/wp-content/uploads/2018/08/NEMT-ROI-Study-Results-One-Pager.pdf and https://mtaccoalition.org/wp-content/uploads/2018/07/NEMT-ROI-Methodology-Paper.pdf

[4] The Stephen Group, *Volume II: Recommendations to the Arkansas Health Reform Task Force Re: Health Care Reform/Medicaid Consulting Services*, October 2015, https://www.stephengroupinc.com/images/engagements/Final-Report-Volume-II.pdf

and states save money, as explained above, forgoing NEMT has been shown to be a barrier to receiving care and maintaining overall health.[5]

For all of these reasons, we support H.R. 3935 and thank you for your leadership on this issue. By codifying NEMT as a required Medicaid benefit, all Medicaid enrollees, including those that we serve, will be able to access this critical health care service that will help them lead healthy, productive lives.

Sincerely,

Emily Stewart
Executive Director
Community Catalyst

Cc: The Honorable Frank Pallone, Chair, House Committee on Energy and Commerce
The Honorable Greg Walden, Ranking Member, House Committee on Energy and Commerce
The Honorable Anna G. Eshoo, Chair, House Subcommittee on Health
The Honorable Michael C. Burgess, Ranking Member, House Subcommittee on Health
The Honorable Tony Cárdenas
The Honorable Tom Graves
The Honorable Sanford D. Bishop Jr.

[5] The Lewin Group, *Indiana HIP 2.0: Evaluation of Non-Emergency Medical Transportation (NEMT) Waiver*, March 11, 2016,
https://www.in.gov/fssa/hip/files/Indiana%20HIP%202.0%20NEMT%20Report%20Updated%203-11-16.pdf

GEORGIANS FOR A HEALTHY FUTURE

January 8, 2020

The Honorable Earl L. "Buddy" Carter
2432 Rayburn House Office Building
Washington, DC 20515

Re: January 8, 2020 hearing on H.R. 3935 by the Subcommittee on Health of the House Committee on Energy and Commerce

Dear Representative Carter:

Georgians for a Healthy Future would like to thank you for sponsoring H.R. 3935, the "Protecting Patients Transportation to Care Act" and express our support. As an organization whose mission is to build and mobilize a unified voice, vision, and leadership to achieve a healthy future for all Georgians, we are acutely aware of how important non-emergency medical transportation (NEMT) is to helping patients access the care they need.

We primarily serve Georgia consumers especially those who experience disproportionate disparities in health care access and care (e.g. low-income Georgians, people of color, Georgians with Medicaid coverage, patients with complex care needs, and others). Without NEMT, Georgians covered by Medicaid would not be able to access critical health services, like dialysis, primary care, preventive care and care for substance use disorders. It is especially important for Georgians living in rural counties where distances to providers are longer and public transportation is scarce. Therefore, we strongly support making NEMT a statutorily mandated Medicaid benefit.

Non-emergency medical transportation is both a critical and cost-effective benefit. In a recent survey of NEMT recipients, 58 percent reported that they would not be able to make any medical appointments without NEMT.[1] By helping patients access routine and preventive care, NEMT helps prevent avoidable medical emergencies and costly hospitalizations. More specifically, while NEMT provides transportation to 10 percent of, or about 7 million, Medicaid enrollees, it only constitutes 1 percent of Medicaid's total budget.[2] Recent data has also shown that NEMT has resulted in a return on investment for both wound care for diabetics and dialysis.[3] Additionally, one Florida study estimated that if just 1 percent of all medical transportation trips prevent a one-day stay in a hospital, the resulting return on investment would be 11:1.[4]

---

[1] Medical Transportation Access Coalition, *The Value of Medicaid's Transportation Benefit – Results of a Return on Investment Study*, https://mtaccoalition.org/wp-content/uploads/2018/08/NEMT-ROI-Study-Results-One-Pager.pdf and https://mtaccoalition.org/wp-content/uploads/2018/07/NEMT-ROI-Methodology-Paper.pdf

[2] Letter from the Congressional Black Caucus to Chairwoman Rosa L. DeLauro and Ranking Member Tom Cole of the House Committee on Appropriations, February 15, 2019

[3] Medical Transportation Access Coalition, *The Value of Medicaid's Transportation Benefit – Results of a Return on Investment Study*, https://mtaccoalition.org/wp-content/uploads/2018/08/NEMT-ROI-Study-Results-One-Pager.pdf and https://mtaccoalition.org/wp-content/uploads/2018/07/NEMT-ROI-Methodology-Paper.pdf

[4] The Stephen Group, *Volume II: Recommendations to the Arkansas Health Reform Task Force Re: Health Care Reform/Medicaid Consulting Services*, October 2015, https://www.stephengroupinc.com/images/engagements/Final-Report-Volume-II.pdf

50 Hurt Plaza SE, Suite 806
Atlanta, Georgia 30303
PHONE 404 567 5016
FAX 404 935 9885
healthyfuturega.org

GEORGIANS FOR A HEALTHY FUTURE

In recent years, both the benefits of NEMT as well as the consequences of not providing NEMT have been demonstrated across states. While providing NEMT has been shown to help patients stay healthy and states save money, as explained above, forgoing NEMT has been shown to be a barrier to receiving care and maintaining overall health.[5]

For all of these reasons, we support H.R. 3935 and thank you for your leadership on this issue. By codifying NEMT as a required Medicaid benefit, all Medicaid enrollees, including those that we serve, will be able to access this critical health care service that will help them lead healthy, productive lives.

Sincerely,

Laura Colbert
Executive Director
Georgians for a Healthy Future

Cc: The Honorable Frank Pallone, Chair, House Committee on Energy and Commerce
The Honorable Greg Walden, Ranking Member, House Committee on Energy and Commerce
The Honorable Anna G. Eshoo, Chair, House Subcommittee on Health
The Honorable Michael C. Burgess, Ranking Member, House Subcommittee on Health
The Honorable Tony Cárdenas
The Honorable Tom Graves
The Honorable Sanford D. Bishop Jr.

[5] The Lewin Group, *Indiana HIP 2.0: Evaluation of Non-Emergency Medical Transportation (NEMT) Waiver*, March 11, 2016, https://www.in.gov/fssa/hip/files/Indiana%20HIP%202.0%20NEMT%20Report%20Updated%203-11-16.pdf

50 Hurt Plaza SE, Suite 806
Atlanta, Georgia 30303
PHONE 404 567 5016
FAX 404 935 9885
healthyfuturega.org

Statement of National Kidney Foundation
In support of H.R. 5534, "Comprehensive Immunosuppressive Drug Coverage for Kidney Transplant Patients Act"

Submitted to the Committee on Energy and Commerce
U.S. House of Representatives

January 8, 2020

The National Kidney Foundation (NKF) is America's largest and oldest health organization dedicated to the awareness, prevention and treatment of kidney disease for the estimated 37 million adults with chronic kidney disease (CKD) and for tens of millions of people at risk of CKD. As an organization that has successfully advocated to improve coverage of immunosuppressive drugs for transplant recipients, NKF applauds the Committee for today's hearing on H.R. 5534, which eliminates Medicare's 36-month post-transplant limit on coverage of immunosuppressive drugs for non-aged, non-disabled kidney recipients. We would especially like to recognize Representatives Burgess and Kind for introducing this legislation, and for their historic leadership on this important issue.

Since 1973, the Medicare program has provided comprehensive coverage for individuals with End Stage Renal Disease (ESRD) who require dialysis, irrespective of their age or disability. While dialysis can be a lifeline for many of these patients, it is also a physically, emotionally and socially limiting treatment option. Kidney transplant is considered the treatment of choice for many patients with ESRD, as they typically enjoy higher quality of life and life expectancy than patients on dialysis.

Organ transplant recipients require life-long immunosuppressive therapy to preserve and maintain their transplant. Unfortunately, for younger, non-disabled patients, the Medicare program only covers immunosuppressive drugs for 36 months following a transplant, after which patients must secure alternative insurance coverage or pay for their drugs out-of-pocket.

Depending on a patient's insurance coverage, a maintenance immunosuppressive regiment represents different levels of cost burden. While the May 2019 Health and Human Services Issue Brief, *Assessing the Costs and Benefits of Extending Coverage of Immunosuppressive Drugs Under Medicare*, used an estimated per-patient-per-year cost of $3,379 and the average Medicare payment per transplant patient per year is $2,340, other reports have estimated costs as high as $2,500 per month, with the average annual expenditure between $10,000 and $14,000.[1,2,3]

---

1 https://aspe.hhs.gov/system/files/pdf/261746/Savings_From_Extending_Coverage_For_Immunosuppressive_Drugs_Final.pdf

This coverage gap has devastating consequences for patients, their families, kidney donors, and for the Medicare program itself. Patients who lack affordable coverage when their Medicare ends must sometimes ration or skip their medications altogether, which inevitably causes the transplanted kidney to fail. As a result, the patient returns to dialysis or requires another transplant, creating significant and preventable expenses for the Medicare program while lengthening the transplant waitlist. Even more troubling, many patients – especially low-income patients -- opt not to pursue or are precluded from pursuing a transplant at all because of their inability to pay for the medications after the 36-month waiting period.

H.R. 5534 addresses this by providing lifelong coverage of immunosuppressive drugs. This legislation – which has been introduced several times in recent Congresses – enjoys strong bipartisan support, but progress has been stymied due to uncertainty about cost. Fortunately, two analyses by the Department of Health and Human Services in May 2019 estimated that providing lifetime Medicare coverage of immunosuppressive drugs would result in a **net savings** to the federal government of up to $300 million over 10 years.

These cost savings are generated by the total cost of Medicare spending on a dialysis patient compared to a kidney transplant recipient. According to the U.S. Renal Data System 2018 Annual Report, Medicare spends almost $90,000 annually on a dialysis patient, compared to $35,000 per year for a kidney transplant recipient after the first year of transplant.[4] Medicare spends only $2,340 per transplant patient on immunosuppressive drugs that are critical to reducing the likelihood of organ rejection, demonstrating the cost effectiveness of the policy.[5]

Many kidney recipients have immunosuppressive coverage through group health plans, under the Affordable Care Act, through Medicaid or the Department of Veterans Affairs, or through other means when their Medicare eligibility expires. However, a considerable number are unable to obtain or afford coverage after 36 months and H.R. 5534 provides a safety net. Under the bill, Medicare would continue only for immunosuppressive medications; all other Medicare coverage would end 36 months after the transplant. The bill also requires group health plans to continue to pay for immunosuppressive drugs if they presently include such a benefit in their coverage, to prevent insurers from passing this obligation to Medicare. This bill will help improve long term transplant outcomes and enable more kidney patients who lack adequate drug coverage to consider

---

[2] *United States Renal Data System. 2018 USRDS annual data report: Epidemiology of kidney disease in the United States. National Institutes of Health, National Institute of Diabetes and Digestive and Kidney Diseases, Bethesda, MD, 2018.*

[3] James, A., & Mannon, R. B. (2015). The Cost of Transplant Immunosuppressant Therapy: Is This Sustainable?. *Current transplantation reports*, 2(2), 113–121. doi:10.1007/s40472-015-0052-y

[4] *United States Renal Data System. 2018 USRDS annual data report: Epidemiology of kidney disease in the United States. National Institutes of Health, National Institute of Diabetes and Digestive and Kidney Diseases, Bethesda, MD, 2018.*

[5] *Ibid.*

transplantation. It is the right thing to do for kidney patients, for living donors, organ donor families, and for the American taxpayer.

In legislation spearheaded by this committee and NKF in 2000, Congress addressed immunosuppressive coverage in the Medicare, Medicaid, and SCHIP Benefits Improvement and Protection Act (BIPA) when it eliminated a similar time limit of immunosuppressive coverage for aged and disabled beneficiaries. It is time for Congress to close that coverage gap for all patients by enacting H.R. 5534.

Once again, NKF applauds the Committee for its attention to this important matter, and looks forward to working with Congressman Burgess, Congressman Kind, and other bill supporters on its swift passage.

ADA American Dental Association®

1111 14th Street, N.W.
Suite 1200
Washington, DC 20005

T 202.898.2400
F 202.898.2437
www.ada.org

January 6, 2020

The Honorable Anna G. Eshoo
Chairwoman, Health Subcommittee
Committee on Energy and Commerce
U.S. House of Representatives
Washington, D.C. 20515

The Honorable Michael C. Burgess
Ranking Member, Health Subcommittee
Committee on Energy and Commerce
U.S. House of Representatives
Washington, D.C. 20515

Dear Chairwoman Eshoo and Ranking Member Burgess:

On behalf of our 163,000 members, we are writing to thank you for holding a hearing on H.R. 1379, the Ensuring Lasting Smiles Act. As the nation's oldest and largest dental professional organization, the American Dental Association (ADA) strongly supports this bipartisan legislation.

As you know, the Ensuring Lasting Smiles Act would require all private group and individual health plans to cover medically necessary services resulting from a congenital anomaly or birth defect. One in every 33 children in the United States is born with a congenital anomaly or birth defect that affects the way they look, develop or function. This legislation is crucial to ensure that children suffering from congenital anomalies and birth defects are able to receive the treatment they need.

Many of these congenital anomalies include severe oral and facial defects such as cleft lip or palate, skeletal and maxillofacial deformities, hypodontia (absence of teeth), and enamel hypoplasia. These anomalies can interfere with a child's ability to breathe, speak, and/or eat in a normal manner. Specialized surgery is needed to correct these anomalies. These procedures are reconstructive in nature and are performed to correct abnormal structures of the body.

Despite this, many insurance companies consider these services to be cosmetic, and while they may cover the preliminary surgeries, they will delay or deny follow-up or corrective procedures, including dental work related to the anomaly. This can further delay a child's developmental milestones.

Passage of H.R. 1379 would help patients with craniofacial anomalies, and would also ensure they have the necessary coverage to restore their ability to function. On behalf of our members and their patients, we would like to thank you for considering this important legislation. Please contact Ms. Natalie Hales at (202) 898-2404 or halesn@ada.org with any questions.

January 6, 2020
Page 2

Sincerely,

Chad P. Gehani, D.D.S.
President

Kathleen T. O'Loughlin, D.M.D., M.P.H.
Executive Director

CPG:KTO:nh

AMERICAN SOCIETY OF PLASTIC SURGEONS®
THE PLASTIC SURGERY FOUNDATION®

Executive Office
444 East Algonquin Road • Arlington Heights, IL 60005-4664
847-228-9900 • Fax: 847-228-9131 • www.plasticsurgery.org

January 03, 2020

The Honorable Anna Eshoo
House Energy and Commerce Committee
2125 Rayburn House Office Building
Washington, DC 20510

The Honorable Michael Burgess
House Energy and Commerce Committee
2125 Rayburn House Office Building
Washington, DC 20510

RE: **ASPS Support for the Ensuring Lasting Smiles Act (H.R. 1379)**

Dear Chairwoman Eshoo and Ranking Member Burgess:

I write on behalf of the American Society of Plastic Surgeons (ASPS) in support of Reps. Collin Peterson's (D-MN-07) and Denver Riggleman's (R-VA-05) legislation, the *Ensuring Lasting Smiles Act*. This important policy will help increase patients' coverage for craniofacial and other birth anomalies. ASPS is the largest association of plastic surgeons in the world, representing more than 7,000 members and 93 percent of all board-certified plastic surgeons in the United States. Our mission is to advance quality care for plastic surgery patients and promote public policy that protects patient safety.

Children with a congenital anomaly or birth defect or disorder who do not receive treatment at an early age face long-term physical and psychological injuries. Despite the ability of reconstructive surgical efforts to improve the outlook for these children, many insurers often claim that these services are "cosmetic" in nature, especially subsequent stage surgeries. However, the American Medical Association defines surgery performed on abnormal structures of the body caused by congenital defects or developmental abnormalities as reconstructive, not cosmetic. Furthermore, insurers frequently overlook the dental and orthodontic needs of these patients – which are essential to their achieving normal form and function – and mislead affected patients and the public when deeming these procedures cosmetic.

This important legislation will address the problem of insurance denials for reconstructive surgery and necessary adjunctive care for children suffering from congenital or development deformities. With your leadership, we can help children suffering from deformities and disfigurement receive coverage for the treatment they need.

For the reasons outlined above, we thank you for your consideration of this legislation and encourage the Committee to pass this legislation. Please do not hesitate to contact Patrick Hermes, Director of Advocacy and Government Relations, at phermes@plasticsurgery.org or (847) 228-3331 with any questions or concerns.

Sincerely,

Lynn Jeffers

Lynn Jeffers, MD, MBA, FACS
President, American Society of Plastic Surgeons

Cc: Members, House Energy and Commerce Committee

January 8, 2020

The Honorable Frank Pallone, Jr.
Chairman
U.S. House of Representatives
Committee on Energy and Commerce
Washington, D.C. 20515

The Honorable Greg Walden
Ranking Member
U.S. House of Representatives
Committee on Energy and Commerce
Washington, D.C. 20515

Dear Chairmen Pallone and Ranking Member Walden:

As the committee prepares to markup health legislation, the Healthcare Leadership Council (HLC) writes to express our support for the following legislation:

- H.R. 2477, The Beneficiary Enrollment Notification and Eligibility Simplification (BENES) Act of 2019; and
- H.R. 3935, The Protecting Patients Transportation to Care Act.

HLC is a coalition of chief executives from all disciplines within American healthcare. It is the exclusive forum for the nation's healthcare leaders to jointly develop policies, plans, and programs to achieve their vision of a 21st century healthcare system that makes affordable high-quality care accessible to all Americans. Members of HLC – hospitals, academic health centers, health plans, pharmaceutical companies, medical device manufacturers, laboratories, biotech firms, health product distributors, post-acute care providers, home care providers, and information technology companies – advocate for measures to increase the quality and efficiency of healthcare through a patient-centered approach.

H.R. 2477, The BENES Act of 2019
HLC strongly supports improving beneficiary outreach and education within the Medicare program. Many Medicare beneficiaries face lifetime penalties, coverage gaps, and other harmful consequences due to complicated enrollment rules and lack of notifications. With a rapid increase of baby boomers aging into the program, more education is needed. Furthermore, it is important that new beneficiaries understand the benefits of Medicare in particular and are not arbitrarily enrolled in fee-for-service Medicare. Individuals who miss their initial Medicare enrollment window may pay lifetime late enrollment penalties, experience lengthy gaps in outpatient health coverage or face unaffordable and unexpected out-of-pocket healthcare costs. This legislation would improve outreach and education by requiring the federal government to send advance notice about the enrollment process to individuals approaching Medicare eligibility and would also reduce confusion by aligning the annual general enrollment period with the annual enrollment period for private Medicare Advantage and Part D prescription drug plans, helping enrollees avoid potentially hefty financial penalties.

H.R. 3935, The Protecting Patients Transportation to Care Act
The barriers and difficulties patients face in accessing healthcare often stem from social determinants, including income, education, and race or ethnicity. These social determinants can hinder patients from attaining the support and social services they need to become, and stay, healthy. Such services can include, but are not limited to, transportation to medical appointments, access to healthy foods, and assistance in securing safe housing.

Each year, Medicaid provides health insurance to approximately 70 million low-income and disabled individuals. Many of these individuals lack access to reliable transportation. Currently, federal regulations require state Medicaid programs to cover non-emergency medical transportation as a mandatory benefit but it is not mandated pursuant to statute. HLC supports this proposed legislation to make this regulation law by adding non-emergency medical transportation services for individuals without other means of transportation to the list of mandatory benefits that every state Medicaid program is required to provide.

Thank you for the opportunity to share our concerns regarding these legislative proposals to improve Americans' healthcare coverage and outcomes. HLC looks forward to continuing to collaborate with you on these important issues. If you have any questions, please do not hesitate to contact Debbie Witchey at (202) 449-3435 or dwitchey@hlc.org.

Sincerely,

Mary R. Grealy
President

MARCH OF DIMES

OFFICE OF GOVERNMENT AFFAIRS

T (202) 659-1800
E advocacy@marchofdimes.org
MARCHOFDIMES.ORG

January 7, 2020

The Honorable Anna G. Eshoo
Chairwoman
Subcommittee on Health
Committee on Energy & Commerce
US House of Representatives
2125 Rayburn House Office Building
Washington, DC 20515

The Honorable Michael C. Burgess
Ranking Member
Subcommittee on Health
Committee on Energy & Commerce
US House of Representatives
2322 Rayburn House Office Building
Washington, DC 20515

Dear Chairwoman Eshoo and Ranking Member Burgess,

On behalf of March of Dimes, the leading non-profit, non-partisan organization fighting for the health of all moms and babies, I write to express our strong support for *The Healthy Start Reauthorization Act of 2019* (HR 4801) and thank you for including the legislation in the January 8 hearing, "Legislation to Improve Americans' Health Care Coverage and Outcomes."

For 30 years, the Healthy Start Program has provided services to promote healthy pregnancies and strong infants in the nation's most challenged communities. Due in part to the success of the program, the US infant mortality rate dropped to an all-time low in 2017.[i] The racial gap in infant mortality rates is narrowing, as well. Despite that progress, however, there is still much more to be done. Infant mortality is higher in the United States than in comparable countries, our rate of infant deaths has declined more slowly than in peer countries, and significant racial disparities in birth outcomes persist.[ii] Non-Hispanic black infants are more likely to be born preterm and more likely to die before their first birthday than non-Hispanic white infants.[iii] Poverty also continues to have a significant impact on birth outcomes.

The United States should be the world's leader on maternal and infant health. In order to do so, we must invest in programs to improve birth outcomes for our most at-risk populations. The Healthy Start Program has a 30-year track record of providing culturally appropriate and effective services to communities with the highest infant mortality rates. March of Dimes strongly supports the reauthorization the Healthy Start Program and offers our endorsement of the *Healthy Start Reauthorization Act of 2019*.

March of Dimes appreciates your leadership on this issue, and we look forward to continuing to work with you to promote the health and well-being of all pregnant women and infants. If we may be of further assistance, please contact Rebecca Abbott, Deputy Director of Federal Affairs for Public Health, at 202.292.2750 or rabbott@marchofdimes.org.

Sincerely,

Stacey D. Stewart
President and CEO

cc:
The Honorable Anthony Gonzalez (R-OH)
The Honorable Tim Ryan (D-OH)
The Honorable Steve Stivers (R-OH)
The Honorable Lauren Underwood (D-IL)

---

[i] Kamal R, Hudman, J, McDermott D. "What do we know about infant mortality in the US and comparable countries?" Peterson-KFF Health System Tracker. October 18,2019. Available at https://www.healthsystemtracker.org/chart-collection/infant-mortality-u-s-compare-countries/#item-start
[ii] Ibid.
[iii] Ibid.

Testimony of John Kahan
Chief Data Analytics Officer of Microsoft / President of Aaron Matthews SIDS Research Guild of Seattle Children's

House Energy and Commerce Subcommittee on Health Hearing
Legislation to improve Americans' health care coverage and outcomes

January 8, 2020

Chairman Eshoo, Ranking Member Burgess and members of the Health Subcommittee, thank you for giving me the opportunity to submit testimony in support of H.R. 2271, Scarlett's Sunshine on Sudden Unexpected Death Act.

On October 6, 2003, the lives of my wife and I were turned upside down when we lost our only son, Aaron Matthew to Sudden Infant Death Syndrome (SIDS). As we started to learn more about SIDS, we were frustrated by what we discovered: it is the leading cause of death in infants, one month to one year of age, in all developed nations. In the United States alone, more than two busloads of children a week – 3,500 a year -- die of SIDS related causes. That's why we have dedicated our lives to ensuring no parent experiences a similar loss or worries their child will be next.

The Aaron Matthew SIDS Research Guild was founded with an innovative approach to solving the medical mystery of SIDS. We bring some of the world's leading data scientists, led by Microsoft, together with some of the world's best medical researchers at the Center for Integrative Brain Research Institute at Seattle Children's. Together they are discovering exciting new avenues of research that are now enable researchers in the field to test their theories using large data sets that were previously unavailable.

The Aaron Matthew SIDS Research Guild is also embarking on its most promising research effort to date – building the first cloud-based genetic database specifically dedicated to SIDS and ultimately infant mortality. This effort, a collaboration between Microsoft and Seattle Children's, promises to bring genetic data from around the world to researchers so they can analyze the genome sequences of babies lost to SIDS for anomalies and clues.

Despite all this promise, we still do not know what causes SIDS nor do we know how to predict or prevent them. All up, SIDS related deaths known as Sudden Unexpected Infant Deaths (SUID) have remained flat since the mid 90s. As medical researchers, data scientists, and business professionals we know what it takes to get us on a path to solve this terrible mystery, and the Scarlett Sunshine on Sudden Unexpected Death Act will help us get there.

H.R. 2271 would strengthen existing efforts to better understand the causes of SIDS by facilitating data collection and analysis to improve prevention efforts. We need to enable researchers to study and find better ways to reduce the incidence of Sudden Unexpected Infant Death (SUID; defined as sudden unexpected deaths in infants between one month and one year) and Sudden Unexplained Death in Childhood (SUDC; defined as death in children between 1 and 18 years that remains unexplained after a thorough investigation, including an autopsy). We need to develop an ongoing system of consistent data collection on all births/deaths that includes data on infants (or children) and both parents. We need to enable our top medical researchers and world class data scientists to succeed. Many of us are parents who have lost children to SUID or SUDC, and we know firsthand the impact on us and on parents everywhere. We have an obligation to turn our technological advances into medical advances that will save many lives.

Scarlett's Sunshine on Sudden Unexpected Death Act takes the following critical steps:

- **Strengthen data consistency and completion** by directing the CDC to authorize grants to state and local agencies to revise standardized case reporting forms for SUID and SUDC.
- **Enables updated data collection guidelines by** authorizing a CDC-commissioned study to advise on the appropriateness of genetic analyses and best practices for testing in these cases.
- **Authorizes funding for essential grants** to support, among other things:
    - Training grants and materials for death scene investigators
    - Grants to states to review of all SUID and SUDC cases; and to support data infrastructure that will enable the leveraging of data to inform prevention experts and clinical care.
    - New HRSA grants for outreach to educate families on safer-sleep practices for infants, to provide low- or reduced-cost products conducive to safer sleep recommendations from national organizations, and for new local grants to support grieving families.
- **Establishes new monitoring measures** by requiring annual reports to the appropriate Senate committees to include the absolute number and incidence of SUID/SUDC, actions undertaken, and any new recommendations.
- **Improve training** to address unsafe sleep practices, a major factor contributing to SIDS.

Those of us who have experienced the tragedy of SIDS personally understand the toll it takes. And no new parent, or their extended families, will rest easy until we have solved it. We believe that we are on the cusp of a breakthrough with researchers closer than ever to finding the answers to this confounding and devastating medical mystery. But we can't get to the finish line without your help. I urge all members of this subcommittee to support H.R. 2271 and for the Committee to favorably report the bill to the full House for consideration, doing so will help bring us all closer to a world without SIDS.

Background

The CDC includes three categories in its definition of Sudden Unexpected Infant Death:

1. SIDS: Sudden Infant Death Syndrome: the sudden and unexplained death of an infant between one month and one year;
2. Accidental suffocation in a sleeping environment; and
3. Other deaths from unknown causes

Infant mortality rates

deaths in the first year of life/1,000 live births, OECD countries, 2013

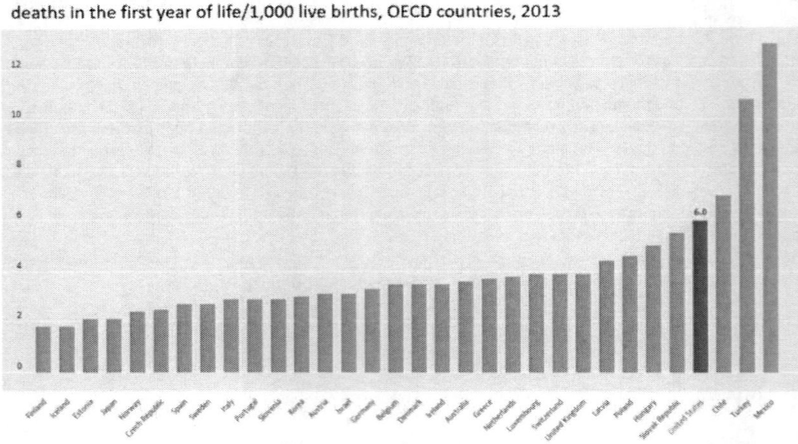

The following data from the Centers for Disease Control shows that while SIDS rates in the U.S. have come down, the overall SUID rate has not improved since the mid '90s. While we have seen great strides in prevention of death due to neonatal preterm birth complications (still the leading cause of death worldwide), there hasn't been a comparable improvement in preventing SUID or SUDC.

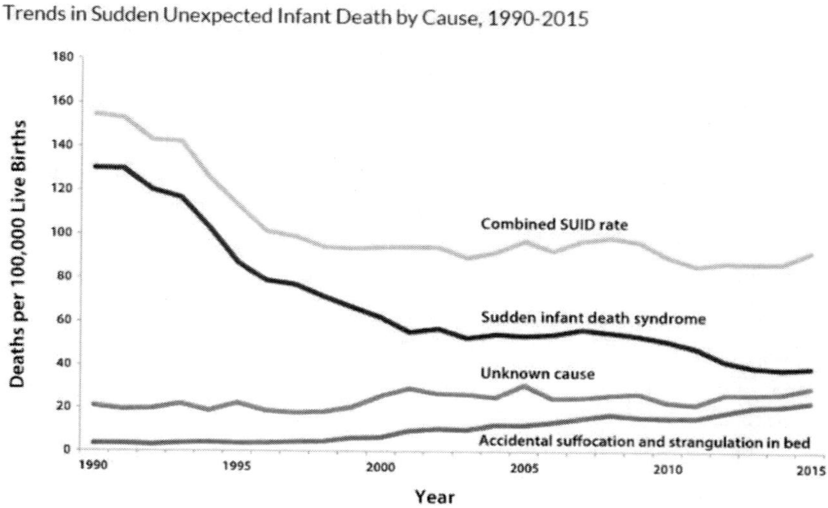

FARE
Food Allergy Research & Education

January 6, 2020

The Honorable Steny Hoyer
Cannon House Office Building, 102
Washington, D.C. 20515

The Honorable Phil Roe
Longworth House Office Building, 1705
Washington, DC 20515

Dear Representative Hoyer and Representative Roe:

FARE (Food Allergy Research and Education) is the nation's leading organization dedicated to food allergy research, education, advocacy and the world's largest private source of funding for food allergy research. We write today to offer our strong support for H.R. 2468, the School-Based Allergies and Asthma Management Program Act, which would ensure that states that require schools to establish allergy and asthma management guidelines are given increased preference in the awarding of relevant grants. This important piece of legislation would improve the safety of children with asthma and food allergies and help ensure the full inclusion of these students in all school activities.

Food allergy is a life threatening, growing public health concern. 32 million Americans have food allergies, including nearly 6 million children. FARE advocates for the adoption of policies that improve the safety and inclusion of students and has been a leader in this area, providing training and resources to school and parents. In 2013, FARE collaborated with the Centers for Disease Control and Prevention in the creation of *Voluntary Guidelines for Managing Food Allergies in Schools and Early Care and Education Programs*—the first national comprehensive guidelines for school food allergy management.

More than six million American children have asthma, a disease that is one of the leading causes of school absenteeism. According to the National Asthma Education and Prevention Program, parents report that students miss 14 million days of school every year due to asthma. While asthma poses serious health and educational threats, with proper treatment and care, asthma can be controlled and does not have to negatively impact a student's access to education.

Guidelines around food allergies and asthma are important for several reasons.

- As 25 percent of first-time anaphylactic reactions occur at school, it is critical that students experiencing an anaphylactic reaction have immediate access to emergency stock epinephrine at school. Research suggests that the majority of fatal food allergy reactions are triggered by food consumed outside one's home.
- More than 15 percent of school-aged children with food allergies have had a reaction in school.
- In a 2013-2014 survey of schools participating in a program to provide undesignated (stock) epinephrine for emergency use, over 600 schools—more than 10 percent – reported at least one case of anaphylaxis.
- Approximately 20-25 percent of epinephrine administrations in schools involve individuals whose allergy was unknown at the time of the reaction.

H.R. 2468 will encourage states to prioritize the development of these guidelines, making millions of children with food allergies and asthma safer. We look forward to working with you, the members of the House Energy and Commerce Committee who will soon consider the legislation, and all members of Congress to pass this ask that all members of the Health Subcommittee support this important piece of legislation. Should you have any questions, please contact Steve Danon at 858-774-1290. We would welcome the opportunity to discuss this bill further with you, as well as our support for H.R. 2117, the FASTER Act.

Sincerely,

Lisa Gable
Chief Executive Officer
FARE

CC: Chairman Rep. Frank Pallone, Chairwoman Rep. Anna Eshoo, Ranking Member Rep. Greg Walden, and Ranking Member Rep. Michael Burgess

Testimony from

American Academy of Allergy, Asthma & Immunology (AAAAI)

for the hearing of the House Committee on Energy and Commerce

Subcommittee on Health

"Legislation to Improve Americans' Health Care Coverage and Outcomes"

January 8, 2020

Chairwoman Eshoo, Ranking Member Burgess, and members of the Subcommittee, thank you for the opportunity to submit testimony on H.R. 2468, the "School-Based Allergies and Asthma Management Program Act," introduced by Majority Leader Steny Hoyer (D-MD) and Rep. Phil Roe, M.D. (R-TN). This important, bipartisan legislation would encourage elementary and secondary schools receiving asthma-related grants to have trained personnel and a comprehensive school-based allergies and asthma management program.

The two most important strategies for preparing schools in the event of an allergy or asthma incident are implementing management plans and ensuring school staff members are ready to assist children experiencing an attack. The "School-Based Allergies and Asthma Management Program Act" would encourage states to adopt these strategies so that schools are better equipped to help students with severe allergies and asthma manage their disease. Such changes in schools will not only will improve child health but will also help students to better focus on learning in the classroom.

Over six million American children have asthma, a disease that is one of the leading causes of school absenteeism. According to the National Asthma Education and Prevention Program, parents report that students miss 14 million days of school every year due to asthma. While asthma poses serious health and educational threats, with proper treatment and care, asthma can be controlled and does not have to negatively impact a student's access to education.

The U.S. Department of Education and the U.S. Department of Health and Human Services (HHS) recommend that schools have comprehensive management plans in place to support children with asthma and ensure that their disorders are under control while at school. Unfortunately, most schools do not have such programs in place. An asthma action plan outlines what medications to take and when and how to increase the doses or add more medication if needed in the case of an asthma attack. If a school does not have an asthma action plan for a child, there is little they can do when that child suffers an asthma attack. They cannot provide medication, even if they have it, without parental authorization. An asthma action plan based on communication with the student's physician enables a school nurse or other designated school staff member to administer a rescue inhaler that can mean the difference between life and death.

In addition, it is important that schools have a similar action plan for students who have a history of a severe allergy to an environmental exposure (e.g., peanut or insect sting). This action plan should follow the same principle as outlined above: affording the school the opportunity to provide life-saving medication (e.g., epinephrine autoinjector) to a student who develops a severe allergic reaction while in school while also providing for an approved management plan including critical contact information for both family members and medical professionals involved in the care of the student.

To ensure that schools have the necessary information and necessary tools to retain and quickly put into action both the asthma and severe allergy action plans for each student, the AAAAI, in collaboration with other stakeholders, developed SAMPRO™, the School-based Asthma Management Program. SAMPRO™ provides a tool-kit at no cost to assist families and schools in creating and maintaining this important health information. SAMPRO™ standardizes recommendations for school-based asthma plans and provides websites and resources useful for the care of children with asthma in the school setting. This also provides the blueprint for a management plan for students with severe allergies.

The "School-Based Allergies and Asthma Management Program Act" would amend the Public Health Service Act to revise the conditions under which HHS, in making asthma-related grants, gives preference to a state. A preference is given to states that require elementary and secondary schools to have:

(1) at least one individual, such as a school nurse or other school staff, trained in the administration of rescue medications for allergies and asthma on the premises during operating hours, and

(2) an allergies and asthma management program that includes a method to identify students with allergies and asthma and an action plan and support system for each such student.

The "School-Based Allergies and Asthma Management Program Act" is supported by the American Academy of Allergy Asthma and Immunology (AAAAI) as well as the American College of Allergy, Asthma, and Immunology, the Asthma and Allergy Foundation of America, the Allergy and Asthma Network, and the National Association of School Nurses.

No child should be at risk in school because there are not systems in place to help them manage their respiratory and allergic disorders. AAAAI urges the Subcommittee to markup this important legislation.

August 22, 2016

The Honorable Orrin Hatch
Chairman, Committee on Finance
U.S. Senate
Washington, DC 20510

The Honorable Ron Wyden
Ranking Member, Committee on Finance
U.S. Senate
Washington, DC 20510

The Honorable Kevin Brady
Chairman, Committee on Ways & Means
U.S. House of Representatives
Washington, DC 20515

The Honorable Sander Levin
Ranking Member, Committee on Ways & Means
U.S. House of Representatives
Washington, DC 20515

The Honorable Fred Upton
Chairman, Committee on Energy & Commerce
U.S. House of Representatives
Washington, DC 20515

The Honorable Frank Pallone
Ranking Member, Committee on Energy & Commerce
U.S. House of Representatives
Washington, DC 20515

Dear Chairman Hatch, Ranking Member Wyden, Chairman Brady, Ranking Member Levin, Chairman Upton, and Ranking Member Pallone:

As former Administrators of the Centers for Medicare & Medicaid Services/Health Care Financing Administration, Republicans and Democrats, we frequently disagree among ourselves about any number of issues. But we all agree on the importance of treating Medicare beneficiaries fairly, efficiently, and as helpfully as possible. That's why we have come together in support of the bipartisan Beneficiary Enrollment Notification and Eligibility Simplification (BENES) Act (S. 3236 and H.R. 5772).

Many of the problems addressed by the BENES Act did not exist when most of us were in the government, but the decoupling of eligibility ages for Medicare and full Social Security benefits, revisions to Medicare Secondary Payor law, and the growing number of Americans working past the age of 65 have, together, substantially complicated the decision making process for eligible individuals and couples in deciding when and how to enroll in Medicare.

Signing up for Part B is not a straightforward task, particularly for the increasing share of Americans who are working longer and delaying retirement. For these individuals, knowing when and whether to enroll in Part B requires understanding complex and varied rules. Enrollment missteps are a common occurrence and often lead to a lifetime of higher Part B premiums. In 2014, 750,000 people with Medicare were paying a Part B Late Enrollment Penalty (LEP) and the average LEP amounted to nearly a 30 percent increase in a beneficiary's monthly premium.[1] Gaps in coverage, higher health care costs, and limited access to needed care are also consequences experienced by those who make honest enrollment mistakes.

To prevent costly enrollment errors among people new to Medicare, the BENES Act provides enhanced notice and education for those approaching Medicare eligibility, aligns and simplifies Part B enrollment periods, and updates existing mechanisms for those seeking reprieve from Part B premium penalties and coverage delays. We encourage you to support the BENES Act.

Thank you.

---

[1] P. Davis, "Medicare: Part B Premiums," (Congressional Research Service: August 2016), available at: https://www.fas.org/sgp/crs/misc/R40082.pdf

Sincerely,

Leonard D. Schaeffer
Administrator
Health Care Financing Administration
1978 – 1980

William L. Roper, MD, MPH
Administrator
Health Care Financing Administration
1986 – 1989

Gail R. Wilensky, Ph. D.
Administrator
Health Care Financing Administration
1990 – 1992

Bruce C. Vladeck, Ph. D.
Administrator
Health Care Financing Administration
1993 – 1997

Nancy-Ann DeParle
Administrator
Health Care Financing Administration
1997 – 2000

Tom Scully
Administrator
Centers for Medicare & Medicaid Services
2001 – 2004

Mark McClellan, MD, Ph. D.
Administrator
Centers for Medicare & Medicaid Services
2004 – 2006

Donald M. Berwick, MD
Administrator
Centers for Medicare & Medicaid Services
2010 – 2011

CC: The Honorable Mitch McConnell, Majority Leader, U.S. Senate
The Honorable Harry Reid, Minority Leader, U.S. Senate
The Honorable Paul Ryan, Speaker, U.S. House of Representatives
The Honorable Nancy Pelosi, Minority Leader, U.S. House of Representatives

**Supporters of the
Beneficiary Enrollment Notification and Eligibility Simplification (BENES) Act
(S. 1280/H.R. 2477)**

1. AARP
2. ACCSES
3. AFL-CIO
4. AgeOptions
5. Aging Life Care Association
6. AHIP (America's Health Insurance Plans)
7. Alliance for Aging Research
8. Alliance for Retired Americans
9. Allies for Independence
10. AMDA – The Society for Post-Acute and Long-Term Care Medicine
11. American Association of Service Coordinators (AASC)
12. American Association on Health and Disability
13. American College of Clinical Pharmacy (ACCP)
14. American Federation of Government Employees (AFGE)
15. American Federation of State, County and Municipal Employees (AFSCME)
16. American Foundation for the Blind
17. American Geriatrics Society
18. American Society on Aging
19. Association of Jewish Aging Services of North America (AJAS)
20. Association of University Centers on Disabilities (AUCD)
21. Autism Society of America
22. B'nai B'rith International
23. Better Medicare Alliance
24. Blue Shield of California
25. BlueCross BlueShield Association (BCBSA)
26. Brain Injury Association of America
27. California Health Advocates
28. Center for Advocacy for the Rights & Interests of the Elderly (CARIE)
29. Center for Elder Law & Justice
30. Center for Independence of the Disabled, NY
31. Center for Medicare Advocacy, Inc.
32. Community Catalyst
33. Community Services Center of Greater Williamsburg
34. Compassion & Choices
35. Connecticut Alliance for Retired Americans
36. CVS Health (formerly Aetna)
37. Dialysis Patient Citizens
38. Disability Rights Education and Defense Fund (DREDF)
39. Disabled In Action of Metro NY
40. Domtar
41. Easterseals
42. Empire Justice Center

43. Epilepsy Foundation
44. Families USA
45. Family & Children Association, Senior Services HIICAP (Nassau County, NY)
46. Gerontological Society of America
47. Humana
48. International Association for Indigenous Aging
49. International Union, United Automobile, Aerospace & Agricultural Implement Workers of America
50. The Jewish Federations of North America
51. Justice in Aging
52. Lakeshore Foundation
53. LeadingAge
54. Lutheran Services in America
55. MAXIMUS
56. Medicare Rights Center
57. Metro New York Health Care for All
58. National Academy of Elder Law Attorneys (NAELA)
59. National Active and Retired Federal Employees Association (NARFE)
60. National Adult Day Services Association (NADSA)
61. National Adult Protective Services Association (NAPSA)
62. National Alliance on Mental Illness (NAMI)
63. National Association for Home Care & Hospice (NAHC)
64. National Association for the Support of Long Term Care (NASL)
65. National Association of Area Agencies on Aging (n4a)
66. National Association of Councils on Developmental Disabilities
67. National Association of Health Underwriters (NAHU)
68. National Association of Nutrition and Aging Services Programs (NANASP)
69. National Association of Social Workers (NASW)
70. National Association of State Head Injury Administrators
71. National Association of State Long-Term Care Ombudsman Programs (NASOP)
72. National Coalition on Health Care (NCHC)
73. National Committee to Preserve Social Security and Medicare
74. National Consumer Voice for Quality Long-Term Care
75. National Consumers League
76. National Council on Aging
77. National Hospice and Palliative Care Organization (NHPCO)
78. National Hispanic Council on Aging (NHCOA)
79. National Multiple Sclerosis Society
80. National Partnership for Women & Families
81. National Patient Advocate Foundation
82. New York Legal Assistance Group
83. New Yorkers for Accessible Health Coverage
84. Partnership to Improve Patient Care (PIPC)
85. Program to Improve Care, Altarum
86. Service Employees International Union (SEIU)
87. Smart Policy Works (formerly Health & Disability Advocates)
88. Social Security Works
89. Southern Tier Independence Center (STIC)

90. The Actors Fund
91. The Arc of the United States
92. Third Way
93. UAW Retiree Medical Benefits Trust
94. United Jewish Organizations of Williamsburg
95. Women's Institute for a Secure Retirement (WISER)

Last Updated December 13, 2019

December 16, 2019

Majority Leader Mitch McConnell
Minority Leader Chuck Schumer
United States Senate
Washington, D.C. 20150

Speaker Nancy Pelosi
Minority Leader Kevin McCarthy
United States House of Representatives
Washington, D.C. 20515

Leaders McConnell, Schumer; Speaker Pelosi and Leader McCarthy:

The undersigned 72 national organizations write to urge you include several important Medicare and Medicaid provisions in the "Extenders" legislative package that is expected to be considered by December 20th, including: (1) relief for those Medicare beneficiaries who, without congressional action this year, would face even higher prescription drug out-of-pocket costs due to the January 1st increase in Part D catastrophic coverage eligibility thresholds from $5,100 to $6,350; (2) making permanent the Medicaid Home and Community-Based Services (HCBS) Money Follows the Person Program (MFP), and Spousal Impoverishment Protections; (3) an extension (preferably with permanent, increased funding) for Medicare low-income outreach and enrollment efforts; (4) needed improvements in the Medicare Part B enrollment process; and (5) an extension of Medicaid funding in US Territories.

Addressing the Scheduled Increase in Medicare Prescription Drug Costs

Under the current Part D program, once Medicare beneficiaries hit an annual out-of-pocket spending threshold they can access catastrophic coverage that allows them to pay significantly less for their prescription drugs. Slightly over 1 million beneficiaries had drug costs above the catastrophic threshold in 2017. However, the threshold is scheduled to jump by an unprecedented $1,250 in 2020, increasing the amount beneficiaries with the greatest prescription drug needs must pay. At a time when these seniors and people with disabilities on Medicare were expecting legislation to pass this year that would decrease their prescription drug costs, for example with a much-needed out-of-pocket cap, they will be surprised and disappointed if their costs increase. According to initial estimates, failure to act would result in increasing prescription drug costs next year by over $2 billion for people with Medicare.

For Americans who are retired or on a fixed income, any increase in their out-of-pocket costs can become a significant financial burden. The average Medicare Part D enrollee takes more than 4 prescriptions per month, and over two-thirds have two or more concurrent chronic illnesses, which often require costly prescription medications. At the same time, most Medicare beneficiaries live on modest incomes, with an annual median income of just over $26,000. Something must be done this year to prevent these beneficiaries from facing the sticker shock of being forced to pay even more for medications they need to live healthier lives.

Making Permanent Programs that Help Medicaid Enrollees Remain in their Communities

We urge that two critical, expiring Medicaid HCBS programs be made permanent, consistent with the bipartisan Senate Finance Committee proposal released on December 6th. The Money Follows the Person (MFP) program provides enhanced funding to assist with the costs of transitioning people back to the community, including identifying and coordinating affordable and accessible housing and providing additional services and supports to make successful transitions. The program has helped over 91,000 people with disabilities and older adults move from institutional settings back to their communities. In the first year of the program, the Centers for Medicare & Medicaid Services (CMS) found an average cost savings of $22,080 in the first year per older adult participant, $21,396 per person for people with physical disabilities, and $48,156 per person for people with intellectual disabilities.

Medicaid's "spousal impoverishment protections" make it possible for an individual who needs a nursing home level of care to qualify for Medicaid while allowing their spouse to retain a modest amount of income and resources. Since 1988, federal Medicaid law has required states to apply these protections to spouses of individuals receiving institutional LTSS. Congress extended this protection to eligibility for HCBS in all states beginning in 2014, so that married couples have the same financial protections whether care is provided in a facility or in the community. Allowing the policy to expire could force people whose needs warrant a nursing facility level of care and who now receive such care in their homes, into more costly institutional care against their wishes. Further, not securing these protections could stall or even reverse progress states have made in helping people with disabilities and older adults remain at home and in the community.

<u>Continuing Medicare Low-Income Outreach and Enrollment Assistance</u>

We urge that a provision also be included to continue funding for Medicare outreach and enrollment efforts to low-income beneficiaries, many of whom are dually eligible for Medicaid. Funding supports community-based efforts through State Health Insurance Assistance Programs, Area Agencies on Aging, Aging and Disability Resource Centers, and a National Center on Benefits Outreach and Enrollment which provides grants to a network of 84 local Benefits Enrollment Centers (BECs) in 43 states. These efforts, originally authorized in 2008 and extended 7 times since then, enable Medicare beneficiaries with the least resources to access assistance for prescription drug coverage and other essential Medicare benefits for which they are eligible. We urge you to extend funding for as long as possible (ideally making the program permanent) and include the funding increase from $37.5 to $50 million that House committees approved.

Almost 3 million beneficiaries eligible for prescription drug low-income subsidies (LIS/Extra Help) are not enrolled. The LIS program helps low-income beneficiaries pay for their rising prescription drug costs. Improving enrollment in this important program is a critical component toward reducing out-of-pocket prescription drug costs for those who can least afford them.

Previous allocations for low-income outreach and enrollment activities have led to important, proven results, including: (1) assisting 2.5 million individuals in need; (2) increasing the number of low-income Medicare beneficiaries enrolled in the Medicare Savings Programs from 6.4 million in 2008 to 9 million as of June 2018; and (3) targeting rural communities and other hard-to-reach populations to improve access to help with Medicare prescription drug costs.

<u>Improving the Part B Enrollment Process</u>

We also support inclusion of the Beneficiary Enrollment Notification and Eligibility Simplification (BENES) Act (S. 1280; HR 2477) in the forthcoming legislation. Currently, far too many people with Medicare are irreversibly harmed due to the cumbersome and confusing Part B enrollment system. The consequences of these missteps can be significant—often leading to a lifetime of higher premiums, substantial out-of-pocket health care costs, gaps in coverage, and barriers to accessing needed services. The bicameral, bipartisan BENES Act aims to prevent these costly mistakes by modernizing, simplifying, and improving the Medicare Part B enrollment process.

Extending Medicaid Funding in US Territories

Finally, we support extending critical funding for the Medicaid programs in US territories including American Samoa, Guam, the Northern Mariana Islands, Puerto Rico, and the US Virgin Islands. The expiration of current enhanced federal funding allotments and matching rates for the territories poses a significant threat to the health and well-being of territory residents who face coverage losses, barriers to access, and cuts to important health care benefits. If these enhanced funds are allowed to expire, territories will revert to the inadequate capped allotment that would devastate their budgets, access to health care, and ultimately, patients' health.

We strongly urge you to take the steps outlined above to protect Medicare beneficiaries against further increases in out-of-pocket costs, improve enrollment, and extend critical Medicaid programs and funding for low-income Americans.

Sincerely,

ADAPT
ADvancing States
Aging Life Care Association
The AIDS Institute
Alliance for Aging Research
Alliance for Retired Americans
AMDA The Society for Post-Acute and Long-Term Care Medicine
American Academy of Physical Medicine & Rehabilitation
American Association on Health and Disability
American Association on Intellectual and Developmental Disabilities (AAIDD)
American Autoimmune Related Diseases Association
American Kidney Fund
American Network of Community Options & Resources (ANCOR)
American Physical Therapy Association
American Therapeutic Recreation Association
The Arc of the United States
Association for Gerontology and Human Development - HBCU
Association of People Supporting Employment First (APSE)
Association of University Centers on Disabilities (AUCD)
Autism Society of America
Autistic Self Advocacy Network
Bazelon Center for Mental Health Law
Brain Injury Association of America

Caregiver Action Network
Caregiver Voices United
Caring Across Generations
Center for Medicare Advocacy
Center for Public Representation
Christopher & Dana Reeve Foundation
Coalition on Human Needs
CommunicationFIRST
Community Catalyst
Disability Rights Education and Defense Fund (DREDF)
Easterseals
Epilepsy Foundation
Family Voices
GO2 Foundation for Lung Cancer
Justice in Aging
Lakeshore Foundation
LeadingAge
Lupus and Allied Diseases Association, Inc.
Lutheran Services in America
Meals on Wheels America
Medicare Rights Center
National Academy of Elder Law Attorneys
National Adult Day Services Association (NADSA)
National Alliance on Mental Illness
National Association for Home Care and Hospice
National Association of Area Agencies on Aging (n4a)
National Association of Councils on Developmental Disabilities
National Association of Nutrition and Aging Services Programs (NANASP)
National Association of Social Workers (NASW)
National Association of State Directors of Developmental Disabilities Services
National Association of State Head Injury Administrators
National Association of State Long-Term Care Ombudsman Programs (NASOP)
National Caucus and Center on Black Aging, Inc.
National Committee to Preserve Social Security and Medicare
National Consumer Voice for Quality Long-Term Care
National Council on Aging
National Council on Independent Living
National Disability Rights Network
National Down Syndrome Congress
National Health Council
National Kidney Foundation
National Multiple Sclerosis Society
National Respite Coalition
Patient Access Network Foundation
Program to Improve Eldercare, Altarum
RetireSafe
Special Needs Alliance
United Spinal Association
The Women's Institute for a Secure Retirement (WISER)

MEDICARE RIGHTS CENTER
Getting Medicare right

Congress Must Streamline and Simplify Medicare Enrollment

The BENES Act (S. 1280/H.R. 2477) Offers Commonsense, Bipartisan Solutions

While most people are automatically enrolled in Medicare Part B—because they are collecting Social Security retirement benefits at age 65—a growing number are not, as they are working later in life and deferring their Social Security benefits. Unlike those who are auto-enrolled, these individuals must make an active Medicare enrollment choice, taking into consideration specific timelines and existing coverage. If this transition is mismanaged, individuals new to Medicare may face lifetime late enrollment penalties, higher health care costs, gaps in coverage, and disruptions in care continuity.

Unfortunately, many individuals do make mistakes—often because they are not informed about their enrollment responsibilities or Medicare's complex enrollment rules. These rules are so complicated that even the most sophisticated Human Resources experts struggle to follow them, and many employers' benefits departments lack the Medicare knowledge to guide their employees and retirees on Medicare enrollment. Clear and simple advice to those approaching eligibility could help prevent enrollment errors, but today the federal government provides virtually no notification to people nearing Medicare eligibility that they may need to actively enroll or how and when to do so. As a result, people with employer-based or other private coverage often bear the full burden of navigating Medicare's complicated enrollment system.

The bipartisan **Beneficiary Enrollment Notification and Eligibility Simplification (BENES) Act** (S. 1280/H.R. 2477), championed by Senators Todd Young (R-IN) and Bob Casey (D-PA) and Representatives Raul Ruiz (D-CA), Gus Bilirakis (R-FL), Brad Schneider (D-IL), and Jackie Walorski (R-IN) includes commonsense solutions to address these challenges.

Enrollment Errors Affect Tens of Thousands of Americans in Every State

The Medicare Rights Center answers nearly three million questions each year through its National Consumer Helpline and educational programs. Year after year, about one in four Helpline calls concerns Medicare enrollment. In 2017, nearly one-third of these calls were from individuals experiencing challenges enrolling in Part B, many because they were navigating a specific hurdle, did not understand enrollment periods, or were confused about Part B costs, eligibility, and other issues. In 2018, about 760,000 people with Medicare were paying a Part B Late Enrollment Penalty (LEP) and the average LEP amounted to nearly a 30% increase in a beneficiary's monthly premium.[1]

The BENES Act Would:

Increase Beneficiary Notification and Education. The BENES Act would direct the federal government to provide advance notice to individuals approaching Medicare eligibility about basic Medicare enrollment rules, filling a long-standing gap in education for older adults and people with disabilities.

Eliminate Harmful Coverage Gaps. The BENES Act would also eliminate needless multi-month coverage gaps in Medicare by mandating that Part B insurance begin the first of the month following one's enrollment during both the later months of their Initial Enrollment Period (IEP) and during the General Enrollment Period (GEP).

Modernize and Align Part B Enrollment Timelines. The BENES Act would also reduce confusion by aligning the annual GEP with the annual enrollment period for private Medicare Advantage (MA) and Part D prescription drug plans. Additionally, the BENES Act would allow the federal government to create a Part B Special Enrollment Period (SEP) for "exceptional circumstances," a provision currently used in MA and Part D when people are not able to sign up for Medicare due to occurrences like hurricanes and other natural disasters.

A Case Study

Throughout their working lives, Mr. and Mrs. G held good jobs with good health insurance. When Mr. G turned 65, Mrs. G was working for a large company whose group health plan covered them both. In late 2015, when Mrs. G was 64, the company she worked for was acquired, and her position was terminated. As part of her termination, the couple was provided two years of continuing enrollment in the company's group health plan, paid for by the company. The coverage for those years was identical to the coverage available to them while Mrs. G was employed.

Planning ahead, before the group health plan coverage was due to terminate in late 2017, the couple went to their local Social Security office to enroll in Medicare. For the first time, they were told that when Mrs. G stopped working, it triggered a change in how her group health coverage was treated under Medicare rules. Because Mrs. G was not "actively" employed within the past eight months, she and her husband were ineligible to enroll in Part B through a Special Enrollment Period.

Mr. and Mrs. G were able to enroll in Medicare Part A immediately, and did so, but that only covered hospitalizations and inpatient care. For outpatient coverage through Part B, Mrs. G and her husband were told they would have to wait for the General Enrollment Period in January 2018 and their coverage would not be effective until July 1, 2018—**meaning Mrs. G and her husband would be without adequate health coverage for nearly a year.**

At the same time, the couple learned that because they delayed Part B enrollment for two full years and did not have employer-sponsored coverage through "active" employment during this time, they will be **required to pay a penalty of 20 percent** (10 percent multiplied by the number of years delayed) on their Part B premium. This amount will be added to their monthly Part B premium **for the rest of their lives.**

Facing a precarious situation, Mrs. G attempted to purchase individual insurance for her and her husband, to fill the coverage gap while waiting for Medicare, and was turned away. So, Mrs. G called the Medicare Rights Center for help. The helpline counselor explained that Medicare law prohibits the sale of policies that offer the same coverage as Medicare to anyone who is enrolled in any part of Medicare. All available avenues to enrollment were explored, to no avail.

Mrs. G expressed her frustration at the lack of information she and her husband had received from her employer, from Social Security, and from Medicare. According to Mrs. G, they did not even realize "Medicare was something we needed to look into as long as we were covered by an excellent medical plan." Mrs. G said being without health coverage for any outpatient medical needs for many months is what worried her most of all. At the time, she told Medicare Rights Center that she was "keeping her fingers crossed" that neither she nor her husband would need any significant health care while in the coverage gap. Unfortunately, this wishful thinking was the only solution available to them.

Had the BENES Act been in place when Mrs. G turned age 65, she would have received information explaining Medicare enrollment rules and considerations. If they had been informed, Ms. G and her husband would not be facing many months without Part B coverage. With 10,000 Americans reaching Medicare eligibility age each day and as people stay in the workforce longer, more individuals will have to actively enroll in Part B, and could face similar challenges. The BENES Act's bipartisan, low-cost solutions are needed now more than ever.

---

[1] Congressional Research Service, "Medicare: Part B Premiums" (April 4, 2019), available at: https://crsreports.congress.gov/product/pdf/R/R40082.

For more information, please contact Lindsey Copeland, Federal Policy Director, Medicare Rights Center at lcopeland@medicarerights.org

The New York Times | https://nyti.ms/2Jk1SjB

THE NEW OLD AGE

Why You Shouldn't Wait to Sign Up for Medicare Part B

By Paula Span

Oct. 26, 2018

Twenty years ago, George Zeppenfeldt-Cestero left his job as a hospital administrator in New York to open a one-person health care consulting firm.

Since he was losing his employee medical coverage, he shopped around and bought a private health insurance plan through Aetna.

It was expensive, with premiums starting at about $1,000 a month, but "it paid for all my doctors' visits and my medications," he said. "I was a satisfied consumer."

But several years ago, Aetna informed him that it was discontinuing that plan, sending him scrambling for another insurer. That's when, applying for coverage through the state marketplace under the Affordable Care Act, Mr. Zeppenfeldt-Cestero learned that he (and, he argues, Aetna) had made a serious error.

He should have signed up for Medicare Part B three years earlier when he turned 65.

By delaying, he had missed the best window — the so-called Initial Enrollment Period — to apply for Part B, which covers much of what we consider health care: doctor visits, tests, injectable drugs (including chemotherapy), ambulances, physical therapy and other non-hospital services. As a result, he has to pay permanently higher premiums, and he had to endure an unsettlingly long period — from December to July — before the coverage actually kicked in.

"It was very nerve-racking," Mr. Zeppenfeldt-Cestero, now 71 and still working. "For six months, I was without any coverage whatsoever."

Such Part B mistakes appear to happen with some frequency. Last year, nearly 700,000 Medicare beneficiaries were paying Part B penalties, according to the Centers for Medicare and Medicaid Services.

"It's one of those issues that has started to snowball," said Fred Riccardi of the nonprofit Medicare Rights Center, which annually fields 20,000 Medicare-related questions on its helpline (800-333-4114) and three million through its online tool Medicare Interactive.

To simplify a complex process, people are supposed to sign up for Part B when they turn 65, unless they are working and have coverage through an employer, or a working spouse's employer.

Yet as people approach age 65, Mr. Riccardi pointed out, "there's no notice that says, 'It's time to enroll in Medicare and if you don't, you could have problems.'"

One factor underlying the confusion, experts say, is the decoupling of Medicare eligibility from the Social Security full retirement age. Both threshold ages used to be 65 but now, the full Social Security retirement age has passed 66 and will gradually rise to 67.

"It's all become far more complicated than it used to be when people turned 65, got their Social Security, got their Medicare, and that was that," said Patricia Neuman, director of the Kaiser Family Foundation Program on Medicare Policy.

Enrollment in Medicare Part A, which covers hospitalization and requires no premiums for most beneficiaries, occurs automatically at age 65 if you're drawing Social Security retirement benefits. You have to take steps to enroll if you delay taking Social Security past age 65.

If you're not yet receiving Social Security benefits, you also have to sign up for Part B, which this year costs $134 a month, more for individuals with incomes over $85,000 a year. The question is when to enroll.

Bear with me as I try to clear a path through the thicket, keeping in mind that I'm talking about Medicare based on age. Younger people with certain disabilities, also insurable through Medicare, contend with different rules.

You have seven months — the month in which you turn 65 and the three months both before and after it — to apply for Part B without penalty. You can apply online at https://www.medicare.gov/sign-up-change-plans/how-do-i-get-parts-a-b or at a Social Security office.

If you're still employed and working at a company or organization with 20 or more employees (or your spouse is), and you're covered by an employee health plan, you may not need Part B yet. Instead of paying premiums, it could make financial sense to hold off. But it's important to know that after losing employee coverage — due to retirement, layoffs or any other reason — you have an eight-month "special enrollment period" to sign up for Part B.

If you miss that window, you have to wait for the general enrollment period, which runs from January 1 through March 31 each year. That creates two problems.

First, Medicare will add a permanent 10 percent penalty to your premiums for each year you delayed. Mr. Zeppenfeldt-Cestero has to pay $187.60 per month now because he waited more than three years to sign up. If he had enrolled when he was 65, his monthly premium would be $134.

"Without good information, people make mistakes and they're costly," Dr. Neuman said. "In this case, it's a cost that continues the rest of your life."

The second problem: the general enrollment period imposes coverage gaps.

The general enrollment period (not to be confused with the Open Enrollment Period currently underway when those already receiving Medicare can change plans) runs from January through March, remember. But coverage doesn't begin until the following July 1.

If you didn't sign up for Part B and recognize your error in March, you can be insured in July. If you figure it out in April, however, you can't enroll until the following January and coverage begins the *following* July.

"It could be well over a year, depending on when you discover the problem," said David Lipschutz, senior policy lawyer at the Center for Medicare Advocacy. "Unfortunately, some people discover it when they get sick."

What causes this predicament? Working seniors may be getting bad information from human resources departments, benefits counselors or insurance brokers. They may be relying on a COBRA plan, in which case Medicare should become their primary insurer at 65.

Or they may have transitioned from employee coverage to a retiree plan. Then, too, Medicare should become their primary insurer, with the other plan the secondary insurer.

"Their retiree coverage looks just the same as when they were working," Mr. Lipschutz said. "But in Medicare's eyes, everything changes when you retire."

An insurance company that belatedly learns it's been paying your medical bills, when Medicare should have been your primary insurer, may try to recoup what it spent.

Because this process involves many exceptions and caveats (if you're a federal employee, say), and remedies for a few people, there's no substitute for consulting with an expert as you near 65. "You need to investigate," Mr. Lipschutz advised.

Given the risks of misinformation from employers, that probably means talking to Social Security by phone or in person, documenting all your conversations with dates and names.

"Very educated, astute folks get caught in this trap," Mr. Lipschutz said. "They're not scofflaws. They tried to play by the rules."

A legislative attempt to fix the mess, the BENES Act (for Beneficiary Enrollment Notification and Eligibility Simplification), would send notices to those approaching age 65, clearly explaining Part B enrollment. The bill has made little headway, despite bipartisan support, but advocates hope it will gain traction after the midterm elections.

Mr. Zeppenfeldt-Cestero has full Medicare coverage now, plus a supplemental Medigap policy. But he's still angry about what he calls "my nightmare."

Over several months, "I spoke to every advocacy and oversight agency out there to try to get this resolved in my favor," he said. He called Social Security and the Centers for Medicare and Medicaid. He tried his senator's office.

"They all said, 'You're out of luck.'"

THE WALL STREET JOURNAL.

https://www.wsj.com/articles/medicare-enrollment-can-be-confusing-and-lead-to-unexpected-costs-11576155600

U.S.

Medicare Enrollment Can Be Confusing and Lead to Unexpected Costs

More Americans are working past 65 and delaying Social Security, which makes enrolling in Medicare complicated

By Anne Tergesen
Dec. 12, 2019 8:00 am ET

As more Americans postpone retirement, a growing number are experiencing Medicare enrollment problems that can saddle them with hefty penalties and monthslong coverage gaps.

The roots of the problem are Medicare's complex rules and a lack of notice from the program explaining the steps older workers must take to enroll once they leave their jobs. In recent decades, Americans have remained in the workforce longer for reasons including concerns about savings and a desire to keep working, with many putting off taking Social Security payments.

That has contributed to a 14% increase in the number of people paying late-enrollment penalties between 2013 and 2017, according to government statistics.

There is a silver lining: From Jan. 1 to March 31 of each year, individuals who missed key Medicare enrollment deadlines can belatedly sign up, though they may face coverage gaps and penalties.

The easiest time to sign up for Medicare is during a seven-month period that starts three months before turning 65, the age most people become eligible for the federal health insurance program.

For those already collecting Social Security, enrollment is generally automatic for Medicare Part A, which covers hospital care, and Part B, which covers doctors' visits and outpatient care. Part A is typically free, while Part B costs between $135.50 and $460.50 a month, depending on an individual's income, this year.

SHARE YOUR THOUGHTS

Have you, or has someone you know, had to choose between leaving an employer's health care or enrolling in Medicare? How was the decision made? Join the conversation below.

For individuals are automatically enrolled when turning 65, said David Lipschutz, associate director at the nonprofit Center for Medicare Advocacy, "their Medicare cards show up in the mail." But people who delay Social Security past age 65 must sign up for Parts A and B on their own.

According to the U.S. Bureau of Labor Statistics, 27% of Americans ages 65 to 74 are in the labor force, up from 17.7% in 1998. For those in that group who delay Social Security, enrolling for Medicare can be complicated.

"Neither Social Security nor Medicare fully explains the rules" or sends them a reminder when it's time to sign up, said Frederic Riccardi, president of the nonprofit Medicare Rights Center.

Enrollment rules can differ depending on whether individuals work for a small or large company. In addition, while most workers with employer-based coverage are allowed to delay Medicare without penalty, they must sign up within eight months of stopping work, even if they keep their employer-based insurance through a retiree medical plan or under Cobra, a federal law that permits workers who leave their jobs to temporarily remain in a former employer's health plan.

A spokesman for the Centers for Medicare and Medicaid Services, which administers Medicare, did not respond to a request for comment. In the past, spokespeople who have responded to questions about difficulties with Medicare's enrollment rules have said the agency is following the laws governing the insurance program.

Those who run afoul of the rules can find themselves without coverage for months—which is what happened to Sarah Truman, 67, of Phoenix. A former teacher's aide, she chose to remain on her husband's insurance through his former employer under Cobra rather than sign up for

Medicare. About two weeks before the couple's Cobra coverage ended on Sept. 30, Ms. Truman visited a Social Security office to enroll in Medicare.

There, Ms. Truman said, she "got the shock of my life" when an agent told her that she would not be able to sign up for Medicare Part B until Jan. 1—and her coverage would not go into effect until July 2020. A diabetic who generally sees her doctor every three months, she says she now has trouble sleeping due to anxiety over what could happen if she has a serious medical problem.

Late enrollment frequently triggers penalties that inflate Part B premiums by 10% of the standard premium amount—currently $135.50 a month—for every year of delay. Ms. Truman expects to pay an additional 10%, or $13.55, to 20%, or $27.10, for Part B each month for the rest of her life.

"I don't feel like I did anything wrong," said Ms. Truman. "I wasn't cheating the system. I had insurance. It makes no sense to me that I am being punished."

Advocates say a growing number of people are in the same situation. According to the Centers for Medicare and Medicaid Services, about 700,000 of the 53.4 million people with Part B paid late enrollment penalties in 2017, up from 609,000 in 2013. The average penalty was a 28% premium increase, which would mean an increase of $37.94 a month above today's standard premium.

"This is one of the top problems we see on our helpline," said Mr. Riccardi.

In May, federal legislators introduced a bill that would require Social Security to notify people age 65 who have yet to claim retirement benefits of Medicare's enrollment rules. The bill, which has bipartisan support, would also allow people who delayed signing up for Part B and must use the enrollment period between Jan. 1 and March 31 to start their coverage the month after they enroll, rather than in July.

"As more and more Americans reach Medicare age, it's clear that we need to simplify the Part B enrollment process," said Rep. Jackie Walorski (R-Ind.), a co-sponsor.

Medicare advocates recommend that people who plan to stay on the job past 65 consult with their State Health Insurance Assistance Programs, which provide free Medicare help, or read the Medicare publication, "Enrolling in Medicare Part A & Part B."

And those who encounter enrollment problems may request what is called "equitable relief," which allows for immediate enrollment in Part B without penalty, from Social Security.

NAVIGATING DELAYED ENROLLMENT

Here are two common scenarios in which people experience Part B enrollment problems—and how to avoid snafus.

If your employer has fewer than 20 workers

If you or your spouse work and receive health insurance on the job, you can choose to enroll in Medicare or remain on the employer's plan.

But workers at firms with fewer than 20 employees must sign up for Medicare Part B at 65 for their primary insurance. Their employer's plan will provide only secondary coverage.

Sue Greeno, an advocate at the Center for Medicare Advocacy, said a client who works for a small company decided not to sign up for Medicare Part B because he assumed he was fully covered under his employer's plan. After having a stroke, he discovered his employer's plan paid only for secondary coverage, forcing him to pay out-of-pocket for the benefits Medicare would have provided.

If you have retiree medical insurance or Cobra coverage

Once an employee stops working, he or she has eight months to sign up for Medicare Part B. Those who miss this window must wait until between Jan. 1 and March 31 to sign up. Their Part B benefits don't go into effect until July. Late-enrollment penalties may apply.

After age 65, Cobra and retiree medical plans generally provide secondary benefits.

To get it, you generally must prove that your failure to enroll was due to an error, misrepresentation or lack of action on the part of a government representative, said Sue Greeno, an advocate at the Center for Medicare Advocacy who recommends keeping track of the names of any government workers you speak with, and the dates of those interactions.

Signing up for a Part D prescription drug plan also generally isn't automatic. Under the rules, individuals can delay signing up for Part D beyond age 65 without penalty if they have "creditable" prescription coverage under another health plan, including under Cobra.

Once that "creditable" coverage is lost, individuals have 63 days to buy a Medicare Part D plan or pay a penalty of 1% of a base premium amount for every month they should have been enrolled. Individuals who miss the 63-day window must wait to enroll between Oct. 15 and Dec. 7. The coverage starts Jan. 1.

Write to Anne Tergesen at anne.tergesen@wsj.com

Joint Statement from Congressman Tim Ryan (OH-13), Congresswoman Lauren Underwood (IL-14), Congressman Anthony Gonzalez (OH-16), Congressman Steve Stivers (OH-15)

Subcommittee on Health
House Committee on Energy & Commerce
2322 Rayburn House Office Building
Wednesday, January 8, 2020 @10:00am

Thank you, Chairman Pallone, Chairwoman Eshoo, Ranking Member Walden, Ranking Member Burgess, and Members of the Committee, for holding this important hearing today. We are thankful the Committee is starting the year off by prioritizing proposals to improve the health of children and for including our bill, the Healthy Start Reauthorization Act (H.R. 4801), in this effort.

According to the Centers for Disease Control and Prevention, for every 1,000 live births in the United States, nearly six babies will not live to see their first birthday. Worse yet, these numbers are twice as high for black infants in our country. Established by President George H.W. Bush in 1991 as a pilot program, the Healthy Start Program is the federal government's primary initiative to reduce infant mortality. The program identifies and supports communities with infant mortality rates that are at least one and a half times the U.S. national average or increasing above the national average.

To carry out these efforts, Healthy Start takes a community-based approach – working with community organizations, universities, and local health departments to deliver services to women and families before, during, and after pregnancy. Over the years, Healthy Start has sought to gradually improve and build off its established infrastructure – adding a greater emphasis on evidence-based practices and the development of facilitation structures to share information and experiences. These strategies have proven to reduce rates of preterm birth, low birthweight, birth defects, maternal complications, prenatal opioid exposure, neonatal abstinence syndrome, and sleep-related deaths. In fact, infant mortality rates in Healthy Start programs are lower than the national average.

Our bill reauthorizes this important program for five years at an annual funding level of $135 million, includes some additional language to encourage coordination with the community in which grantees are located, expands the criteria used to evaluate Healthy Start projects, and instructs the U.S. Government Accountability Office to report back to Congress on this program.

At a time when the need in our communities is so great, we must do all we can to give every child, in every community, a healthy start in life. This vital funding supports our states' most vulnerable communities and ensures more mothers and babies have access to the care they need to reach their fullest potential. Thank you.

Congress of the United States
Washington, DC 20515

October 17, 2017

The Honorable Greg Walden
Chairman
Committee on Energy and Commerce
2125 Rayburn House Office Building
Washington, D.C. 20515

The Honorable Frank Pallone, Jr.
Ranking Member
Committee on Energy and Commerce
2322A Rayburn House Office Building
Washington, D.C. 20515

Dear Chairman Walden and Ranking Member Pallone:

We are writing to express our concern about legislation (H.R. 1394) that would allow states to eliminate Medicaid non-emergency medical transportation (NEMT) for patients that are blind, elderly, or disabled.

As you may be aware, NEMT is an essential component of our nation's health care delivery system, especially in rural areas. According to a recent Kaiser study (see attached chart), over half of Medicaid transportation services are utilized by patients with the highest burden of chronic diseases, including those diagnosed with cancer, HIV, mental health and substance abuse disorders, and end-stage renal disease requiring kidney dialysis three times a week.

NEMT is utilized by roughly 10% of Medicaid enrollees and accounts for only 1% of total Medicaid spending. It is reserved for beneficiaries who have no other means of transportation to and from their medical appointments. State programs help to ensure the benefit is accessible only to those in need.

We believe that the elimination of NEMT would adversely impact both beneficiaries and state budgets. Studies have shown that the benefit has a significant return-on-investment as, over time, health care costs are reduced when patients have appropriate, non-emergency access to care. We would be grateful if you would oppose any attempt to eliminate or undermine Medicaid NEMT and hope that you would support the requirement for States to offer transportation to all Medicaid patients that have no other means to access health services.

Sincerely,

Rep. Sanford D. Bishop, Jr.

Rep. Jim Cooper

Rep. Charlie Crist

Rep. Henry Cuellar

Rep. Vicente Gonzalez

Rep. Josh Gottheimer

Rep. Daniel Lipinski

Rep. Tom O'Halleran

Rep. Collin C. Peterson

Rep. David Scott

Rep. Kyrsten Sinema

Congress of the United States
Washington, DC 20515

February 15, 2019

The Honorable Rosa L. DeLauro
Chairwoman
Subcommittee on Labor, Health and Human Services, Education, and Related Agencies
House Committee on Appropriations
H-305, The Capitol
Washington, D.C. 20515

The Honorable Tom Cole
Ranking Member
Subcommittee on Labor, Health and Human Services, Education, and Related Agencies
House Committee on Appropriations
H-305, The Capitol
Washington, D.C. 20515

Dear Chairwoman DeLauro and Ranking Member Cole:

We are writing to express our concern about a soon-to-be proposed change in a Medicaid regulation that for the first time would allow states to eliminate Medicaid non-emergency medical transportation (NEMT) for patients that are blind, elderly, or disabled. The Medicaid rule, which is expected to be promulgated in May 2019, would repeal long-standing regulations (CFR §431.53) that have been upheld in the courts requiring State plans to include necessary transportation to and from providers.

As you may be aware, NEMT is an essential component of our nation's health care delivery system, especially in rural areas. According to a recent Kaiser study (see attached chart), over half of Medicaid transportation services are utilized by patients with the highest burden of chronic diseases, including those diagnosed with cancer, HIV, mental illness, substance abuse, and end-stage renal disease. In fact, NEMT is vital to many of our constituents who are Medicaid patients. Without this help, they could not access chemotherapy, dialysis, and other services that allow them to remain at home and out of the hospital. NEMT also helps them to travel to their pharmacists to obtain their drug prescriptions and medical supplies.

Currently, NEMT is utilized by roughly 10% of Medicaid enrollees and accounts for only 1% of total Medicaid spending. It is reserved for beneficiaries who have no other means of transportation to and from their medical appointments. State programs help to ensure the benefit is accessible only to those in need.

The elimination of Medicaid NEMT would have an adverse impact both on beneficiaries and state budgets. As members of the Congressional Black Caucus, we respectfully request that the Fiscal Year 2020 Labor-HHS Appropriations bill contain the following legislative language to block implementation of this unwise policy:

> *None of the funds appropriated in this bill or otherwise made available to the Department of Health and Human Services shall be used to publish the proposed regulation in the Fall 2018 Unified Agenda of Regulatory and Deregulatory Actions relating to the Medicaid Nonemergency Medical Transportation benefit for Medicaid beneficiaries expected to be published for comment in May 2019 and promulgated in Fall 2019 (RIN:0938-AT81).*

We would be grateful if you would include this important legislative language in the FY2020 Labor-HHS Appropriations bill and join us in blocking any attempt to eliminate or undermine Medicaid NEMT. It is essential that we retain the requirement for States to offer transportation to all Medicaid patients that have no other means to access health services.

Thank you for your kind attention.

Sincerely,

Rep. Sanford D. Bishop, Jr.

Rep. Alma S. Adams

Rep. Colin Z. Allred

Rep. Karen Bass

Rep. Joyce Beatty

Rep. Lisa Blunt Rochester

Rep. Anthony G. Brown

Rep. G.K. Butterfield

Rep. André Carson

Rep. Yvette D. Clarke

Rep. William Lacy Clay

Rep. James E. Clyburn

Rep. Danny K. Davis

Rep. Val Butler Demings

Rep. Marcia L. Fudge

Rep. Alcee L. Hastings

Rep. Steven Horsford

Rep. Hakeem S. Jeffries

Rep. Henry C. "Hank" Johnson, Jr.

Rep. Brenda L. Lawrence

Rep. Barbara Lee

Rep. Lucy McBath

Rep. Emanuel Cleaver

Rep. Elijah E. Cummings

Rep. Antonio Delgado

Rep. Dwight Evans

Rep. Al Green

Rep. Jahana Hayes

Rep. Sheila Jackson Lee

Rep. Eddie Bernice Johnson

Rep. Robin L. Kelly

Rep. Al Lawson, Jr.

Rep. John Lewis

Rep. A. Donald McEachin

Rep. Gregory W. Meeks

Rep. Gwen Moore

Rep. Joe Neguse

Rep. Eleanor Holmes Norton

Rep. Ilhan Omar

Rep. Donald M. Payne, Jr.

Rep. Stacey E. Plaskett

Rep. Ayanna Pressley

Rep. Cedric L. Richmond

Rep. Bobby L. Rush

Rep. David Scott

Rep. Robert C. "Bobby" Scott

Rep. Terri A. Sewell

Rep. Bennie G. Thompson

Rep. Lauren Underwood

Rep. Marc A. Veasey

Rep. Maxine Waters

Rep. Bonnie Watson Coleman

Rep. Frederica S. Wilson

List of organizations supporting H.R. 3935:

AIDS Action Baltimore
AIDS Alabama
AIDS Alabama South
AIDS Foundation of Chicago
Allies for Independence
American Academy of HIV Medicine
American Association of People with Disabilities
American Association on Health and Disability
American Federation of County and Municipal Employees
American Kidney Fund
American Network of Community Options and Resources
American Public Transportation Association
American Therapeutic Recreation Association
Amida Care
The ARC of the United States
Association of Programs for Rural Independent Living (APRIL)
Autistic Self Advocacy Network
Center for Autism and Related Disorders
Center for Public Representation
Children's Health Fund
Community Catalyst
Community Transportation Association of America
Dialysis Patient Citizens
Disability Rights Education and Defense Fund
Easterseals
Epilepsy Foundation
Equality NC
FamiliesUSA
First Focus Campaign for Children
Global Alliance for Behavioral Health and Social Justice
Greater WI Agency on Aging Resources, Inc. (GWAAR)
HIV Dental Alliance
HIV Medicine Association
Hudson Valley Community Services
Lakeshore Foundation
Los Angeles LGBT Center
Lutheran Services in America
Medical Transportation Access Coalition
Medicare Rights Center
Mental Health America
Michael J. Fox Foundation for Parkinson's Research
National Adult Day Services Association (NADSA)
National Alliance on Mental Illness
National Association for Children's Behavioral Health

National Association of Area Agencies on Aging (n4a)
National Association of Directors of Developmental Disabilities Services
National Association of Nutrition and Aging Services Programs (NANASP)
National Consumer Voice for Quality Long-Term Care
National Council on Aging
National Healthcare for the Homeless Council
Nevada Disability Coalition
Pennsylvania Council on Independent Living
Schizophrenia And Related Disorders Alliance of America
SKIL Resource Center
The Transportation Alliance
Treatment Action Group
Treatment Communities of America
United Spinal Association
WI Association of Mobility Managers (WAMM)

Last Updated January 7, 2020

Non-Emergency Medical Transportation: Findings from a Return on Investment Study

Americans with low incomes may lack access to reliable transportation, and lack reliable of transportation can lead to missed medical appointments and poor health outcomes. To check this problem, Non-Emergency Medical Transportation ("NEMT")—free or low-cost transport to medical appointments for beneficiaries who need it—has been a mandatory Medicaid benefit since the program's inception in 1966. It is codified in regulation.[1] States can limit its availability through federal waivers. The Trump Administration's budget would allow states to limit the benefit without seeking a waiver.[2] Indiana and Iowa do not provide the benefit to a most beneficiaries within their Medicaid expansion populations, and Kentucky and Massachusetts plan to do so.[3]

We face an unusual moment where NEMT is being expanded across multiple health insurance markets even as it faces curtailment in Medicaid.[4] Perhaps this is because we lack strong evidence of the financial benefit of NEMT, although a few studies have offered positive savings frameworks.[5] Because there is limited research on the financial benefit of NEMT, the Medical Transportation Access Coalition commissioned Faegre Baker Daniels Consulting, Wakely Consulting Group, and Patricia Salber, M.D., to conduct a first of its kind study to examine NEMT's return on investment. The findings suggest that NEMT more than pays for itself as part of a care management strategy for people with chronic diseases, resulting in a total positive return on investment of over $40 million per month ($480 million annually) per 30,000 Medicaid beneficiaries. The methodology used to conduct the study and calculate disease specific results is detailed below.

Methodology Used to Calculate ROI

The financial benefit of NEMT is likely to be shown most clearly in the costs avoided due to increased utilization of lower cost medical services (i.e., physician appointments) to increase adherent treatment care. The theory goes: missed medical appointments lead to deviations from clinical guidelines which, in turn, lead to complications and increased expensive medical services, such as hospitalizations. Therefore, for each disease and corresponding treatment, our ROI methodology involved: (1) determining the present-state treatment volumes of NEMT users and expected future-state treatment volumes if NEMT were not provided; (2) calculating the difference in total medical costs at the present-state and future-state treatment volume levels; (3) subtracting the cost of NEMT from change in total medical costs; and (4) extrapolating the per member per month ROI to the appropriate disease population.

[1] See: https://www.healthaffairs.org/do/10.1377/hblog20180608.971229/full/ . See also: 42 CFR § 431.53: "Assurance of transportation. A State plan must—(a) Specify that the Medicaid agency will ensure necessary transportation for recipients to and from providers; and (b) Describe the methods that the agency will use to meet this requirement."

[2] Per the President's budget: "Make Medicaid Non-Emergency Medical Transportation Optional: Under current regulations, states are required to provide Non-Emergency Medical Transportation to all Medicaid beneficiaries. The Budget commits to using regulatory authority to change provision of this benefit from mandatory to optional." See also: https://www.hhs.gov/sites/default/files/fy-2019-budget-in-brief.pdf

[3] Iowa, Indiana, and Kentucky eliminate the benefit for most non-medically frail adults covered by Medicaid expansion; Massachusetts and Arizona may implement similar cuts.

[4] See: https://www.healthaffairs.org/do/10.1377/hblog20170920.062063/full/

[5] A 2008 study conducted by Florida State University concluded that if only 1 percent of the medical trips funded resulted in the avoidance of an emergency department visit, the payback to the State would be 1108 percent. A 2013 study in the *Journal of Health Economics and Outcomes Research* examined the high costs of ambulance transportation and suggested that greater use of public transportation and NEMT might save as much as $1 billion a year.

Calculating Medical Costs by Treatment Volumes

Six diseases and corresponding treatments were identified as potentially having sufficient monthly treatment volumes to be evaluated for this study: (1) wound care for diabetic wounds, (2) dialysis for kidney disease, (3) treatment for bipolar disorder, (4) treatment for schizophrenia, (5) adult day care for dementia, and (6) treatment for substance use disorder. We reviewed 2014 and 2015 Medicaid claims for each type of treatment using the Truven Health MarketScan® Database. For each disease and treatment, medical claims, pharmacy claims, and long-term care claims for members[6] enrolled during the 24-month period were processed based on the following logic:

1. Members were identified based on an initial indicator claim and the earliest date of treatment was recorded (the "identification date"). Members whose identification date was after August 31, 2015, were excluded from the analysis. This restriction was included to ensure that an adequate number of months were used to determine the monthly adherence rate (defined below).

2. Adherence events occurring after the identification date were counted and recorded, and members were segmented by the number of days containing an adherence event post-identification divided by the member months post-identification (the "monthly adherence rate").

3. All medical costs for each monthly adherence rate segment were summed together and divided by the total number of member months for the segment to determine the average total medical costs per member per month for the segment.

4. Finally, monthly adherence rate segments were combined based on clinical treatment protocols and medical cost changes, and very low volume treatment segments were excluded.

Additional parameters were used for dialysis and diabetic wound care. Members identified as having had a kidney transplant were removed from the analysis at the date of transplant. Members with wound care treatments spanning fewer than sixty days were not included in this study and the observation window used to calculate the monthly adherence rate for the remaining members was limited to sixteen weeks during the 24-month period after the initial treatment, since regular treatment for a wound is generally limited to 16 weeks. We did not find credible population sizes or claims for bipolar disorder, schizophrenia, and adult day care for dementia. Hence, these diseases were dropped from the analysis. The following charts show the average total medical costs for each of the remaining conditions by monthly adherence rate categories.

[6] We use the term "members" in this paper in the interest of conforming with common health insurance industry terminology (i.e., per-member per-month). Use of this term is not meant to imply that this study controlled for a managed care delivery system. Rather, both the claims dataset and survey included a mix of fee-for-service and managed care enrollees.

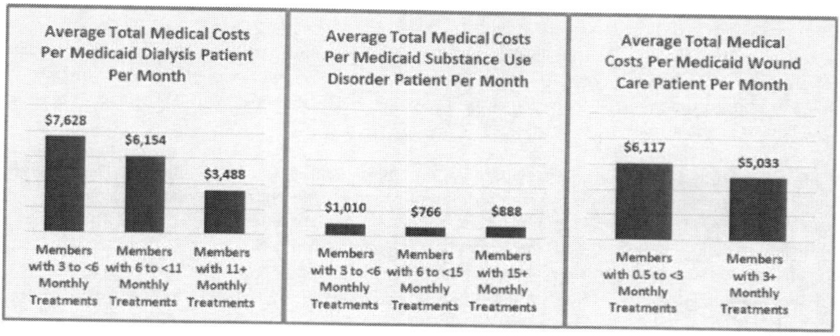

Survey to Determine Treatment Volumes with and without NEMT

To determine the present-state treatment volumes of NEMT users and expected future-state treatment volumes if NEMT were not provided, we surveyed Medicaid beneficiaries who use NEMT to attend their medical appointments. We surveyed Medicaid beneficiaries in New Jersey, Louisiana, and Michigan who use NEMT services provided by LogistiCare, the nation's largest NEMT broker.

We asked survey participants the following questions: what disease treatment he or she uses NEMT to attend; whether he or she has access to public or private transportation; what type of NEMT he or she uses; how many treatments he or she attends per month and uses NEMT to attend; how many treatments he or she would attend per month absent the availability of NEMT; how his or her health has been affected by NEMT; and what would happen if NEMT were not provided.

The survey vendor collected 460 surveys from respondents who self-identified as dialysis patients, 311 who self-identified as substance use disorder patients, and 206 who self-identified as diabetic wound care patients. We then calculated the self-reported average treatment volumes with and without NEMT per disease/treatment. See the averages and standard deviations below. (Note: nearly all survey respondents reported that they used NEMT to attend all of their treatments.)

Dialysis			Treatment for SUD			Wound Care		
Survey Count	Average Treatments per Month with NEMT (SD)	Average Expected Treatments per Month without NEMT (SD)	Survey Count	Average Treatments per Month with NEMT (SD)	Average Expected Treatments per Month without NEMT (SD)	Survey Count	Average Treatments per Month with NEMT (SD)	Average Expected Treatments per Month without NEMT (SD)
460	12.0 (1.5)	4.1 (5.3)	311	16.4 (6.1)	4.3 (7.2)	206	5.5 (3.7)	1.3 (2.7)

Overall, 58% of respondents reported that they would make none of their treatments if NEMT were not provided, 22% reported that they would make all of their treatments if NEMT were not provided, and

20% reported that they would make less than all but more than none of their treatments if NEMT were not provided. Importantly, in open-ended response to the question "what would happen if you did not have the transportation ride services you currently receive," 103 respondents (10%) reported that they would die or probably die.

We found limited variation in the survey data by different demographics. No significant variations were found between members in different states, different genders, different marital statuses, different ethnicities, different living environments (urban/rural/suburban), or different age ranges. The only significant variations were found between members that responded "yes" or "no" to the question "do you have access to public or private transportation. "Yes" respondents were approximately two times higher on average than "no" respondents in projecting the number of expected treatments per month without NEMT.

Specific Disease Results

A positive ROI was found for both dialysis for kidney disease and wound care for diabetes. The study failed to determine a positive ROI for SUD, though we believe our methods were ill-suited for SUD treatment and might have had better results under different study parameters.

Survey respondents reported attending 12.0 dialysis treatments per month on average with NEMT and would expect to attend 4.1 treatments per month without NEMT. The Medicaid cost analysis shows that dialysis patients who attend 3 to 6 dialysis treatments per month incur on average $4,140 more per month in total medical costs than dialysis patients who attend 11+ dialysis treatments per month.[7] The cost of the average round trip of NEMT for dialysis patients (based on private broker data) is $60.24, so the average cost of NEMT per survey respondent per month for dialysis is 11.9[8] x $60.24 = $717.25. Therefore, the Medicaid cost avoided due to NEMT per survey respondent per month is $4,140 – $717.25 = $3,423. Assuming that the survey represents at least 10,000 like Medicaid members, the ROI of NEMT for treating kidney disease with dialysis per 10,000 members per month is $34,229,448.

Survey respondents reported attending 16.4 treatments for SUD per month on average with NEMT and would expect to attend 4.3 treatments for SUD per month without NEMT. The Medicaid cost analysis shows that SUD members who attend 3 to 6 treatments per month incur on average $123 more per month in total medical costs than SUD members who attend 15+ SUD treatments per month. The cost of the average round trip of NEMT for SUD patients (based on private broker data) is $20.47, so the average cost of NEMT per survey respondent per month for SUD is 16.3 x $20.47 = $333.71. Therefore, the Medicaid cost avoided due to NEMT per survey respondent per month is $123 – $333.71 = ($211). Assuming that the survey represents at least 10,000 like Medicaid members, the ROI of NEMT for treating SUD per 10,000 members per month is ($2,109,779). While our analysis does not yield positive ROI for SUD transportation, we believe different study parameters, i.e., a longer claims analysis period, relapse rates, quantification of social costs (e.g., increased employment and productivity, less law enforcement and judicial system costs, less strain on child services agencies and foster care system), likely would have led to positive ROI.

---

[7] We note that alignment with the survey results with the similar average bucket is a simplifying assumption as the distribution may be non-normal. However, given data limitations, we believe this assumption is appropriate.

[8] The average NEMT round trips per member per month (11.9) is slightly less than average treatments per member per month for dialysis (12) since a few dialysis survey respondents reported that they used NEMT to attend less than all of their treatments.

For diabetic wound care, survey respondents reported attending 5.5 wound care treatments per month on average with NEMT and would expect to attend 1.3 treatments per month without NEMT. The Medicaid cost analysis shows that wound care patients who attend 0.5 to 3 wound care treatments per month incur on average $1,084 more monthly medical costs than wound care patients who attend 3+ wound care treatments per month. The cost of the average round trip of NEMT for wound care patients (based on private broker data) is $53.25, so the average cost of NEMT per survey respondent per month for wound care is 5.5 x $53.25 = $291.96. Therefore, the Medicaid cost avoided due to NEMT per survey respondent per month is $1,084 – $291.96 = $792. Assuming that the survey represents at least 10,000 like Medicaid members, the ROI of NEMT for attending diabetic wound care treatments per 10,000 members per month is $7,920,635.

Disease/ Treatment	Average Treat. per Month with NEMT	Average Monthly Medical Cost with NEMT	Average Treat. per Month without NEMT	Average Monthly Medical Cost without NEMT	Average Monthly Medical Cost Increase without NEMT	Average Cost per NEMT Round Trip	Average NEMT Round Trips PMPM	Total Cost of NEMT PMPM	Avg. ROI of NEMT PMPM	ROI Per 10,000 Members Per Month
Dialysis for Kidney Disease	12.0	$3,488	4.1	$7,628	$4,140	$60.24	11.9	$717.25	$3,423	$34,229,448
Treatment for Substance Use	16.4	$888	4.3	$1,010	$123	$20.47	16.3	$333.71	($211)	($2,109,779)
Wound Care for Diabetes	5.5	$5,033	1.3	$6,117	$1,084	$53.25	5.5	$291.96	$792	$7,920,635

For all conditions, the total ROI per month is $40,040,304 (per 30,000 members; 10,000 in each condition).

Policy Implications

The significant positive ROI associated with dialysis and wound care transport demonstrate that, at least for these conditions and presumably others (such as asthma and heart disease), curtailing NEMT is penny-wise, pound-foolish. While our analysis does not yield positive ROI for SUD transportation, we believe that speaks to study limitations rather than the value of the benefit. The data presented above offers a strong indication that NEMT more than pays for itself as part of a care management strategy for people with chronic diseases within and outside of Medicaid.

To learn more about this study, contact: Tricia Beckmann Tricia.Beckmann@faegrebd.com.

Study Authors: Michael Adelberg; Patricia Salber,M.D.; Taylor Pruisner, FSA, MAAA;, Michael Cohen, PhD.; Aaron Dobosenski, JD

The authors thank the Medical Transportation Access Coalition for supporting this research. We also thank Tricia Beckmann and Kacey Stotler for their important contributions to this project.

CVSHealth

CVS Health Applauds Introduction of Key Legislation Ensuring Kidney Transplant Patients Can Maintain Medicare Coverage of Immunosuppressive Drugs

WOONSOCKET, R.I., [January 8, 2020] — CVS Health issued the following statement today regarding the introduction of the *Comprehensive Immunosuppressive Drug Coverage for Kidney Transplant Patients Act of 2019* in the United States Congress:

Tens of thousands of people in the United States have kidney transplants each year and taking immunosuppressant medications is key to the success of each patient's journey. Unfortunately, when kidney patients are without health coverage, they too often stop taking these medications and in turn, redevelop kidney failure. CVS Health applauds reintroduction of the *Comprehensive Immunosuppressive Drug Coverage for Kidney Transplant Patients Act of 2019*, legislation that ensures kidney transplant patients can maintain access to Medicare Part B coverage for immunosuppressant drugs after it currently expires, if no other coverage is available.

As a company committed to patient-centric and clinically-optimal kidney care, we support policies like these that have the potential to improve the lives of kidney disease patients. CVS Health is focused on reshaping the patient experience through CVS Kidney Care and will continue to advance new kidney disease management programs while also developing new technologies to treat kidney failure. We applaud Representatives Michael Burgess (R-TX) and Ron Kind (D-WI) for championing this important legislation.

About CVS Health

CVS Health is the nation's premier health innovation company helping people on their path to better health. Whether in one of its pharmacies or through its health services and plans, CVS Health is pioneering a bold new approach to total health by making quality care more affordable, accessible, simple and seamless. CVS Health is community-based and locally focused, engaging consumers with the care they need when and where they need it. The Company has approximately 9,900 retail locations, approximately 1,100 walk-in medical clinics, a leading pharmacy benefits manager with approximately 102 million plan members, a dedicated senior pharmacy care business serving more than one million patients per year and expanding specialty pharmacy services. CVS Health also serves an estimated 38 million people through traditional, voluntary and consumer-directed health insurance products and related services, including rapidly expanding Medicare Advantage offerings and a leading standalone Medicare Part D prescription drug plan. The Company believes its innovative health care model increases access to quality care, delivers better health outcomes and lowers overall health care costs. Find more information about how CVS Health is shaping the future of health at https://www.cvshealth.com.

# # #

AMERICAN SOCIETY FOR HISTOCOMPATIBILITY & IMMUNOGENETICS
1120 Route 73 • Suite 200 • Mt. Laurel, NJ 08054
Phone: 856.638.0428 • Fax: 856.439.0525 • Web site: www.ashi-hla.org • E-mail: info@ashi-hla.org

ASHI
AMERICAN SOCIETY FOR HISTOCOMPATIBILITY & IMMUNOGENETICS

January 8, 2020

The Honorable Anna Eshoo
Chair
House Committee on Energy and Commerce
Subcommittee on Health
U.S. House of Representatives
2125 Rayburn House Office Building
Washington DC 20515

The Honorable Michael Burgess
Ranking Member
House Committee on Energy and Commerce
Subcommittee on Health
U.S. House of Representatives
2322-A Rayburn House Office Building
Washington DC 20515

Dear Chairwoman Eshoo and Ranking Member Burgess:

On behalf of the American Society for Histocompatibility and Immunogenetics (ASHI), we appreciate the Subcommittee's work to improve Americans' health care coverage and outcomes by highlighting current deficiencies in Medicare coverage of immunosuppressive drugs for kidney transplant patients.

ASHI is a professional association of clinical and research professionals dedicated to advancing the science and application of histocompatibility and immunogenetics. The compatibility testing performed by ASHI members is an integral component of successful kidney transplantation, and the organization strongly supports policies strengthening the continued success of these transplants by decreasing the likelihood of preventable rejection. H.R. 5534, the *Comprehensive Immunosuppressive Drug Coverage for Kidney Transplant Patients Act of 2019*, would provide this vital support by permanently removing the harmful 36-month Medicare coverage limit on immunosuppressive drugs post-transplant.

Given the significant number of patients awaiting transplants and the limited supply of transplantable kidneys, ASHI encourages the Subcommittee to support and advance H.R. 5534 to bolster the long-term success of kidney transplants. If ASHI can be of any assistance, please contact Katherine Giovetsis at kgiovetsis@ashi-hla.org.

Thank you for work on this important issue.

Sincerely,

Medhat Askar

Medhat Askar, MD, PhD, D(ABHI)

DENVER RIGGLEMAN
5TH DISTRICT, VIRGINIA

COMMITTEE ON
FINANCIAL SERVICES

1022 LONGWORTH HOUSE OFFICE BUILDING
WASHINGTON, DC 20515
(202) 225-4711

686 BORKMAR CIRCLE
CHARLOTTESVILLE, VA 22901
(434) 973-9631

308 CRAGHEAD STREET
SUITE 102-D
DANVILLE, VA 24541
(434) 791-2596

Congress of the United States
House of Representatives
Washington, DC 20515–4605

January 8, 2020

Chairwoman Anna Eshoo
House Committee on Energy & Commerce
Subcommittee on Health
2125 Rayburn House Office Building
Washington, DC 20515

Ranking Member Michael Burgess
House Committee on Energy & Commerce
Subcommittee on Health
2322 Rayburn House Office Building
Washington, DC 20515

Dear Chairwoman Eshoo and Ranking Member Burgess,

I write today to thank you for your leadership in recognizing a loophole in our nation's health system that impacts the lives of patients suffering from congenital anomalies and their families. H.R. 1379, the Ensuring Lasting Smiles Act, is a bipartisan bill I introduced with Congressman Collin Peterson (D-MN) to ensure that all health plans cover medically necessary services, including reconstructive surgeries and oral-related procedures, resulting from congenital anomalies or birth defects. I strongly support this bill and urge the committee to support it.

Approximately 4 percent of children born in the United States have congenital anomalies or birth defects that affect the way they look, develop, or function, often with repercussions that affect them for the rest of their lives. Many born with congenital anomalies suffer from severe oral and facial defects such as a cleft lip or palate, skeletal and maxillofacial deformities, hypodontia, and enamel hypoplasia. The patients who do not have their craniofacial and other anomalies treated often face long-term physical and psychological injuries.

Many health plans provide coverage for congenital anomalies, and many states require insurers to provide coverage of any health services related to congenital anomalies or birth defects. Despite this, health plans systematically and routinely deny claims and appeals for any oral or dental related procedures – such as reconstructive surgery for a cleft palate – under the pretense that such service is merely cosmetic or covered under separate dental plans. This is common practice across the country and leaves families with the burden of paying for treatment or procedures that are necessary for their child to function. Additionally, when private insurance denies a patient's reconstructive surgery, families may end up turning to Medicaid, SCHIP, or other state-sponsored programs for coverage, increasing costs for taxpayers.

The Ensuring Lasting Smiles Act will close the loopholes and unintended coverage gaps that health insurers use to bypass state congenital anomaly laws. It will ensure they meet their contractual obligations to approve claims for medically necessary treatments of congenital anomalies and make sure children suffering from birth defects and anomalies get the treatment they need.

Thank you again for your leadership on this important issue, and I urge the committee to support the Ensuring Lasting Smiles Act.

Sincerely,

Denver Riggleman
Member of Congress

Attachments—Additional Questions for the Record

Subcommittee on Health
Hearing on
"Legislation to Improve American's Health Care Coverage and Outcomes"
January 8, 2020

Lee Savio Beers, M.D.
President Elect
American Academy of Pediatrics

The Honorable Gus M. Bilirakis (R-FL)

1. Dr. Beers - According to the CDC, for every 1,000 live births in the United States, nearly 6 babies will not live to see their first birthday. Additionally, 1 in 10 babies is born premature, the leading cause of infant death. Statistics get even worse when racial and other disparities are accounted for. However, infant mortality rates in Healthy Start programs are lower than the national average.

   a. *How is Healthy Start achieving this critical mission to protect our youngest, most-vulnerable citizens – our infants?*

   Healthy Start aims to screen all pregnant women and families for risk factors such as physical and behavioral health, employment, housing, and potential for domestic violence. Healthy Start connects women, children, and families at high risk with continuous access to essential health care and support services that help reduce infant mortality rates, leading to a rate that is lower than the national average. The program offers key support services including case management, home visitation, enhancement of parenting skills, transportation, child care, breast feeding and nutrition support.

   Healthy Start also attempts to alleviate racial and ethnic disparities among maternal and infant birth outcomes by providing intensive and culturally sensitive parent support. Furthermore, the program helps remove barriers to accessing health care by facilitating enrollment of eligible women and children in Medicaid or exchange plans.

      i. *Why is it important to deliver services to women and families not just during pregnancy, but also pre and post-pregnancy?*

      Delivering high quality health care and social services at all stages of pregnancy, including prenatal and postpartum, as well as preconception care, is critical for the health of both mother and baby. Appropriate preconception, prenatal and primary care can help women minimize potentially preventable risk factors for poor pregnancy and birth outcomes, including chronic disease management, avoidance of addictive behaviors and environmental exposures (i.e.: smoking, alcohol, and chemicals), and preventive health measures (i.e.: immunizations, dental hygiene, and vitamins). Additionally, prenatal services can help provide education to women and families on what to anticipate during pregnancy and also provide specialized education for those who may be at higher risk for complications, such as women with genetic disorders.

Furthermore, postpartum care and services help monitor the health and development, including physical, social, and psychological well-being, of both the infant and the mother during the period following childbirth. Lactation counseling or connection to treatment for maternal depression, for example, are some of the critical services that can be provided during the postpartum period.

b. *What is the average first year cost of care for babies born premature?*

In 2007, the Institute of Medicine reported that the cost associated with premature birth in the United States was $26.2 billion each year ($51,600 per infant annually) through the age of 5. These costs included $16.9 billion in medical and health care costs for the baby ($33,200 per infant), with 85% or $28,500 of these costs occurring in the first year of life. The remaining $1.9 billion encompassed the labor and delivery costs for mothers, totaling $3,800 per infant.

A 2014 Centers for Medicare and Medicaid Services report indicated that state Medicaid programs are paying for an increasing proportion of births and costly complicated births, and a September 2017 *Pediatrics* study noted that, in 2013, employer-sponsored plans spent $2 billion on care of infants. Eight percent of those were born prematurely but cost 1/3 of the aggregate sum.

i. *What is the long-term cost of medical and social services provided to premature babies?*

For preterm infants, the 2007 Institute of Medicine report indicated an associated $2.535 billion total in medical and health care costs, or $4,980 annually after the first year of life on average. These costs include:

- $611 million for early intervention services ($1,200 per infant), which are programs for children from birth to age 3 with disabilities and developmental delays. These services teach families strategies and interventions that help children acquire physical, cognitive, language, social and self-help skills to their full potential.
- $1.1 billion for special education services ($2,200 per infant) that are specifically designed for children with disabilities ages 3 through 21.
- Benefits from the Supplemental Security Income (SSI) program, which are provided to adults and children with disabilities who have limited income and resources.

The cost of medical care beyond early childhood is not reflected in the above numbers. Conditions that are more common in children who were born prematurely include but are not limited to the following

- Behavioral and emotional problems
- Attention deficit hyperactivity disorder (ADHD)
- Cerebral palsy
- Chronic lung disease – abnormal lung development due to premature birth and/or to oxygen therapy and ventilator support that predisposes them to more severe respiratory diseases throughout childhood

- Asthma
- Intestinal problems, e.g. due to necrotizing enterocolitis, a potentially lethal neonatal complication with lifelong implications on nutrition and growth due to short gut and/or impaired gut function
- Dental problems
- Vision or hearing impairment

Responses to Additional Questions for the Record by Kenneth Mendez
President and CEO
Asthma and Allergy Foundation of America
February 27, 2020

Subcommittee on Health
Hearing on
"Legislation to Improve Americans' Health Care Coverage and Outcomes"
January 8, 2019

The Honorable Lisa Blunt Rochester (D-DE)

1. H.R. 2468, the School-Based Allergies and Asthma Management Program, would create a preference within the CDC's National Asthma Control grant program for states that meet a specific set of standards. What are the benefits of taking the AAFA's Honor Roll findings into account when the grant preference standards are being developed?

AAFA's State Honor Roll report tracks state requirements related to asthma and allergy in schools. Our original standards were developed in consultation with a team of experts to reflect key steps that are reasonable for states to protect school-aged children. Over the years, we have seen some remarkable gains. In 2013, only eight states were on AAFA's State Honor Roll, having met at least 18 of our 23 standards; today, 15 states are on the State Honor Roll, and many others have added requirements. We produce the State Honor Roll report to measure and incentivize progress in state policies, and we believe it has made a difference.

H.R. 2468 establishes certain criteria for school asthma and allergy control programs in order for states to qualify for a preference in National Asthma Control Funding. We understand that CDC would likely flesh out the specific parameters of these requirements. Many of the standards in AAFA's State Honor Roll report provide a guide to meet some of the requirements in H.R. 2468. We hope that AAFA's past work in this area can serve as a helpful resource for CDC and states in this process.

2. Despite the progress you've seen in the number of states making the honor roll over the past few years, your testimony mentioned that there are still gaps that should be addressed. What are some of those gaps?

There is indeed still significant room for improvement in many states' approaches to asthma and allergy in schools. For example:

- **Only 27 states require schools to have emergency protocols for asthma.**
- **Only 36 states require emergency protocols for anaphylaxis.**

- **Only 24 states require schools to maintain allergy and asthma incidence reports.**
- **Only 12 states require schools to have indoor air quality management plans.**
- **Only eight states set a minimum nurse-to-student ratio for schools, despite the central role school nurses play in helping manage and respond to asthma and allergy in schools.**

These gaps concern us, but we believe that the many states that have led the way on these and other indicators have laid the groundwork for other states to follow.

The Honorable Michael C. Burgess (R-TX)

1. Can you share how you measure a state's progress in addressing either asthma and allergies within its populations, and what challenges states are facing in implementing plans to address this growing epidemic?

AAFA measures a state's progress in addressing either asthma or allergies within its populations in a variety of ways. For example, AAFA publishes the Asthma Capitals report each year to raise awareness about the nationwide impacts of asthma and to help people who live in Asthma Capitals recognize, prevent and manage asthma symptoms. AAFA's Asthma Capitals™ 2019 Report analyzes data from across the continental United States and ranks the 100 largest cities where it is challenging to live with asthma. The report ranks cities by the most critical of health outcomes – asthma prevalence, emergency department visits due to asthma attacks and asthma mortality. The report also identifies risk factors that influence health outcomes.

The ranking is based on analysis of data from the 100 most populated Metropolitan Statistical Areas (MSAs) in the contiguous 48 states. The three individual factors analyzed for the 2019 rankings are: estimated asthma prevalence; crude death rate from asthma; and emergency department visits due to asthma. For each factor, AAFA used the most recently available calendar year(s) data. Weights are applied to each factor; factors are not weighted equally. Total scores are calculated as a composite of all three factors, and cities are ranked from highest total score (city rank #1) to lowest total score (city rank #100).

Another way that AAFA measures a state's progress in addressing either asthma or allergies within its populations is through our annual State Honor Roll report of Asthma and Allergy Policies in Schools report. AAFA's 2019 State Honor Roll of Asthma and Allergy Policies for Schools ranks the states with the best public policies for people with asthma, food allergies, anaphylaxis and related allergic diseases in U.S. elementary, middle and high schools. The report checks to see how every state compares against 23 key measures that affect people with asthma and allergies in schools. States make the honor roll when they meet 18 of 23 core policies.

In addition to our analysis and reports, AAFA works with volunteers and stakeholders across the country to track state laws and policies and to provide valuable assistance to state and local governments implementing asthma and allergy policies. AAFA's four

regional chapters work with volunteers, health care providers, and local government and leaders to track and report on states' progress in addressing asthma and allergies.

Despite this work, many states face challenges implementing plans and policies that address asthma and allergies. Ten people per day lose their life to asthma. Although older adults are at the highest risk of fatality, asthma disproportionately affects children from low-income families. Some of the top risk factors for asthma that may impact a state's success in effectively addressing asthma in their state include poverty, lack of health insurance for state residents, poor air quality and anti-smoking laws, to name a few.

To address the challenges faced by states trying to address the growing burden of asthma, states should:

- **Track asthma rates and the effectiveness of control measures so continuous improvements can be made in prevention efforts**
- **Improve asthma care through policies and funding that promote and support:**
  - **Free asthma screening programs**
  - **Influenza (flu) and pneumonia vaccination for people with asthma**
  - **Preexisting conditions coverage protections**
  - **Medicaid and Medicare expansion to cover poor, uninsured people**
  - **Affordable drugs and copayments**
  - **Asthma education and intervention programs**
  - **Asthma management plans in schools**
  - **Nurses in every school**
  - **Promote improvements in indoor air quality for people with asthma through measures such as smoke-free air laws and policies, healthy schools and workplaces, home improvements and remediation for low income housing**
- **Support policies that reduce air pollution and improve outdoor air quality**
- **Implement tobacco prevention programs and vaping/e-cig interventions for teens and children**
- **Support and fund primary, secondary and tertiary asthma prevention research**
- **Include people with asthma in all levels of planning for asthma-related interventions and**

- **Oppose step therapy for drug coverage that does not have adequate patient protections and may force patients to take a drug that is not designed to treat their specific health circumstances, negatively impacting care.**

Finally, while certainly not the only way to address broader systemic challenges, increased funding for the CDC's National Asthma Control Program (NACP) could go a long way toward helping states address some of the challenges they face with asthma. NACP awards competitive grants to states for efforts aimed at reducing the number of asthma deaths, hospitalizations, and visits to the emergency room; reducing the number of missed school and workdays; and helping people with asthma be active without limitation. AAFA believes strongly that this grant program provides valuable support and expertise to states and that the program should receive expanded funding and be expanded to all fifty states.

In addition to asthma, states face significant challenges addressing the burden of allergies. An allergy could result from something you eat, inhale into your lungs, inject into your body or touch. For example, nearly 32 million people are affected by food allergies in the United States alone. Between 2005 and 2014, there was a nearly 200 percent increase in food allergy-related emergency department visits among children 5-17 years old. Having asthma also puts a child with food allergies at higher risk of fatal outcomes. Additionally, indoor environmental exposure to allergens, such as dust mites and mold, is a common trigger of asthma symptoms in children. These allergens are common in schools. To address these challenges, states should:

- **Continue efforts to require stocking of both epinephrine auto-injectors and quick-relief asthma medication in schools.**
- **Make sure schools are equipped to obtain the medicine and know how to use it. Increase the number of school nurses.**
- **Remove barriers to putting these laws into practice, whether that means more funding, awareness or training.**
- **Refresh or develop programs to improve air quality, both for indoor air pollution and outdoor air pollution in the school environment.**
- **Encourage innovation and partnerships between government and private companies (public-private partnerships)**
- **Ensure that their school's policies are in line with federal and state laws that protect all who live with food and other allergies.**

a. Would legislation such as H.R. 2468, the School-Based Allergies and Asthma Management Program Act address these problems without additional federal costs?

Yes. H.R. 2468 would create an incentive for states through an existing competitive grant program, the National Asthma Control Program (NACP). The bill would not authorize any additional funds, but would simply instruct CDC to create a preference within the NACP program for states that meet certain criteria related to asthma and allergy in schools.

It is also important to note that many free resources are available to assist states, districts and schools in establishing school-based allergy and asthma programs. For example, the American Academy of Allergy, Asthma and Immunology has developed the School-Based Asthma Management Program (SAMPRO™), a comprehensive toolkit that addresses asthma management, staff education, school environment, and other components of a school-based response to asthma.[1]

The Honorable Gus M. Bilirakis (R-FL)

The Department of Education and the Department of Health and Human Services have recommended that schools have comprehensive asthma management programs; however, many schools do not have such programs in place.

1. How does the School-Based Allergies and Asthma Management Program Act encourage states to implement these programs so that schools are better equipped to help students with asthma manage their disease?

The School-Based Allergies and Asthma Management Program Act (H.R. 2468) would encourage states to implement comprehensive asthma programs by creating a preference within the National Asthma Control Program, or NACP. The NACP is an existing CDC program that funds a broad range of state asthma activities. The NACP is a competitive grant program, and the bill instructs the CDC to develop a preference for states that meet certain criteria, including having "a comprehensive school-based allergies and asthma program that includes—

"(I) a method to identify all students of such school with a diagnosis of allergies and asthma;

"(II) an individual student allergies and asthma action plan for each student of such school with a diagnosis of allergies and asthma;

"(III) allergies and asthma education for school staff who are directly responsible for students who have been identified as having allergies or asthma, such as education regarding basics, management, trigger management, and comprehensive emergency responses with respect to allergies and asthma;

---

[1] AAAI, "School-Based Asthma Management Program (SAMPRO™)." Available at https://www.aaaai.org/conditions-and-treatments/school-tools/SAMPRO

"(IV) efforts to reduce the presence of environmental triggers of allergies and asthma; and

"(V) a system to support students with a diagnosis of allergies or asthma through coordination with family members of such students, primary care providers of such students, and others as necessary."

To receive a preference in applications for NACP funding, states would have to meet these components, and require schools to have a nurse or other personnel trained to administer asthma and allergy medication onsite during operating hours.

AAFA believes that these elements are crucial components of a comprehensive school response to asthma. We do strongly support increased appropriations to the NACP, to provide funding not only for school-based asthma activities, but for all of the crucial asthma control work taking place at the state level.

Attachments—Additional Questions for the Record

Subcommittee on Health
Hearing on
"Legislation to Improve American's Health Care Coverage and Outcomes"
December 4, 2019

Frederic Riccardi
President
Medicare Rights Center

The Honorable Gus M. Bilirakis (R-FL)

1. **What is credible coverage and does Medicare recognize all forms of health insurance coverage as credible coverage?**

"Creditable coverage" is a specific term with applicability to Medicare Part D. It refers to prescription drug coverage that is expected to pay, on average, as much as the standard Medicare prescription drug coverage.[1]

Creditable coverage can be from job-based insurance or from other sources such as federal programs or retiree plans. Every year, health plans must notify enrollees whether their drug coverage is creditable.

This classification is important because those who maintain enrollment in creditable drug coverage can avoid a late enrollment penalty (LEP) for delaying Part D. They can also access a two-month Special Enrollment Period (SEP) to enroll in a Part D plan.

Similarly, though there is no "creditable coverage" under Part B, certain Medicare-eligible individuals can access a Part B SEP that allows them to sign up outside of the normal enrollment timelines without being subject to the LEP that would normally accrue.

The Part B SEP is only available to people with coverage from current employment (from their job, their spouse's job, or sometimes a family member's job) who have been continuously insured since becoming eligible for Medicare. The Part B SEP begins when the individual is in their first month of Part B eligibility and ends eight months after they lose coverage from current work.[2]

[1] Medicare Rights Center, Medicare Interactive. "Creditable drug coverage," https://www.medicareinteractive.org/get-answers/coordinating-medicare-with-other-types-of-insurance/coordination-of-benefits-basics/creditable-drug-coverage.
[2] Medicare Rights Center, Medicare Interactive. "Enrolling in Medicare with job-based insurance," https://www.medicareinteractive.org/get-answers/coordinating-medicare-with-other-types-of-insurance/job-based-insurance-and-medicare/enrolling-in-medicare-with-job-based-insurance.

Mr. Frederic Riccardi
Page 2

However, just because someone has access to this enrollment pathway doesn't mean they should delay Part B in reliance on it. Before making this decision, those who qualify for the Part B SEP must also endeavor to understand Medicare's intricate coordination of benefits requirements. These rules govern how other types of insurance works with Medicare. Specifically, which pays first, or primary, and which pays secondary.

The rules are different for each type of insurance. For employment-based coverage, the coordination depends on the size of the employer: small employers (fewer than 20 employees) pay secondary to Medicare, while large employers (20+ employees) pay primary.

Understanding these interactions is critical because when Medicare is primary, the other insurance may not pay until Medicare does, whether the individual is enrolled in Part B or not. Accordingly, if an individual has secondary insurance—such as a small employer-based plan—and does not enroll in Part B, it is as if they have no outpatient coverage at all.

To avoid being functionally uninsured, those with secondary coverage should typically sign up for Medicare when they are first eligible, even if they could use the Part B SEP to do so later.

a. How does the growing bloc of seniors working later in life impact the number of Medicare beneficiaries exposed to possible late-enrollment penalties?

While most beneficiaries are still automatically enrolled in Medicare Part B at age 65 because they are receiving Social Security benefits, a growing number of Americans are not. In 2016, only 60% of Medicare-eligible 65-year-olds were taking Social Security, compared to 92% in 2002.[3] Many of these individuals are working later in life and deferring their retirement benefits, though they may not realize that doing so impacts their Medicare coverage.[4] Others may choose—appropriately or not—to delay signing up for Medicare because they have another source of coverage, such as an employer-based plan.

Unlike those who are auto-enrolled in Part B, these individuals must actively do so, taking into consideration specific enrollment periods, existing coverage dynamics, and complicated Medicare rules. This process is so confusing that even sophisticated Human Resources experts have trouble with it, and many employers' benefits departments lack the Medicare knowledge to effectively guide their employees and retirees. Further, the federal government provides virtually no notification to people who are nearing Medicare eligibility about their responsibilities, including if they must actively enroll.

As a result, many people bear the full burden of navigating Medicare's arduous enrollment process. If this transition is mismanaged, they can face severe consequences, including lifetime late enrollment penalties, higher health care costs, and gaps in coverage.

---

[3] Medicare Payment Advisory Commission, "Report to the Congress: Medicare and the Health Care Delivery System" (June 2019), http://www.medpac.gov/docs/default-source/reports/jun19_medpac_reporttocongress_sec.pdf?sfvrsn=0.
[4] Johnson, R.W., Urban Institute, "Older Workers: Opportunities and Challenges" (July 2010), http://www.urban.org/UploadedPDF/412166-older-workers.pdf.

Mr. Frederic Riccardi
Page 3

Unfortunately, many people do make mistakes. Year after year, among the most frequent calls to Medicare Rights' National Consumer Helpline are those from or on behalf of people with Medicare who inadvertently and through no fault of their own failed to enroll in Part B on time and are living with the repercussions.[5]

The demographic[6] and employment[7] trends that have so significantly changed how people experience their initial Medicare eligibility show no sign of abating. As a result, more and more beneficiaries will face complex Part B enrollment decisions—and experience the pitfalls of the current system. These pressures mean the BENES Act's commonsense solutions are needed now more than ever.

b. Can you discuss the benefit of aligning the annual general enrollment period with the annual enrollment period for private Medicare Advantage and Part D prescription drug plans?

Medicare Advantage and Part D, as well as commercial and job-based insurance plans, generally conduct enrollment from October to December of each year, with coverage beginning the following January. This is a time of heightened outreach and awareness for many people, as well as a familiar timeframe. Medicare's General Enrollment Period (GEP) runs from January through March with coverage beginning July 1, making it a confusing outlier. This divergence can cause beneficiary confusion and enrollment mistakes that lead to lifelong financial penalties, heightened health care costs, and harmful gaps in coverage.

c. Under the BENES Act, the federal government can create a Part B Special Enrollment Period for "exceptional circumstances." Is this provision currently used anywhere else and why is it necessary?

Special Enrollment Periods (SEPs) for "exceptional circumstances" are currently available in Medicare Advantage (MA) and Part D. CMS relies on this statutory authority to provide some enrollment relief for beneficiaries who are impacted by natural disasters.

This flexibility allows CMS to account for situations that may leave people unable to meet enrollment deadlines, obtain necessary paperwork, or access assistance. Since this authority was established, CMS has granted MA/Part D exceptional circumstances SEPs only three times—for Hurricane Sandy in 2012, for those affected by snowstorms in New York in 2014, and due to the hurricanes and wildfires in 2018.

However, similar administrative flexibility does not currently exist in Part B. Because that statute significantly pre-dates the creation of Medicare Parts C and D, it lacks the clarity of and parity with the newer language. As a result, Medicare rules do not reflect the reality that this enrollment

---

[5] Medicare Rights Center, "Medicare Trends and Recommendations: An Analysis of 2017 Call Data from the Medicare Rights Center's National Helpline" (April 2019), https://www.medicarerights.org/pdf/2017-helpline-trends-report.pdf.
[6] Administration for Community Living, "A Profile of Older Americans: 2018" (April 2018), https://www.acl.gov/aging-and-disability-in-america/data-and-research/profile-older-americans.
[7] Mitra Toossi and Elka Torpey, Bureau of Labor Statistics, "Older Workers: Labor Force Trends and Career Options" (May 2017), https://www.bls.gov/careeroutlook/2017/article/older-workers.htm.

relief is just as necessary for people with Part B as it is for people with MA or a prescription drug plan.

This asymmetry leads to enrollment relief being inconsistently applied. It allows people with Part B to be treated differently than people with MA or Part D, despite living in the same area and experiencing the same natural disaster. For example, CMS did not view Hurricane Sandy as justifying a special enrollment period for Part B, but did grant one for MA and Part D.

The BENES Act would correct this misalignment by extending the Secretary's authority to issue an exceptional circumstances SEP to Part B. This would help avoid future conflicting policy interpretations and better ensure all people with Medicare have the opportunity to make optimal, timely coverage choices.

The Honorable Larry Bucshon (R-IN)

1. **If the NEMT benefit is eliminated, unintended consequences will include people skipping their medical treatments until they can arrange transportation. Have any experts examined the potential cost implications of this?**

A number of studies have demonstrated the vital role that NEMT plays in ensuring that people with Medicaid can attend medical appointments, comply with treatment plans, and receive needed care. For example, the National Academies of Sciences published the "Cost-Benefit Analysis of Providing Non-Emergency Medical Transportation" which found that NEMT increased attendance at appointments, reduced the length of hospital stays, and led to fewer emergency room visits.[8] Similarly, a separate study found that Medicaid beneficiaries with chronic conditions were significantly more likely to attend their routine appointments if they used NEMT.[9]

Medicaid NEMT facilitates access to medical services for low-income beneficiaries who have no other means of transportation, allowing them to receive routine and preventive care they might otherwise go without. Due to the program's strict eligibility requirements, those who qualify tend to have higher and more complex health needs than the general population.[10] Mental health problems, hypertension, heart disease, asthma, chronic obstructive pulmonary disease, diabetes, and end-stage renal disease are especially prevalent. But because these conditions are particularly responsive to appropriate care—including regular and sustained physician visits[11]—NEMT plays an outsize role in helping these individuals build and maintain their health, as well as avoid more costly medical emergencies, hospitalizations, and institutionalizations. In so doing, the program lowers individual and system-wide health care costs.[12]

[8] National Academies of Sciences, Engineering, and Medicine, "Cost-Benefit Analysis of Providing Non-Emergency Medical Transportation," The National Academies Press, p. 14 (2005), https://doi.org/10.17226/22055.
[9] Michael Adelberg & Marsha Simon, "Non-Emergency Medical Transportation: Will Reshaping Medicaid Sacrifice An Important Benefit?," Health Affairs Blog (September 2017), https://www.healthaffairs.org/do/10.1377/hblog20170920.062063/full/.
[10] National Academies of Sciences, Engineering, and Medicine, "Cost-Benefit Analysis of Providing Non-Emergency Medical Transportation," The National Academies Press, p. 34 (2005), https://doi.org/10.17226/22055.
[11] *Id.*, p. 61.
[12] Kara E MacLeod, et al., "Missed or Delayed Medical Care Appointments by Older Users of Nonemergency Medical Transportation," Gerontologist, 55(6), pp. 1026–1037 (December 2015), https://www.ncbi.nlm.nih.gov/pmc/articles/PMC4668763/.

Mr. Frederic Riccardi
Page 5

Absent access to NEMT, multiple studies suggest health outcomes would plummet while expenses would rise. One recent review found that for the estimated 3.6 million people who miss or delay medical care each year due to lack of transportation, NEMT is a cost-effective way for them to manage their conditions.[13] Another found that adults who lack transportation to medical care are more likely to have chronic health conditions that can escalate to a need for more costly emergency care if not properly managed.[14] And another concluded that NEMT yields impressive returns on investment, providing a "payback of 835%, or $8.35 per each dollar invested in these [transportation] programs."[15] Were Medicaid beneficiaries who rely on NEMT, for example beneficiaries on dialysis, forced to forgo or delay the care the benefit allows them to receive, their conditions would likely worsen.

2. **As a representative from a rural region and state, I recognize the value of the NEMT benefit to Medicaid beneficiaries who lack access to transit and who must travel great distances for many medical appointments. I would welcome your thoughts as to the potential impact on transportation access and on the transportation infrastructure in rural regions were the federal guarantee to this benefit to go away.**

Medicaid NEMT and broader community transportation services are interdependent. They are commonly provided by the same transportation agencies, especially in rural communities. To achieve efficiencies, these operating agencies often "commingle Medicaid NEMT with other essential services, including para-transit for people with developmental and physical disabilities, senior rides for older adults, and services for other vulnerable citizens who rely on public transportation to get to work, grocery stores, vocational training, and other destinations necessary to maintaining community engagement."[16]

As a result of this interdependence, "cuts to Medicaid NEMT would undermine entire communities'—not just Medicaid beneficiaries'—access to transportation." Localities already experiencing transportation funding challenges, as many rural areas are, would be particularly hard hit.[17] Eliminating the program entirely would only amplify these impacts.

3. **The recently passed appropriations package calls for the Department of Health and Human Services (HHS) to freeze any new regulation until MACPAC completes a study on the NEMT benefits. Do you know when this study will be completed, or when HHS' rule-freezing will be implemented?**

We do not have an official timeline for the completion of the MACPAC study but look forward to its conclusion as the appropriations language asks the commission to "examine, to the extent data are available, the benefits of NEMT from State Medicaid programs on Medicaid beneficiaries, including beneficiaries with chronic diseases including end stage renal disease

---

[13] National Academies of Sciences, Engineering, and Medicine, "Cost-Benefit Analysis of Providing Non-Emergency Medical Transportation," The National Academies Press, p. 14 (2005), https://doi.org/10.17226/22055.
[14] Richard Wallace, et al., "Access to Health Care and Nonemergency Medical Transportation: Two Missing Links," 1924 Transportation Research Record: Journal of the Transportation Research Board, pp. 76-84 (2005), http://www.researchgate.net/publication/39967547_.
[15] Michael Adelberg & Marsha Simon, "Non-Emergency Medical Transportation: Will Reshaping Medicaid Sacrifice An Important Benefit?," Health Affairs Blog (September 2017), https://www.healthaffairs.org/do/10.1377/hblog20170920.062063/full/.
[16] Michael Adelberg & Scott Bogren, "The Hidden Risk of Cutting Medicaid NEMT: An Examination of Transportation Service Interdependency at the Community Level," https://mtaccoalition.org/wp-content/uploads/2020/01/NEMT-Co-dependency-final.pdf.
[17] *Id.*

(ESRD), substance abuse disorders, pregnant mothers, and patients living in remote, rural areas, and to examine the benefits of improving assisted transportation services" and "directs HHS to take no regulatory action on availability of NEMT service until the study is completed."[18]

Currently, the OMB unified agenda indicates that CMS plans to begin the rulemaking process with a request for information at any time.[19] Given the devastating impact changes to NEMT could have on people with Medicaid, we agree that it is important to wait for MACPAC's study and other relevant data before considering whether any regulatory actions are appropriate.

---

[18] Division A—Departments of Labor, Health, and Human Services, and Education, and Related Agencies Appropriations Act, 2020, https://docs.house.gov/billsthisweek/20191216/BILLS-116HR1865SA-JES-DIVISION-A.pdf.
[19] Office of Management and Budget, Office of Information and Regulatory Affairs, "Request for Information: Assurance of Medicaid Transportation (CMS-2481-NC)," https://www.reginfo.gov/public/do/eAgendaViewRule?pubId=201910&RIN=0938-AT81.

Chapter 2

Examining Pathways to Universal Health Coverage*

Committee on Oversight and Reform

Tuesday, March 29, 2022
House of Representatives,
Committee on Oversight and Reform,
Washington, D.C.

The committee met, pursuant to notice, at 9:05 a.m., in room 2154, Rayburn House Office Building, and via Zoom; Hon. Carolyn B. Maloney [chairwoman of the committee] presiding.

Present: Representatives Maloney, Norton, Lynch, Connolly, Krishnamoorthi, Raskin, Khanna, Mfume, Ocasio-Cortez, Tlaib, Porter, Bush, Brown, Davis, Welch, Johnson, Sarbanes, Kelly, DeSaulnier, Gomez, Pressley, Comer, Jordan, Foxx, Hice, Grothman, Cloud, Sessions, Keller, Biggs, Clyde, LaTurner, Herrell, and Donalds.

Also present: Representatives Jayapal, Omar, Bowman, and Jones.

Chairwoman MALONEY. The Committee will come to order. I am told we need to restart the opening because of the stream was not there.

Today, I am convening the Committee on Oversight and Reform to examine a subject that touches the lives of every person in the United States, our Nation's healthcare system and Americans' access to affordable, high-

* This is an edited, reformatted and augmented version of Hearing before the Committee on Oversight and Reform, House of Representatives, One Hundred Seventeenth Congress, Second Session, Serial No. 117–73, dated March 29, 2022.

In: Healthcare Coverage
Editor: Anne Winter
ISBN: 979-8-89113-564-2

quality medical care. Democrats in Congress have spent decades fighting, and succeeding, to expand access to healthcare in the United States.

In 2010, under the leadership of President Obama, we passed the Affordable Care Act, a landmark law that made affordable healthcare accessible to more than 30 million people across the United States. That includes 14 million people with lower incomes who finally received high-quality health insurance, thanks to the Affordable Care Act's Medicaid expansion. This also includes millions of people who had previously experienced obstacles to obtaining healthcare, including people with preexisting conditions, older Americans, and women.

Unfortunately, my colleagues on the other side of the aisle not only opposed this law, but over the last decade, they have voted more than 60 times to repeal it or weaken it. Republican Attorney Generals sued in Federal court, trying to strike it down, and the Trump administration refused to defend the ACA in court. Despite these relentless attacks and thanks to the tireless work of patients, caregivers, and community advocates, the ACA still stands.

Since President Biden took office, congressional Democrats have continued to strengthen and enhance the ACA to make healthcare more affordable and accessible for every person in the United States. Last year, we passed President Biden's American Rescue Plan, sweeping legislation that expanded the ACA's financial assistance for patients and families working to make ends meet.

But our work is not done yet. Today, more than 27 million people in the United States remain uninsured, and even for some who do have insurance, it is not enough to insulate them from the significant cost of getting healthcare in this country. congressional Democrats have proposed and advanced many different reforms to close these coverage gaps and move our Nation toward universal health coverage. We have voted on legislation to close the coverage gap left by Republican States that failed to expand Medicaid under the ACA, as well as legislation to expand Medicare benefits for older Americans and to further reduce out-of-pocket costs for patients with commercial coverage.

And more than 100 of us have cosponsored the Medicare for All Act, as proposed by my colleague Congresswoman Pramila Jayapal and championed by numerous members on this committee. Medicare for All, a comprehensive proposal to transition our healthcare system to a national single-payer model, offers a bold vision for an America where no patient is denied necessary medical care because it is too expensive and no family has to decide between putting food on the table or paying their medical bills. This proposal fulfills a promise that I have long fought for, the promise that healthcare is a human right.

Medicare for All would contain skyrocketing costs across our healthcare system and provide a sustainable path to more equitable and accessible healthcare, especially for communities where access has historically been pushed out of reach. I have proudly supported Medicare for All since it was first introduced in Congress nearly two decades ago, and I will continue to push for this vision of the American healthcare system.

At the same time, my Democratic colleagues and I will continue to fight for every bit of progress we can make in moving our Nation toward universal coverage. While Republicans raise barriers to affordable healthcare, Democrats will continue working tirelessly to ensure that no person's financial circumstances keep them from obtaining quality healthcare.

Let me conclude by taking a moment to recognize the leadership of several of our committee members in bringing renewed energy and urgency to the fight for universal coverage. Congresswoman Cori Bush, Ayanna Pressley, Alexandria Ocasio-Cortez, and Rashida Tlaib, all members of this committee, have been some of the most powerful voices in Congress for an America where healthcare is a human right, and I am grateful to partner with them.

Before I recognize the distinguished Ranking Member for his opening remarks, I would like to recognize Congresswoman Bush for an opening Statement.

You are now recognized, Congresswoman Bush.

Ms. BUSH. St. Louis and I thank you, Chairwoman Maloney, for your partnership in convening this historic hearing on the urgent need for comprehensive and universal health coverage in the United States. The committee's exemplary leadership, tireless advocacy, and commitment to genuine health equity will rightfully bring this conversation back to the forefront of public health policy.

I must acknowledge the tremendous work and contribution of Senator Sanders and Rep. Jayapal for putting forth the boldest legislative proposal to date, the Medicare for All Act, and to my sisters in service on this committee for their partnership and steadfast leadership in our effort to protect healthcare as a human right.

Thank you to our seeing witnesses, a comprehensive range of patients and researchers, healthcare professionals, who have come together today to passionately advocate for universal healthcare.

Medicare for All is transformational policy change that would implement a national single-payer universal healthcare system that guarantees comprehensive healthcare coverage to every person in America and end the for-profit, privatized broken system we have in place now.

I have personally bore witness to the stark inequities faced by uninsured and underinsured patients during my tenure as a registered nurse. For some people, it is hard to imagine rationing expensive medication like insulin, skipping dialysis appointments, forgoing surgical procedures, or refusing medical care entirely. People are having to choose between their life or a lifetime of medical debt, and that is not OK.

And I know because I am one of those people. Until I was sworn in as a Member of Congress, I was uninsured for over a week, and actually, I have spent the better part of my adulthood lacking access to health coverage, overburdened by medical debt, and unable to receive regular preventive and routine medical care. It shouldn't have taken a job for me to be able to access affordable medical care. Healthcare is a human right, and we should guarantee it for everyone.

Providing every single person in the United States with healthcare is a powerful anti-poverty mechanism. Medicare for All would help low-income households save over $38 billion annually on medical out-of-pocket expenses like deductibles, copays, co-insurance, and self-payments. Research has proven universal coverage will help reduce poverty rates by over 20 percent.

In St. Louis, our communities are facing systemic threats to their health from all angles—from poverty, substandard housing conditions, environmental destruction, overdose and mental health crises, pollution, to over policing. Lack of affordable healthcare has resulted in millions of preventable deaths before the pandemic, and the situation continues to rapidly deteriorate as COVID–19 claims over 1 million lives and counting.

While Democrats have a majority in the House, Senate, and the executive branch, it is imperative lawmakers seize this narrow opportunity now to enact transformational public health policy and poverty-reductive policies like Medicare for All. Taking strides toward universal healthcare coverage is the only path forward to reversing troubling trends in U.S. population health.

I urge my colleagues on both sides of the aisle to earnestly consider the lethal consequences of continuing to prioritize big pharma profits over human life and health.

Thank you, and I yield back.

Chairwoman MALONEY. The gentlelady yields back.

I now recognize the distinguished Ranking Member, Mr. Comer, for an opening Statement.

Mr. COMER. Thank you, Chairwoman Maloney, and I want to thank our witnesses for your testimony here today.

Keeping with the majority's pattern this Congress, today's hearing is not an oversight hearing. It is not a hearing that will bring transparency or accountability to the executive branch. It is not a hearing to find ways to save taxpayer dollars, especially as Americans toil under inflation.

Instead, today's hearing is an attempt to find more ways to spend taxpayer dollars and expand the reach of the Federal Government. It is a hearing to grow massive entitlement spending, this time by pushing for Government-run healthcare.

With inflation at a 40-year high, Americans are struggling to afford essential items like food and medicine. Since day one of this administration, President Biden's policies have crippled America's energy independence. Gas prices have skyrocketed. In California, gas prices are over $6 a gallon.

Meanwhile, fentanyl is streaming across the Southern border unchecked. According to the Centers for Disease Control, fentanyl overdoses are now the leading cause of death for adults age 18 to 25. Children are also being hit hard by the fentanyl crisis with reports daily about accidental overdoses.

Yet my Democrat colleagues refuse to look into any of these issues. The mission of the Oversight Committee is to root out waste, fraud, abuse, and mismanagement in the Federal Government, but Democrats keep finding new ways to use the tools of the committee to spend even more taxpayer dollars.

Instead of looking for ways to expand Government, Oversight Committee Republicans have been conducting our own investigation in the healthcare space on Medicaid improper payments. And what we have found is very disturbing. Documents obtained during the investigation show that Democrat policies, such as Medicaid expansion and removing eligibility checks, have increased improper payment rates in the program.

In fact, improper payments are so rampant, the most recent data shows that more than 1 out of every 5 Medicaid payments are improper. That is about $87 billion in taxpayer money being misused in one Fiscal Year alone. Why aren't we holding a hearing on that?

Instead, this hearing is about further expanding Obamacare and moving the United States closer to socialized medicine. Medicare for All will gut quality healthcare coverage in favor of waiting lines, rationed care, and stalled medical innovation. Medicare for All will cancel first-rate health plans for millions of workers, children, and seniors in favor of giving D.C. politicians unlimited control of your healthcare.

Evidence around the world shows socialized medicine causes long lines for treatment, decreased innovation, and empowers the Government to decide who lives and who dies. It also enables systems that benefit the rich who can afford private insurance to bypass Government waitlists.

Democrats have seen the polling and know the American people don't want Medicare for all. So Democrats have worked to hide their end goal from the American people, using terms like "Medicare for all who want it" and "public options," when, in reality, these are just steppingstones to socialized medicine. But no amount of Washington spin can change the fact that socialized medicine is a bad deal for the American people.

Americans recognize the frightening attempts at Government takeover of healthcare for what they are, bans on good healthcare plans that work, eradicating Medicare for seniors as we know it, and doubling everyone's taxes. And voters will reject it. When they do, Republicans stand committed to working together to improve the broken status quo and lower healthcare costs for families and small businesses.

Republicans, through the Healthy Future Task Force, are already working to develop common sense proposals to increase competition, encourage investment in new cures and therapies, protect access to care for all Americans, and ensure patients remain in control of their care. But Republicans know centralizing control in D.C. and continuing to limit access and choice for patients is an awfully bad starting point for Democrats.

Republicans will continue to fight Democrats' takeover of healthcare through common sense solutions to increase the availability of affordable care for all Americans while ensuring we remain the global leader in healthcare innovation.

And with that, Madam Chair, I yield back.

Chairwoman MALONEY. The gentleman yields back.

We have very important witnesses today, and I want to focus on getting to their testimony. Let me briefly say that President Biden has unified our allies in Asia and Europe. He has restored trust in American leadership. He has swiftly acted to move against the aggression of Russia against the Ukraine. After the COVID crisis, he has taken steps to help our economy and has had record employment, the most ever in the history of our country.

I would like to place into the record a list of all the Federal hearings that we have had in Oversight and address the other attacks on the Biden administration and respond very simply to the claim that our hearing today is too expensive.

The truth is we cannot afford our current healthcare system. We pay more for healthcare than any other comparable nation, nearly 20 percent of our GDP and rising yearly. Americans go bankrupt because they don't have health insurance, and that is a national disgrace. And studies show that the reforms we are discussing today would actually save money over time.

I would like to submit for the record a study from the University of California San Francisco, which analyzed 22 single-payer proposals and found that every single one would result in long-term financial savings.

Without objection.

Chairwoman MALONEY. If my Republican colleagues were really worried about inflation, they would support policies that bring down healthcare costs instead of voting 60 times against the Affordable Care healthcare plan that has expanded healthcare to 30 million Americans.

Finally, in terms of the deficit, I don't hear my Republican colleagues complaining when President Trump pushed through $1.9 trillion in tax cuts for the very well off. I invite my Republican colleagues to stop playing politics and let us work together on real solutions, all kinds of ideas that we will be discussing today, real solutions so that working families can get the healthcare they so justly deserve at an affordable price.

And before we move on, I would like to ask unanimous consent that Representatives Omar, Bowman, Jones, and Jayapal be allowed to participate in today's hearing.

Without objection, so ordered.

Now we are going to introduce our distinguished first panel of witnesses who are all patient advocates. The first panel will not be taking questions, but we welcome their experience, their perspective.

I now recognize Ms. Bush to introduce the first witness.

Ms. BUSH. I am proud to represent a witness in this hearing from St. Louis, Mr. Christopher Willcox, who will share his testimony as both an underinsured patient and a relentless advocate for Medicare for All.

Chris is currently the mutual aid and policy advocate at A Red Circle, where he helps connect St. Louis County residents with community resources. As a social worker who is passionate about healthcare, housing, and freedom from police violence, Chris has extensive experience helping patients navigate a fragmented healthcare system.

I am confident his testimony will lay bare the true human cost of the brutal for-profit healthcare industry.

Chairwoman MALONEY. Thank you.

Our next witness will be Nikki Lyons, who is a pre-med student from my district in New York.

After that, we will hear from Chris Briggs, who is a patient advocate from Woodburn, Virginia.

I now recognize Ms. Tlaib to introduce our next witness.

Ms. TLAIB. Thank you so much, Chairwoman Maloney, for your incredible courage in having this hearing and, of course, to all of my other sisters in service for helping us bring so many of our families into the halls of Congress as they express the dismay of our broken healthcare system.

I have the honor of introducing Bishop Walter Starghill from Inkster, strong in Thirteenth congressional District. The bishop has already had personal experiences himself, almost going blind because of our broken healthcare system, but he also serves in one of my amazing federally accredited clinics. He serves as the vice chair of an all-volunteer board of directors of Western Wayne Family Health Centers, whose goal is to provide high-quality, affordable care for all of our residents and our communities, regardless of insurance status.

I want to thank him so much for his courage and for him providing this testimony that is so critical. As the bishop will tell you, in our district, we are not about just surviving. We are also about thriving. And that is why we need to get closer to passing Medicare for All.

Thank you so much, Chairwoman. I yield.

Chairwoman MALONEY. I now recognize Ms. Pressley to introduce our final witness.

Ms. PRESSLEY. Thank you, Madam Chair, for your leadership and heeding our calls, working with my colleagues and I to hold this critically important, historic, and timely hearing. It has been a long time coming.

I thank Rep. Jayapal for being undeterred in this justice fight, and of course, I want to recognize my colleague and sister in service, Representative Bush, for spearheading this effort.

The fight to make Medicare for All a reality is intrinsically a fight to center people with disabilities once and for all, and that is why I am proud to introduce Leslie Templeton, constituent of the Massachusetts Seventh, a resident of Boston, who from a young age has navigated the world as a disabled person and uses her experiences to advocate for others.

Thank you, Leslie, for your tireless dedication to advancing disability justice in the Commonwealth and across the United States. You make the Massachusetts Seventh and the movement very proud.

Chairwoman MALONEY. The gentlelady yields back.

The witnesses will be unmuted so that we may swear them in. Please raise your right hands.

Do you swear or affirm that the testimony you are about to give is the truth, the whole truth, and nothing but the truth, so help you God?

[Response.]

Chairwoman MALONEY. Let the record show that the witnesses answered in the affirmative.

Thank you. And without objection, your written Statements will be made part of the record.

With that, Mr. Willcox, you are now recognized for your testimony. Mr. Willcox?

Statement of Christopher Willcox, Msw, St. Louis, Missouri

Mr. WILLCOX. Great. Thank you for the kind introduction and thank you for inviting me to speak.

My name is Chris Willcox. I'm an organizer with St. Louis Mutual Aid, and I work for A Red Circle, which is a nonprofit that serves North St. Louis County.

My history with healthcare systems in America comes from the perspective of those receiving services and from providing them. I was first diagnosed with anxiety and depression in college before I graduated in 2011 at the peak of the Great Recession. Getting treatment for depression suddenly made a lot of struggles in my life make sense.

The thing about depression is that the simplest things, such as getting out of bed, can feel incredibly difficult, and it can be hard to even imagine that there is anything worth getting up for. Adding to that, failing to overcome challenges makes it all the easier to gather what feels like a cumulative body of evidence of your own worthlessness.

We deal with arbitrary disruptions in healthcare because of our dependence on private health insurance companies and struggles with precarious employment. I've had to change therapists at least three times because the ones I was working with was no longer in network.

When I was temporarily uninsured or had to start with a new insurer, I've had to go through withdrawals multiple times because of denials or delays, prior authorizations, or any other bureaucratic headaches we spend hours and hours of unpaid time dealing with.

In my experience working in social services, the limitations of existing public health insurance left many of my clients' needs unmet. Many agencies operate by churning as many billable services as possible from underpaid and poorly supported staff. Imagine being worried about making your numbers while trying to be present for a client that is telling you about their suicidal ideation.

One client I work with is particularly ill-served. She had to borrow money from her brother to get her medications while she waited on Medicaid to establish her coverage. I was advised to reschedule her appointments so that I could pick up others to get my numbers up because she would frequently have to reschedule. Understandable for someone needing treatment for serious mental health challenges.

The very day I was given this advice, this same client texted me a call for help as she was struggling with suicide. After I intervened, she went to the hospital for the second time for suicide before she was finally granted coverage by Medicaid. This was while I was having my own thoughts about suicide related to the conditions of my job, but I had put off seeing a therapist for several months because during that time, I was hired late in the year, and I would have to pay entirely out-of-pocket, have the deductible reset in January.

These problems exist simply because we choose not to make the commitment to care for every person who needs it. This may be even more the case in mental illness, which can be every bit as lethal. It takes courage and resolve just to seek treatment, as fear of being seen as weak or as making it up in your head only adds to the barriers we already put between people and care.

Without getting the care I needed, I might not even be alive today, let alone speaking to Congress about finally getting the support our people need and deserve. We know what we need to do to make sure that everyone gets the care that they need, Medicare for All now.

Thank you.

Chairwoman MALONEY. Thank you. The gentleman yields back. Ms. Lyons, you are now recognized for your testimony. Ms. Lyons?

Statement of Nicole Lyons, New York City, New York

Ms. LYONS. Hi. OK, thank you so much for giving me the opportunity to speak today, members of the House committee.

Just give me one second. I'm having a little technical difficulty right now.

So, as the speaker said, my name is Nikki Lyons. I'm here to speak today because the second time in my 20's, I am waiting for an organ transplant due to kidney failure.

This loss of control regarding so many aspects of my life and waiting for an organ transplant has had me thinking many times about what I would say to you guys with the power to make changes in this place where decisions are made. Like so many Americans, Medicare for All would have changed the course of so many aspects of my life and provide comfort for my future.

The first time I found out I was sick, I was at a hospital in the middle of college midterms week and waking up from an emergency appendectomy. The diagnosis was not adequately explained, and there is no followup care that one would expect.

As a struggling college student, I didn't have the luxury to see a doctor anywhere besides the emergency room. Because of this, I didn't know how truly sick I was, and because of my illness, I ended up failing out of school, which further delayed my career and cost thousands and thousands of dollars.

Years later, I found out at that time I already should have been looking for a transplant because I was in the end stages of kidney failure, not told just to watch my sodium—or not just to watch my sodium, as I was told. Had I had regular access to healthcare, blood tests, anything like that, the extent of my organ failure could have been stalled or even prevented, had it been caught early enough.

While waiting for my first transplant, instead of resting and conserving the little energy I did have, I was working 50-plus hours a week on my feet at a bar and at a gym to afford my doctors' appointments and medication. For those who don't know, potential transplant patients are evaluated for stability as to not waste the gift of an organ. They look at your housing, your economic status, your compliance with doctors. Not being able to afford medication or appointments could have disqualified me for the organ I needed to live at any point.

Medicare for All would have meant not deciding if I needed to skip meals to qualify for a kidney. I wouldn't have had to work myself to the bone while incredibly sick.

I was lucky enough to receive a transplant in 2016, but I am again in organ failure. This round of organ failure I can say with 100 percent certainty would have been prevented by Medicare for All. I wasn't able to get regular transplant checkups because of the resources I had allotted for healthcare went toward mitigating the symptoms of long-term COVID. Because of the lack of care, I had no idea my body was rejecting my transplant as a complication of said long-term COVID.

I haven't been able to properly work or attend class adequately since winter of 2020. The COVID symptoms transitioned into kidney failure symptoms so seamlessly to the point I didn't realize what was happening. All I had needed was a simple blood test, and the rejection would have been caught earlier. When rejection is caught quickly, it is very treatable.

I, unfortunately, wasn't that lucky. It was amazing I was alive for the second time in my life. Since June, I have had six long-term hospital stays, with the longest being seven weeks; travel 12 hours a week 3 times—12 hours 3 times a week for dialysis for 3 1/2 hours; blood transfusions, chemicals similar to chemo to try and save the kidney and prevent anything from getting worse, and that just ends up making me feel significantly worse. I've had days I'm only able to be awake for four hours. There's no way for me to work, finish school, or thrive at all in this condition.

On top of this, I had no insurance when this first started until Medicare kicked in, which took six months from the time I applied. I was told their online system never got my application several times, and then after that, several times the local office had lost my paperwork and never filed it.

So, for those six months, I couldn't access care unless I went to an ER. I ended up going into heart failure as well during this time, which took four ERs to catch. But had I been able to see a cardiologist for something as simple as an ultrasound of the heart or an echo, it would have been spotted immediately.

I was also told peritoneal dialysis would have been a much better option than the standard hemodialysis that I had to endure because no surgeon would place the right catheter if I didn't have insurance to pay for said surgery. So I have spent the past six months getting the entirety of my blood taken out through a tube in my neck, cleaned, and returned to my body while often going into shock when there's a loss of fluids because it makes your heart unable to pump blood through the body, having horrible insomnia, deep pain, and fatigue.

Six months of suffering due to a lack of access to care for a medical situation that should have been prevented in the first place. Medicare eventually kicked in, and now 229 days after my first dialysis session, I am finally switched over to in-home peritoneal dialysis that I should have gotten in the first place. Two hundred twenty-nine days of my life were robbed from me for reasons out of my control, but preventable for the next person by the elected officials sitting in this room.

The experiences I briefly shared are but a drop in the bucket compared to my full story. I wanted to take the time to thank everybody for listening to me, and I implore you to take the time to fully absorb what the words I said meant.

This situation is happening across the country, and Medicare for All would prevent it. It is inhumane to present any human being in a situation where they must choose between eviction, a lack of food, or their healthcare.

Thank you.

Chairwoman MALONEY. Thank you.

Mr. Briggs, you are now recognized.

Statement of Chris Briggs, Woodburn, Virginia

Mr. BRIGGS. Chairwoman Maloney, Ranking Member Comer, members of the House Committee on Oversight and Reform, please allow me to thank you to testify before you today. And just a point of correction, I do, in fact, live in Northern Virginia, and I am a patient advocate, but I also am public affairs counsel for Independent Institute, which is a think tank in Oakland, California.

In November 2015, my wife got the most dreadful call a parent can get. The doctor knew why our daughter, Colette, then 2 1/2, hadn't been feeling well. Bloodwork had revealed leukemia, cancer. We raced Colette to Inova Fairfax Hospital, the only one in Northern Virginia, where we live, that treats pediatric cancer and got there just in time.

Thanks to Obamacare, we were already in difficult straits regarding healthcare. In 2014, that law had eliminated a plan we had had for years.

Before the ACA went into effect, the private marketplace consistently and reliably had offered us a wide variety of inexpensive plans that covered specialist care even out of State. After the ACA went into effect, however, all that was left were increasingly costly plans with fewer benefits, including fewer doctors and fewer hospitals.

Thanks to Obamacare, we were, and still are to this day, basically restricted to medical facilities within a short radius of our zip codes. Obamacare, in a word, has made us into medical serfs. We're tied to the land on which we live, unable to leave it, even to save a little girl dying from cancer. Which is why, when we tried to take Colette to Johns Hopkins, just up the road in Baltimore, we were denied. Under our pre-ACA plan, which didn't geofence sick children from the care they deserve, she would have been admitted.

Our predicament was made all the more painful by swelling premiums, as well as by skyrocketing deductible and maximum out-of-pocket expenses. They can go as high as $16,500, as it has been for my family.

But things were about to get much worse than expensive for our family. In mid–2017, President Trump merely suggested the scrapping of the massive Obamacare payments to insurance giants, which were delivering worse care at ever greater cost. And in response—because Obamacare, for some reason, permits this—every insurer in Northern Virginia with a family plan, including the one we had, pulled out for the following year, 2018.

Except one. Cigna Connect, however, wouldn't cover my daughter at Inova Fairfax, the one hospital in Northern Virginia, as I say, with a pediatric cancer ward. So under Obamacare, our daughter was effectively without coverage for cancer. Not the common cold or a broken bone, but cancer.

We went through another terrifying event in 2020. In mid-March of that year, with COVID sweeping the country, Anthem, the plan we had for that year, announced suddenly that on April 1, it would no longer cover not the hospital this time, but the clinic where she received most of her doctor-administered chemotherapy. So we called the marketplace. Perhaps it would grant us a waiver to buy the Cigna plan still available for sale in our zip code. Not a chance, we were told.

The failure of the ACA to cover our daughter battling a terminal illness was not considered, we were told, a "qualifying event." So once again, thanks to the ACA, we were left without coverage for our daughter, recovering from cancer at the clinic, the only one she could go to in Northern Virginia.

Now in both cases of systems collapse, we were forced to turn to the author of these failures that is to the Government, to all of you. Specifically, we had called Senator Mark Warner for Virginia, one of our Senators, so he could bully a private company—Cigna in the first instance and Anthem in the second—into covering, respectively, the hospital and the clinic. And in both cases, the threats from the State drove the insurance giants back into the marketplace.

But I do hope all of you can see how these successes that I achieved were actually failures. Ad hoc exercises of Government power to ensure proper functioning of the ACA means we are not dealing, despite the rhetoric, with a marketplace, but rather with a closed web of insurance companies and medical providers at the mercy of the police powers of a complicit government.

Now perhaps to solve the instability of Obamacare, which is inherent to it, the Government could just take over all medical facilities. But everybody in the country at that point would be at the mercy of the same Government bureaucracy that has been brutalizing my daughter and her parents for years.

The high costs of Obamacare would go higher. The rationing of care that we've already experienced would be even more pronounced, and here is why. It's very simple. Bad ideas don't get better just because you make them bigger. They get worse.

Twice in a three-year period, the most important problem that we faced wasn't high costs, bad as they were, but the terrifying reality that high prices in a planned, closed economy always signify that we are on the way to scarcity. Twice in three years we found ourselves with no insurance product to buy for any amount of money that could save a little girl battling cancer.

And here's the thing that's the main point of what I want to say. Scarcity doesn't go away under universal coverage or single-payer, whatever word we want to use this week or next week to describe it. Under full Government control of the body, that is under full Government control of the body by all of you, scarcity wouldn't be, as it is in my case now, circumstantial. My family was effectively a canary in the coal mine.

Scarcity under such authoritarian medicine becomes policy, and by that, I mean this. Those long wait times that everyone can read about for cancer screenings in Great Britain or Canada, that is scarcity made institutional, universal, but in a very bad way. And if you want an example closer to home, try the Government-run hospitals of the Veterans Administration, where people die in line waiting for care.

In other words, if we unfortunately get more managed care from all of you, the Government, my daughter will be everyone's daughter. And every mother and father will experience what my wife and I have experienced. We watched our daughter battle cancer while the institutions of medicine, thanks to the ACA, colluded with the disease against her.

There is one correct long-term answer in my view. We must prohibit the Government, that is to say all of you, from further interfering in the acquisition by private citizens of their preferred medical care, and we do that by repeal of the ACA and placing back into the hands of Americans real, actuarially sound, automatically renewable insurance products curated to individual needs. That is the kind of universal coverage this country deserves because it's the only kind that works.

And now a word for my Republican friends. Obamacare, as you may know, has very little to do with actual insurance. It is essentially a giant scheme. Some would say, I would say a giant Ponzi scheme to pay for each other's medical bills. And since my daughter, thanks to the ACA, got very, very sick under a non-insurance regime, she is now permanently uninsurable.

If we ever come to our senses in this country and give back to the citizens real insurance, my daughter will never be able to have one, and here is the logic. You cannot buy auto insurance after the car accident. My daughter managed to get sick with cancer. She's had that accident. She is permanently uninsurable.

However, if I had been allowed to keep my pre-ACA plan, as President Obama promised, things would be very different. My daughter today would have insured, durable access to medical care. In essence, Obamacare turned an insurable illness, one as grave as cancer, into a permanent preexisting condition from which my daughter will never escape.

But my daughter is not alone. Millions of persons have gotten sick under Obamacare, and everybody in this room, in this entire country, will someday suffer a serious illness, such as we'll call it fate for the purposes of this discussion. And soon enough, the number of permanently uninsurable will be so large that you won't be able to repeal Obamacare.

Obamacare, in a word, is creating right now a nation of preexisting conditions. The Democrats know this. All they have to do is wait, and we will be forced to go full State takeover of the body. So how about it? When you Republicans get into the majority, you win both houses and possibly get the presidency back, will you give us back our bodily autonomy and repeal this law?

Your doing so, however, won't help my daughter. For her, it is too late. She and the other victims of Obamacare will need Government healthcare for the rest of their lives. But the rest of us and for those yet unborn, it is not too late.

And to put this another way, and this may sting, but when you come back into power, please, for the love of God, no more Paul Ryan-style tax cuts, which the other side will just eliminate or destroy by inflation as they're doing now. The State takeover of the human person by authoritarian control of medicine is far more worthy of your attention than any tax cut, no matter how deep.

I thank both sides for the time given me to air my concerns.

Chairwoman MALONEY. Thank you.

Mr. Starghill, you are now recognized for your testimony.

Statement of Bishop Walter Starghill, Jr., Detroit, Michigan

Mr. STARGHILL. Well, thank you for allowing me to be part of this testimony and this great information that needs to be given out.

I'm Bishop Walter L. Starghill, Jr., Eastern Michigan pastor of Face-to-Face Outreach Ministries. Thank God for Congresswoman Tlaib allowing me to be a part of the solution or the answer to bear witness what has happened to me.

One of the things back in 2009, I was uninsured, pastoring. During the great migration out of the Michigan area, my membership dwindled. So, therefore, we didn't have the proper funding to make sure that I had insurance. So, therefore, I was uninsured.

I had a condition which is called shingles that I didn't know I had, and at the time, I was feeling very bad. I went to actually one of the major hospitals at about 1 or 2 in the morning, which was an emergency, and I told them I didn't have insurance.

They saw me, but they gave me the bare minimum. They checked my pulse. They checked my blood pressure and told me I may have shingles. But after that, they gave me a bill of $800. Now I couldn't afford it. It took me almost 6 to 7, 8 months just to pay that money back.

But as a friend of mine told me that they had a clinic, which is the Western Wayne Family Health Center. It's a federally funded clinic, and could you possibly come up to them and see what they can do for you? So as I got worse and worse and as a person that didn't have insurance, you are very susceptible to just worry, worry, worry. And I was worried. So that made the condition even worse.

So I finally went up to the clinic and filled out all the paperwork that they had to do for me, and they gave me a $20 copay. So as they were doing that, filling out my paperwork, I had—over the time from the emergency room to the actual clinic, I had rashes all over the right side of my face, all the way going down my nose, and my eye, my right eye started to close. I was like Worf from Star Trek. I was in a bad situation.

And as they gave me a shot, immediately that actual shot started to move everything back. So I thank God for that. And before that happened was, like I say, if I didn't have that clinic, I might have lost the sight in my eye. Yes, sight in my eye.

Again, I had a scenario as a pastor. We went to Niagara Falls with our church. Fifty-six people went there, and we enjoyed ourselves. The weather was quite hot that day, and on the way back, one of the mothers fell ill. So we called 911—we were in Canada— and they came, picked her up in the ambulance, took her to the hospital, and ran every test that they had to run. And as they were doing that, we started to wonder how much the bill was going to be.

And after they got her stabilized and everything up and running so she was able to travel back with us, I asked the doctor, well, how much is this going to be? The doctor said, as I was holding my breath, that it was $70 Canadian, which was $40 American. I quickly paid the $40 and got back on the road.

Now, I don't know. America is the greatest country in the world. Yes, we do have some issues with affordable healthcare. Yes, we need to fix it. That's why we're here today.

But the bottom line is I am one of the 30 million people that was not insured. I'm not talking about underinsured, but actually had no insurance. Now I'm able to live life and go to the doctor, go to the dentist, go to specialists now. So, therefore, I can live a confident, great life, yes, myself. But the bottom line is that we got to look at doing things better for the people.

I thank you for this time, and I want you—I feel for the man that his daughter had these issues. But again, that's why we're here today is to talk about both sides where you can come with solutions that will help all of us obtain affordable healthcare.

Thank you for my time.

Chairwoman MALONEY. Thank you. The gentleman yields back.

And we now hear from Ms. Templeton. You are now recognized for your testimony. Ms. Templeton?

Statement of Leslie Templeton, Boston, Massachusetts

Ms. TEMPLETON. Good morning, everyone, and thank you for having me.

My name is Leslie Templeton, and it's a pleasure to be here. I am a 25-year-old disabled person, and some of my diagnoses include epilepsy, kidney disease, ADHD, familial hypercholesterolemia, and depression.

Being 25 and sick is extremely funny. While many of my friends are worried about their careers, finding life partners, and what they're doing next week, I have the added worry about what my future holds regarding my health. I wonder if I'll always be able to access my healthcare and treatments. If, heaven forbid, something goes wrong, and I don't have access to healthcare, what will happen to me?

Sitting before you, I'd be lying if I said there aren't nights I cry about this, scared of it all—of my diseases, of my future, of losing my healthcare. With Medicare for All, these wouldn't be concerns I'd have to live with every day of my life.

I'm fortunate enough to be able to access the lifesaving healthcare I need right now. That is a privilege that has given me the ability to be here today. Before I was able to access treatment, I struggled to do most things or fully participate in life.

I don't know if you'll understand how deeply I mean this, but having access to healthcare has allowed me to be a 25-year-old. My Wellbutrin, an antidepressant, has given me the ability to enjoy life. My kidney medication is slowing, if not preventing, further progression of my kidney diseases, ensuring I feel well enough to live my life the way I want to.

And there's so much more. I am fortunate enough to be able to afford these interventions currently due to my income level, a privilege not everyone has. Being sick is expensive, and that expense makes treatment inaccessible to so many people. Being able to access healthcare is not enough. It's being able to afford it, too.

As long as I can always have access to healthcare and I can afford it, I will be able to hopefully live a long life. I'll get married. I'll see my kids graduate from college. I'll grow old and watch my body age gracefully. Without Medicare for All, that outcome is not guaranteed, just as it's not guaranteed for millions of Americans right now.

What people don't talk about enough is the cost of staying alive. My ability to live is based on whether I can afford it or not, and that thought keeps me up at night. So many people are in a similar situation to me. Just look at GoFundMe. People shouldn't have to rely on charity to stay alive.

To put it bluntly, I don't want to die. I want to live a long life without constant worry of whether I will be able to afford my meds each month or I'll have insurance to cover my doctors' visits. Medicare for All would give every American that peace of mind, especially those who rely on the healthcare system the most in order to stay alive.

No one should go broke because they have a life-threatening illness. No mother should have to choose between getting her medication or her kids'. No child should have to watch their parents suffer through pain and ailments because they are not insured.

We Americans are counting on you to change this reality for us because, again, to put it bluntly, we don't want to die.

Thank you.

Chairwoman MALONEY. Thank you, and I would like to thank all of the witnesses for their powerful testimony today. You are now excused, and we will welcome our second panel. Thank you so much.

We will pause a moment as we make a transition.

[Pause.]

Chairwoman MALONEY. I would like to introduce our second panel of witnesses.

Our first witness today is Dr. Uché Blackstock, who is an emergency physician and is the founder and CEO of Advancing Health Equity.

Then we will hear from Dr. Sara Collins, who is the Vice President of Health Coverage and Access at the Commonwealth Fund. Next we will hear from Grace-Marie Turner, who is the President of the Galen Institute.

Next we will hear from Dr. Jeffrey Sachs, who is the Director of Columbia University's Center for Sustainable Development and is the President of the United Nations Sustainable Development Solutions Network.

Next we will hear from Dr. Jamila Michener, who is an associate professor at Cornell University and is the Co-director of Cornell's Center for Health Equity.

Finally, we will hear from Ady Barkan, who is the founder of Be A Hero.

The witnesses will be unmuted so we can swear them in. Please raise your right hands.

Do you swear or affirm that the testimony you are about to give is the truth, the whole truth, and nothing but the truth, so help you God?

[Response.]

Chairwoman MALONEY. Let the record show that the witnesses answered in the affirmative.

Thank you. Without objection, your written Statements will be made part of the record.

With that, Dr. Blackstock, you are now recognized for your testimony. And please, let us all try to keep within our five minutes.

Dr. Blackstock, you are now recognized.

Statement of Uché Blackstock, M.D., Emergency Physician, Founder and Chief Executive Officer, Advancing Health Equity

Dr. BLACKSTOCK. Hi, can you hear me? OK, hi, everyone.

Thank you, Chairwoman Maloney, Representatives Bush, Pressley, Tlaib, Ocasio-Cortez, and all of the members of the House Oversight Committee here today. It's an honor to be invited to testify during this very important hearing, a key step toward addressing racial health inequities in our country.

I'm Dr. Uché Blackstock, an emergency medicine physician with over 17 years of clinical experience, a second-generation black woman physician with lived experience with injustice, and the founder of an organization dedicated to advancing health equity. I have worked for years in communities where far too many of my patients were either uninsured or underinsured, mostly black and brown Americans who have sadly been disregarded by our country.

They are not only dealing with mental and physical health issues, but also with systemic afflictions like bias and racism, housing insecurity, economic instability, and lack of access to reliable transportation. These are what we call the social determinants of health, the factors which influence the health and health outcomes of communities and people.

Lack of access to healthcare is one of the primary social determinants of health. I've taken care of thousands of patients over the years, many I could never forget.

The 40-year-old black man with a history of high blood pressure who came into my ER unconscious on a stretcher after he collapsed at home in front of his family. The paramedics were performing CPR on him. The CAT scan of his head showed a brain bleed, a complication of untreated high blood pressure. He had been unable to afford to pay out-of-pocket for his blood pressure medication since he lost a job a year prior and, as a result, his health insurance.

The 55-year-old Latina woman who came into my ER complaining of bleeding and swelling from her left breast for several months. She explained that she did not have health insurance and did not have a primary care physician.

After we spoke, I examined her and found a foul-smelling mass protruding from her left breast. It was advanced breast cancer.

As Black people and people of color, just living in this country is an act of survival, let alone being able to access quality and culturally responsive health care. The ongoing COVID–19 pandemic and the country's presumed reckoning with racism has only exposed the deep preexisting fissures in our health care and public health system.

Despite advances in health care innovation and technology over the last 75 years, Black men still have the shortest life expectancy, Black women have the highest maternal mortality rates, and Black babies have the highest infant mortality rates.

Overall, Black Americans have a six-year life expectancy gap compared to white Americans, the widest gap since 1998 and widened even more by the pandemic. This pandemic should have been a wake-up call to help us understand the urgency of identifying a path toward making universal health care a reality, among other critical strategies to improve health equity.

I have had a front row seat to the tragic loss of Black and brown life from COVID–19 and racism. During the height of the pandemic in New York City, I noticed my patients' demographics quickly shifted to more racially and socioeconomically diverse patient population to mostly Black and brown patients.

They were essential workers, service workers. Some had underlying medical problems. Others were left with no choice but to use public transportation and many live in crowded multi-generational housing.

I vividly remember an elderly Black man who came into my urgent care with shortness of breath and fever. He was in a wheel-chair and his oxygen level was shockingly low. He lived alone.

I was very worried that he had COVID pneumonia and asked if I could call an ambulance to bring him from urgent care to the closest ER. He refused. He didn't want to die in the ER, he told me. He didn't think he would receive good care because he didn't have health insurance. He felt safer at home.

For many years, I worked in two ERs in New York City, Bellevue Hospital, the oldest public hospital in the country, and Tisch Hospital, a private institution that is part of NYU Langone Medical Center, among the wealthiest hospitals in the country that have gotten hundreds of millions of dollars richer after Federal bailouts.

At these two ERs that, literally, sit next door to each other, I experienced firsthand deep inequities in our health care system, one that is separate and unequal. Patients were divided up based on insurance and race.

Nationally, at private academic medical centers, Black patients are two to three times less likely than white patients to receive care, while uninsured patients overall are five times less likely than patients with insurance coverage to be treated.

In cities across this country the top-ranked hospitals do not treat as many patients of color as white patients, even when they are located in diverse communities.

This is the definition of systemic racism. People who look like me are living this every day. But it should not fall solely on us to always have to call out when something is wrong.

Now is the time to protect our most vulnerable and underserved communities and identify a pathway to ensuring universal health care for all Americans. We must work to break the cycles of trauma and injustice, to foster generational progress for more people, especially people of color because it is cruel to talk about an American dream when only a select few live to see it.

Thank you.

Chairwoman MALONEY. Thank you so much, Dr. Blackstock.

Now we will hear from Dr. Collins. You are now recognized for your testimony.

Dr. Collins?

Statement of Sara R. Collins, Ph.D., Vice President of Health Coverage and Access, the Commonwealth Fund

Dr. COLLINS. Thank you, Chairwoman Maloney, Ranking Member Comer, and members of the committee for this invitation to testify on past universal coverage.

My comments will focus on gains in coverage since the passage of the Affordable Care Act, the effects of the pandemic and Federal relief efforts on coverage and policy options to cover the remaining uninsured, and lower consumer costs.

The ACA brought sweeping change to the U.S. health system, expanding comprehensive and affordable health insurance to millions of lower and middle income Americans and making it possible for anyone with health problems to buy insurance.

The number of uninsured people fell by nearly half after the ACA became law, dropping from 49 million people to a low of 28 million in 2016. There has been a slight uptick since then.

Research shows that the ACA lowered financial barriers to care and improve people's ability to afford health insurance and get needed care. Despite expectations that the pandemic would leave millions uninsured, the latest Federal data indicate that the uninsured rate is actually declining. This decline is due in part to the ACA's coverage expansions which provided safety net coverage for those who lost insurance and Federal COVID–19 relief bills that provided enhanced marketplace subsidies and a requirement that States keep people in Medicaid continuously enrolled in exchange for enhanced Federal matching funds.

The result was record enrollment of nearly 15 million people in the marketplaces and nearly 84 million in Medicaid and the Children's Health Insurance Program.

There are four risk factors that could reverse these gains and limit the ability of Americans to afford their health care. The end of the Medicaid continuous enrollment requirement and the enhanced marketplace subsidies could trigger extensive enrollment losses in Medicaid as States redetermine enrollee eligibility and in the marketplaces as subsidies decline.

Twelve States have yet to expand eligibility for Medicaid. Millions of people are eligible for the ACA's coverage expansions but are not yet enrolled. Growth in health care costs is outstripping growth in median income, leaving millions of people under insured and with growing premium burdens.

There are several targeted policy options that might mitigate these risks including extending the marketplace subsidy enhancements at the end of the public health emergency; requiring States to conduct Medicaid eligibility redeterminations gradually; fill the Medicaid coverage gap; maintain aggressive, targeted, and consistent outreach enrollment efforts to reach the remaining uninsured and keep people covered; enable people to automatically enroll in coverage; address the high provider prices that drive most of the health spending growth in private insurance and, by extension, growth in worker premium contributions and deductibles, such as through a public option.

Allow more workers in expensive employer plans to access marketplace subsidies. Fix the family coverage glitch. Rein in deductibles and out-of-pocket costs and marketplace plans. Ban non-ACA compliant policies like short-term plans.

But how can the U.S. reach universal coverage? Can we get there by building on the ACA or will it take a single-payer approach? This question was debated during the 2020 Presidential election. The Urban Institute tackled it at the time by modeling reforms that built on the ACA in two versions of a single-payer approach.

The ACA approach included auto enrollment and a public option that lowered provider plant prices close to Medicare rates. Urban found that it was possible to reach near universal coverage with this ACA approach as well as with the two single-payer approaches.

They also found that the ACA approach and one of the singlepayer approaches reduced national health expenditures, even though nearly everyone is covered. This is because both approaches reduce private insurance prices paid to providers closer to Medicare rates.

The debate at the time focused not on this fact but on the increase in Federal costs under a single-payer approach. But what commentators failed to point out was that this higher Federal cost was not because the single-payer approach was so much more expensive than our current system but that all of the responsibility for financing that spending shifted away from employers, households, and State governments to the Federal Government.

We need to have reasonable discussions as a country about how to share our healthcare spending responsibilities. But it is not just about who pays but also about how much we pay and why and what we are getting for our spending.

The U.S. has one of the most expensive health systems in the world and, yet we rank last among high income countries on most measures of health system performance, including access to care.

Prices paid to providers in private insurance is one of the primary reasons we spend so much more. As we consider strategies to expand health insurance coverage and lower consumer costs, and as we weigh the benefits of those strategies against their Federal costs, it is critical that the prices paid to providers in private insurance be part of the discussion. Thank you.

Chairwoman MALONEY. Thank you, Dr. Collins.

Ms. Turner, you are now recognized for your testimony.

Statement of Grace-Marie Turner, President, Galen Institute

Ms. TURNER. Thank you, Chairwoman Maloney, Ranking Member Comer, and members of the committee and Representative Jayapal—lovely to see you again—for your sponsorship of the legislation we are considering today.

So I would like to emphasize what I believe are widely shared goals for health reform and achieving universal access to care, coverage that is affordable, protecting the—protecting quality and choice, and especially providing a strong safety net for the most vulnerable.

There is no question that Americans are frustrated with our current health care system. Millions remain uninsured, and even for those who do have insurance, coverage and care cost too much. Many face deductibles that are so high that they say they might as well not be insured.

But the more government gets involved, the more that we see the health sector is forced to comply with countless rules and regulations rather than innovating to respond to more choices of more affordable care and coverage for patients.

Wharton Professor Mark Pauly, University of Pennsylvania, explains that the government exerts great control over our health sector with government affected spending, totally nearly 80 percent and part of that, of course, is actually the government direct spending, which is nearly 60 percent, on public programs. Medicare for All and its derivatives such as Medicare buy-in or a Federal public option would take us further toward government control of our health sector with fewer choices and where, I believe, vulnerable patients, as we see in so many other countries, with the greatest health care needs would have to fight even harder to get access to the care that they need.

In proposing policy solutions, I believe it is important to begin by clearly defining the problem that we want to solve. The Congressional Budget Office reports that 29.8 million people were uninsured in 2019, two-thirds of whom were eligible for existing public or private coverage but were not enrolled. Most of the remaining one-third were not lawfully present in the United States, a problem for immigration and citizenship policy, rather than health policy.

Medicare for All also would mean that virtually everyone would lose the plans they have now and there would be no choice but the one government-run health plan for 173 million Americans who value their employer-based health insurance including millions of union workers and 64 million seniors with Medicare, including 26 million with private Medicare Advantage plans.

The CBO found that establishing a single-payer system would be a major undertaking that would be complicated, challenging, and potentially disruptive, and that the changes could significantly impact the overall U.S. economy.

Three States—Vermont, Colorado and, recently, California, as I describe in my testimony—came to similar conclusions in shelving their plans for single-payer.

So rather than dramatically expanding the role of government through new or expanded taxpayer-supported programs, I believe we need targeted approaches to address the specific needs of those who are uninsured, underinsured, and especially focusing on those of marginalized communities.

Uninsured rates continue to be higher in certain populations, as we have as we have heard other witnesses say, including Latinos, Blacks, those with incomes below the poverty level, and residents in States that have not expanded Medicaid.

Tragically, it is often the most vulnerable who are left behind when demand for services outpaces resources. Just five percent of the population accounts for more than half of U.S. health spending. Those who are the sickest with the greatest health care needs are most often disadvantaged, as political leaders inevitably have to balance then in between them and the great majority of healthier constituents.

Medicare for All will restrict access to new medicines and treatments, lead to dramatic increases in Federal spending, and really turn back the clock, I believe, on innovations in personalized care.

I concluded my written testimony and will conclude here describing the experience of Janet, a patient from Colorado with multiple health challenges. Janet received coverage under the ACA but said her access to care was far worse than the State-run high risk pool that she had participated in before, even though her premiums and co-payments were much higher.

I worked with a number of policy experts through the Health Policy Consensus Group to focus on policy recommendations for patient-centered reform and I also commend the Healthy Future Taskforce that is underway here with a number of solutions to, again, move toward solutions but in a patient-centered way.

I would welcome the opportunity to work with you to achieve the goals of access to more affordable coverage for everyone, better protection for the vulnerable through targeted solutions.

And thank you for your invitation to testify. I look forward to questions.

Chairwoman MALONEY. Thank you, Ms. Turner.

Dr. Sachs, you are now recognized for your testimony, and I understand you are testifying from Berlin.

Statement of Jeffrey D. Sachs, Ph.D., Director, Columbia University Center for Sustainable Development, President, United Nations Sustainable Development Solutions Network

Dr. SACHS. I am, indeed, Chairwoman. We have multiple crises in the world and one of them, unfortunately, is nearby here.

Let me proceed expeditiously for you. Thank you for the hearings. If you could move to the next slide.

[Slide.]

Dr. SACHS. The U.S. system is completely broken. This is the main point. We are spending a fortune, unlike every other country, and we are getting worse outcomes. This is what needs to be understood beyond the ideology, beyond the anecdotes. We are going broke from a system out of control, and this is from the wonderful Commonwealth Fund report. I think you are going to have a witness from Commonwealth Fund. They do great work.

And what you see is the top line is the U.S. spending percent of GDP. This goes up to 2019, about 18 percent of GDP. Now we are almost 20 percent of GDP in the most recent data.

Look at all the rest of the countries, all of them. We are broken. If you move on, it is the same story. We are broken. Here, all of the other countries have higher life expectancy than the United States and the gap is widening dramatically. We are broken. We spend far more on health care, we get far less, because we don't even have a healthcare system. We have a hodgepodge of private overpriced monopolies, whether for profit or not for profit. I will say a word about that later on. But this is a broken, unfair, out of control costs system that doesn't deliver.

Next, please.

[Slide.]

Dr. SACHS. So I referred to the Commonwealth report. You could go on to the next slide.

[Slide.]

Dr. SACHS. We rank last—last—in our health system performance and we rank last in access to care, last in administrative efficiency, last in equity, last in health care outcomes.

Let us stop with the individual anecdotes and just look at our system compared to the rest.

Next slide, please.

[Slide.]

Dr. SACHS. This, again, we spend more—that is on the horizontal axis. On the vertical axis is performance. The U.S. is that little dot on the bottom right, expensive and poorly performing. All the rest of the countries less expensive and better performing.

Next, please.

[Slide.]

Dr. SACHS. We spend a fortunate in administrative costs. When you go into a doctor's office or a hospital, you spend hours, in the end, either before or during or after, filling out forms trying to get reimbursed, trying to figure out what is covered, who is in the network, who isn't in the network. I can tell you even with a physician and Master's of Public Health, Ph.D. degrees, it is almost impossible to navigate the U.S. system now and the result is administrative costs out of control, unlike any other country.

Next slide, please.

[Slide.]

Dr. SACHS. Again, we are spending 10, 15, even 20 percent of outlays on administration, people that are working—hundreds of thousands of people employed to move between different accounts because it is private this, it is private that, who is going to reimburse this, who pays for that. It is unbelievable the amount of time we are burning in order to run this ramshackle nonsystem.

Next, please.

[Slide.]

Dr. SACHS. The expenditures continue to soar, and in 2020 we reached almost 20 percent of GDP, basically, twice what other high income countries are spending that are getting the same or better outcomes than in the United States.

This is what I would plead for the committee. Look at the rest of the world. Not at our own internal, ideological, bizarre discussion, but at the comparison with what is happening elsewhere because there are so many solutions abroad.

Next.

[Slide.]

Dr. SACHS. Life expectancy stopped rising a decade ago. It is falling in the United States. When will we understand we are falling apart in this country and our health system doesn't deliver? It doesn't deliver preventative health.

This tragic story of Dr. Blackstock of the patient who comes in with advanced breast cancer who couldn't afford to be seen beforehand, that is a system? That is the United States of America?

It is shocking and it shows up in the most basic measure of societal performance. No, not GDP, life expectancy, which is falling in the United States because we are becoming completely dysfunctional.

Next, please.

[Slide.]

Dr. SACHS. We are at the top of avoidable deaths. Again, from the Commonwealth Fund, if you look in detail at what the cause of deaths are, these are preventable deaths. But the United States has the most of them and it has the least reduction of them of all of our peer countries.

Next, please.

[Slide.]

Dr. SACHS. Costs for low income populations. Well, we have heard this repeatedly—out of control, unlike all of our peer countries. We are the country all the way to the right hand side. We look different from all of the rest of the countries.

Next, please.

[Slide.]

Dr. SACHS. We have, as you know, an epidemic even before COVID of deaths of despair. We have soaring deaths from suicide, from substance abuse, opioid overdoses, and so forth, for people who are battling economically as well, and so you see the biggest rises for the white population with no college degree. This is an absolute shocking epidemic in the United States of America without a health system to address it.

Next, please.

[Slide.]

Dr. SACHS. We have vast differences across the States. Typically, as is true in U.S. politics, the States farthest behind are the ones most defending the status quo. Very sad. But this is how our politics is absolutely upside down.

Instead of a system that could work, we have an opposition to State control, as if we have a functioning market system.

Next, please.

[Slide.]

Dr. SACHS. What we have is a scam going on. Please understand. We have the most high-priced high-cost system and we have a system that is filled with its sense of success because they are making a fortune.

This is what I clipped from the Wall Street Journal list of our CEOs of our pharmaceutical industry. What do you want, $20 million salary? Twenty-five million a year salary? Thirty million a year salary? That is the game of the United States of America health care system.

Chairwoman MALONEY. Dr. Sachs——

Dr. SACHS. Yes?

Chairwoman MALONEY.—you are way over time. It is fascinating. Way over time.

Dr. SACHS. I am sorry. Can I come quickly to an end? I will come—just next slide. I will come very quickly to an end.

[Slide.]

Dr. SACHS. Our not for profit hospital administrators are making millions and millions of dollars.

Next, please.

[Slide.]

Dr. SACHS. I will just do—forgive me, Chairperson. I just want to make two more points.

Chairwoman MALONEY. Please—OK. All right.

Dr. SACHS. This is an incredibly profitable industry. That is where the high prices go.

Next slide.

[Slide.]

Dr. SACHS. This is the biggest lobbying industry. I don't have to say this in congressional testimony. Everybody knows it. This industry lobbies a fortune and makes a fortune. It is a scam, and we should compare with the rest of the world and see what we are getting. We are wasting a trillion dollars a year that is going into administrative costs——

Chairwoman MALONEY. Thank you.

Dr. SACHS [continuing]. High costs for products, for prices, for devices——

Chairwoman MALONEY. Thank you.

Dr. SACHS [continuing]. For hospital care. Thank you very much, Chairwoman.

Chairwoman MALONEY. Thank you. Thank you. The gentleman yields back.

And now, Dr. Michener, you are now recognized for your testimony.

Statement of Jamila Michener, Ph.D., Associate Professor, Cornell University Department of Government, Co-Director, Cornell University Center for Health Equity

Dr. MICHENER. Thank you, Chairwoman Maloney, and the members of the Oversight Committee and everyone who is here today.

My name is Jamila Michener. I am an Associate Professor of Government and Public Policy at Cornell and also co-director of Cornell Center for Health Equity. I am going to focus today in my comments on underscoring the role of universal health insurance coverage, particularly in addressing racial health inequities, but also in terms of strengthening our democracy.

So health equity has never been a reality for people of color in the United States. It has never been a reality for Black, Latinx, or indigenous people in the United States. Notwithstanding changes that have happened over time and some improvements that have occurred, we have seen persistent and continual disparities.

Consider just a few examples that are striking and contemporary. Black and indigenous Americans live for fewer years, on average. Black and indigenous Americans are more likely to die from treatable preventable conditions. They are more likely to die when there is no need for them to die on account of a lack of access to health coverage and health care.

Black people are at a higher risk for chronic health conditions like diabetes and hypertension. They are more likely to die from breast cancer and colon cancer. Importantly, this is particularly because of late stage diagnosis and differential treatment.

Black and indigenous women are more likely to die during or after pregnancy, to suffer serious pregnancy-related complications and they are more likely to lose children in infancy.

All of these things, of course, were exacerbated and became worse during the pandemic, and the few disparities that I just discussed are only the tip of a much, much larger iceberg, an iceberg that this country has been crushed under since before it was even the United States.

Crucially, these inequities are a product of systemic forces, not individual choices. This isn't about people being able to choose. In fact, it is about the lack of options, the lack of ability to have equitable access, and much of this lack is grounded in systemic racism.

Systems of racial stratification shape whether you live in a neighborhood that will promote your health, whether you have access to resources like health insurance to sustain your health, whether you have daily experiences with things like discrimination that might undermine or threaten your health, and importantly— and I will address this shortly—whether you have influence over the political processes that can be activated to protect your health.

Inequitable health insurance is a key factor that contributes to this range of disparities. So the fact that people of color have lower access to health insurance is a significant, life-threatening, policyaltering problem. Unequal, unstable, unaffordable, and constrained access to health insurance contributes to people of color experiencing their healthcare system as profoundly discriminatory and difficult to navigate.

People of color are more likely to delay care or forego treatment. They are less likely to and struggle to adhere to prescribed medication and treatment regimes and, again, these disparities are not lessening. If anything, they are widening.

Access to health care is an ethical and human rights principle. It means that everyone has a fair—health equity, rather—it means that everyone has a fair and just opportunity to be as healthy as possible and, of course, access to health insurance is a critical determinant of whether health equity could be a reality.

I want to spend the last bit of my time here pointing something really important and often overlooked out. Over and above the noted material and health benefits of having access to health coverage, which we have heard quite a bit about today, that access would provide people who receive that coverage with a strengthened position in our democracy. It would reinforce their civic status and reinforce our promise as a country, as a polity, of full inclusion for all. This connection is not obvious.

But social scientists—political scientists, in particular—have established that health and health policy are crucial for democratic— full democratic participation. Medicaid is a perfect example. Medicaid expansion is associated with boost in voter turnout.

Disenrollment is associated with declines in rates of voting. Medicaid beneficiaries and their ability to participate in politics is a function of their experience with the program.

This is not about partisan politics or electioneering. It is about ensuring that people with the most at stake, with the most to lose here, many of the people we have been using in our anecdotes, that they actually have meaningful influence over the political processes that determine their ability to thrive and survive, and we know that that influence happens when, in fact, they have access to the resources that they need to allow them to be full and equal members of our democratic polity.

I want to end with words from a Medicaid beneficiary from systematic qualitative research that I did. This is a woman from Georgia named Lucy. She says, I think a lot of people on Medicaid and without insurance are scared that their voice is not going to be heard, at the end of the day, that no matter how much you protest or how much you call on those in higher upper seats, it is as if our voices don't matter. And people think, why should I even say anything? It is not going to change.

But in actuality, it might just be that one vote that pushes us to change everything. But to us sitting down here, looking at those up there, it is like our voice—what is my little voice going to do?

Lucy and other people who are fighting for health equity, especially racial health equity, in this country have voices that we ought to be responsive to. Universal health coverage is part and parcel of precisely that responsiveness.

Thank you.

Chairwoman MALONEY. Thank you, Dr. Michener.

And Mr. Barkan is our last panelist and you are now recognized for your testimony.

Statement of Ady Barkan, Jd, Founder, Be a Hero

Mr. BARKAN. Good morning, Chairwoman Maloney, Representative Bush, and members of the committee. Thank you for holding this hearing and inviting me to testify.

My name is Ady Barkan and I am the co-executive director of Be A Hero, an organization whose mission is to win health justice in America.

As you can see, I am currently in bed. I live in California and it is rather early here, and because I am living with the neurological disease ALS, which has left me almost completely paralyzed, it takes me a very long time to get ready in the morning. So I am grateful for your grace in permitting me to participate from bed.

But I am even more grateful that it is my bed in my bedroom, in the home I share with my wife and our two young children. I am able to live at home because I have 24-hour home care. Without it I would be forced to live in a nursing home separated from the people I love.

I don't know if that would be a quality of life that I would be willing to tolerate. Home care is, literally, keeping me alive.

Three years ago, I came to the Capitol to testify in the Rules Committee as the first ever hearing about Medicare for All. I was emaciated, weighing about 100 pounds, down from 160. I had trouble breathing and was sweating even though the room was cold. Every month, my body deteriorated further. I felt like I was dying.

Later that year, I had to decide whether to get a tracheostomy, a procedure to implant a breathing tube into my windpipe to compensate for my failing diaphragm. But I didn't know how I would be able to pay for the care that would allow me to stay alive.

My insurance had already denied me a ventilator, stating that it was experimental, and then two weeks after that, they rejected access to an FDA-approved ALS drug. Even good health insurance, which I have, does not cover the long-term home care I need to survive. Paying out of pocket would have left my family bankrupt quickly.

And so for too long after my diagnosis, my wife, Rachel, and I tried to get by without homecare, which put the burden on her to care for both my young son and me.

We eventually secured 24-hour home care after suing my health insurance company in Federal court. Home care has been life changing, allowing me to participate in my family's life in ways I thought were no longer possible for me.

My daughter, Willow, was born six months after I gave my testimony and now I am a father to two beautiful wild children. But it shouldn't take a seasoned activist, a team of lawyers, and the generosity of strangers and friends to get the health care you need to survive. The reliance on crowdfunding to afford healthcare is a uniquely American tragedy. My outcome is the exception. But the challenges we face fighting insurance companies for services we are rightfully owed are not.

We spend such absurd amounts on health care and we get such bad outcomes for our money. The high cost of care and infuriating bureaucracy burdens all of us, including nurses and doctors, working families and small businesses.

The only people who benefit from this absurd system are the corporate executives who profit off of our pain and spend inordinate amounts of money trying to stop you from making life much better for your constituents.

We have allowed greedy health care corporations to set the parameters of what we can expect of our health care system, and because of it, we have been forced to normalize the fate of bankruptcy, illness, and death.

It is shameful that in the richest country in the world we choose to inflict so much suffering. Since that first hearing about Medicare for All, our country has been through the worst public health crisis in a century.

The pandemic has revealed and exacerbated the existing inequalities in our profit-driven health care system. It has hit hardest on disabled people, poor people, Black, Latino, and indigenous people, and especially people who live at the intersections of these categories, and one out of three COVID–19 deaths in the U.S. are related to gaps in health insurance.

Nearly a million Americans have already died from the coronavirus. How much more is necessary to shock our legislators into action? When we lost 3,000 lives on September 11th, we responded by reorganizing our national security system, launching a global war on terror, and conducting two massive invasions and occupations.

Three hundred times more people have died in this pandemic but we have not marshaled our national energy to build a better health care system. It is a scandal and it is a shame.

But in the last two years, we have also seen glimmers of what is possible when our government takes action to prioritize people over profits and works to guarantee care for all.

Congress subsidized the Affordable Care Act marketplace plans, leading to unprecedented enrollment, and paid States to keep millions more people on Medicaid. As a result, more Americans have health insurance than ever before.

Taxpayers funded vaccine research and then our government made vaccines easily accessible to all at no cost, and recently, our government made rapid test kits available to all Americans who requested them free of charge.

These programs and many others are at risk of ending if Congress does not fund them and when the pandemic emergency policies expire. Instead of returning to the status quo, which fails all of us and especially our most vulnerable communities, we should build on the progress we have made during the pandemic.

The American people deserve so much more and so much better. Our seniors and disabled children and adults deserve to live at home, not be warehoused in institutions. Working people deserve high quality care, regardless of their income or their employer marital status.

The people of rural America deserve good mental health care options, good community clinics, good accessible hospitals, and so do the residents of poor urban America and the people who live on Indian reservations. And seniors on Medicare deserve care also for the parts of their body above their necks, which means their teeth and eyes and ears and minds.

We can and must do better. We know what the solution is, a system that brings everyone in and abandons no one, where we are patients and people, not opportunities for profit. The road to reach the better world of our imagination may be long and there are many obstacles in our way.

But our North Star is clear. It is time for America to guarantee comprehensive, affordable health care to all. The best way to do that is by enacting Medicare for All. If each one of us continues to demand better, if, together, we build an even more powerful movement for health justice, then I know that someday we will get there. Thank you.

Chairwoman MALONEY. Thank you so much for your testimony. I now recognize myself for five minutes for questions.

In 2010, President Obama signed the Affordable Care Act into law, laying the groundwork for over 30 million people to achieve affordable and available health care. Republicans not only opposed this law, but in the past decade have voted over 60 times to repeal or weaken it.

Dr. Blackstock, you gave very moving examples of health care challenges. As an emergency physician who sees patients directly, how does access to health care coverage affect a person's health?

Dr. BLACKSTOCK. Thank you, Chairwoman. Well, I mean, access to health care coverage is key. Unfortunately, what I often see in the emergency department, especially working in the communities that I work in, are people who, because they do not have insurance, will come to the ER sometimes for treatment of chronic medical problems or come for issues like advanced cancer, as I described with the patient that I had, with preventable diseases that have essentially become chronic and even late stage.

And so they are at the point in their disease process where, you know, it is very costly for them to even be able to afford to pursue treatment. And so access to care, essentially, results in improved health for my patients and enables them to——

Chairwoman MALONEY. Thank you. Reclaiming my time——

Dr. BLACKSTOCK [continuing]. Utilize primary services.

Chairwoman MALONEY.—because I want to get to Dr. Michener. You have studied the relationship between access to coverage, health equity, and racial justice. How did coverage gains under the Affordable Care Act advance health justice in the United States?

Dr. MICHENER. Well, coverage gains advance health justice, in particular, in relationship to racial justice by allowing more Black and Latino people to have health coverage than had before and we see this in particular in Medicaid expansion States where the increases in terms of access to health insurance were most striking among Black and Latino Americans. And so that is a key factor. Of course, it is more challenging in nonexpansion States. So that gives us like a kind of primary lens into the importance of access.

Chairwoman MALONEY. Thank you so much. And in this Congress, I was proud to join over a hundred of my colleagues in reintroducing Congresswoman Jayapal's Medicare for All Act, which would transition the United States to a national single-payer health care system.

So, Dr. Sachs, how would the Medicare for All Act expand access to health care while controlling skyrocketing costs that you pointed out in your testimony?

Dr. Sachs?

Dr. SACHS. Chairwoman, ACA expanded coverage but it did not control prices. We need Medicare for All to do both, to ensure coverage and to ensure a system in which highly concentrated highly monopolized service providers don't charge an arm and a leg—literally, don't charge prices that are twice what other countries pay.

For each procedure—diagnostic, medicines—we are out of control in price. So Medicare for All would ensure coverage, control prices, and, by my estimates, save about a trillion dollars a year for the U.S. economy.

In my world, a trillion dollars a year is not small change. We could use the savings.

Chairwoman MALONEY. Thank you so much. Let me conclude with you, Mr. Barkan, and thank you for your bold advocacy and for your powerful testimony before us today. You remind us all why we are all in this fight.

Why is it so crucial that we achieve universal coverage in the United States?

Mr. Barkan?

Voice. OK. Just a minute while he writes his answer.

[Pause.]

Voice. OK. He is writing.

Chairwoman MALONEY. He is writing it. It takes him a few minutes, if everybody understands.

Mr. BARKAN. We deserve dignity and health. Because we deserve dignity and health.

Chairwoman MALONEY. Thank you. Thank you for your Statement for equity in health. And, in conclusion, as we will hear today, Democrats have proposed a number of different policies to move us toward a universal coverage, including Medicare for All.

Our party has a diverse set of ideas on how to reach this goal. But we stand unified in pushing to make healthcare more affordable and available for every person in the United States.

I thank all of our witnesses for their testimony this morning. I yield back, and now I yield to the gentleman from Georgia, Mr. Hice.

Mr. Hice?

Mr. HICE. Thank you, Madam Chair. We all realize this is a complicated issue but the solution is not government takeover of the health care. It is returning power to the patients, not overwhelming doctors and hospitals with regulations. This is a disastrous pathway to go down.

Ms. Turner, I would like to begin with you, if I may. And I realize it is extremely difficult to try to take the cost issue out of the debate discussion, but I want to try. OK.

So if we were in some magical land where money was no object, in spite of that, are there still problems that exist with a government socialized healthcare system?

Ms. TURNER. Congressman, there will always be resource constraints. That is the world we live in. There are only so many physicians, so many hospitals. They have to be paid. The people that I worry about most in a system like that are the most vulnerable.

I had a father write to me after Medicaid was expanded in his State and he said that there is so many people now on Medicaid that it is almost impossible for him to find a urologist to treat his daughter with multiple health problems. He has to wait sometimes six months for an appointment.

So when you see the people who are most vulnerable having to struggle the most for care, it is because of resource constraints. The studies that have been done on Medicare for All, Congressional Budget Office said that we would likely see physicians paid 40 percent less, hospitals 30 percent less. Many of them wouldn't be able to keep their doors open.

The American Medical College says that they expect at least to have 120,000 fewer physicians. So when we think about putting everybody in the same system, the people who need care the most are the ones who have to fight the hardest for it because the resources are constrained.

Mr. HICE. And what would happen to those who currently have coverage that they like.

Ms. TURNER. I think that is really a major issue. We are a diverse country and your health—our health sector really represents that diversity. And as I said in my testimony, about 175 million people have employer coverage, either employees, retirees, or dependents, they value, including many union workers, 64 million people on Medicare, including about 26 million with Medicare Advantage plans that they have chosen, among many others.

So the disruption of having one single plan following the same set of rules, I think, would find—as diverse and often complicated as our current system is it is because people are responding to top-down rules rather than responding to patients and what they want and I think they want choice and control and diversity.

Mr. HICE. So there is a problem on both sides of the equation. So is it fair to say, in your opinion, that even those who would be— that those currently who need health care that they themselves through the long lines, the waiting periods, all these things—some of the things you mentioned a moment ago—would they be satisfied with a government-run socialized health care system?

Ms. TURNER. Well, you see in the Medicaid program today too many people are forced to go to hospitals—hospital emergency rooms for even routine care and that is because often physicians are paid so little for providing care for Medicaid patients.

I had a physician write to me one time and he said he had taken care of a patient with relatively complex pulmonary problems. When he got his check from Medicaid, after going through all the paperwork, he got a check for $0.06. He said, I can only see so many Medicaid patients.

Mr. HICE. Wow. OK. And there are problems with this type of system all around the world where it has been attempted. What about right here in America in Vermont? What went wrong with Vermont's attempt?

Ms. TURNER. So Vermont wanted so much to be able to be the first State to be able to produce the single-payer system and they invested an enormous amount of time, energy, and money in coming up with the—with a plan they thought could work for their State.

And, ultimately, it was rejected because they realized, as happened also in Colorado, that it was really going to tank the economy with the taxes and the resource-forced constraints and that people were going to have fewer choices than they do today.

Mr. HICE. And it will tank our economy if we go that path and provide fewer choices as well. So I thank you for your testimony. I appreciate it a great deal.

And with that, Madam Chair, I yield back.

Chairwoman MALONEY. The gentleman yields back.

The gentlelady from the District of Columbia, Ms. Norton, is now recognized.

Ms. NORTON. Thank you, Madam Chair. This is a very useful hearing. We are learning what the Affordable Health Care Act has achieved so that we can evaluate what more needs to be done to improve it until we get universal health care. This is, certainly, far less than what it is that we want in the long run.

When I look at last year, 11 million people used the ACA marketplace. Fourteen million people—and this one is particularly important—have enrolled in Medicaid as a result of the ACA's Medicaid expansion, and I think it is important to note that millions of people have benefited from the ACA's protections for people with preexisting conditions. So it has done a great deal.

But, Dr. Collins, let me ask you how the ACA has improved the economic security of families in the United States, particularly those who have historically struggled for access to health care.

Dr. COLLINS. Thank you very much, Congresswoman. Lots of research has shown that we have not only—the ACA has not only led to enhanced insurance coverage and dramatically reducing uninsured rates but it is also lowered financial barriers to care, reduced people's medical debt burdens, reduced out-of-pocket spending for a lot of people who have had preexisting conditions, for example, prior to the Affordable Care Act's reforms.

So this has been a substantial change both for coverage rates but also for reducing—for improving people's financial security.

Ms. NORTON. How much, Dr. Collins, have people in the United States saved in out-of-pocket healthcare costs since the passage of ACA?

Dr. COLLINS. It varies quite a bit by States and the type of coverage people have. But there has been a significant improvement in premiums, what people faced prior to the Affordable Care Act.

When you went to get coverage in the individual market you had to pay the full premium. You do not have to do pay the full premium anymore. There are subsidies to help you if your income is under 400 percent of poverty.

Medicaid expansion has been substantially important for people with very low incomes, reducing premium costs to zero, very low— very low out-of-pocket spending and cost exposure in those two expansions.

Ms. NORTON. Finally, Dr. Collins, you could help us a great deal. What steps can Congress take to build on the ACA and move where we want to go to universal coverage?

Dr. COLLINS. The Urban Institute has analyzed a set of proposals that shows that we can get to universal coverage by building on the Affordable Care Act: Medicaid expansion in every State, an autoenrollment mechanism, public options addressing the high provider prices that I talked about in my testimony.

We can get to universal coverage by the building on the Affordable Care Act. It is critically important that we have a way of autoenrolling or people have a way of auto-enrolling in coverage.

Keeping people on the Medicaid experience of the last—during the pandemic shows how much more enrollment you can get in Medicaid if people can stay on Medicaid rather than having to get on and off all the time. So but it is, certainly, possible to get there by building on the law.

Ms. NORTON. Well, we do know that if it weren't for the ACA millions more people would face catastrophic medical debt or the choice between paying for their medical care or, perhaps, for groceries.

But I do think it is time to build on the progress Democrats secured with the ACA by enacting policies that move us toward universal coverage. That is where we need to go.

Thank you very much, Madam Chair, for this hearing and I yield back.

Chairwoman MALONEY. The gentlelady yields back.

The gentleman from Wisconsin, Mr. Grothman, is recognized for five minutes.

Mr. GROTHMAN. Thank you. There, obviously, are many reasons for the high cost of health care in this country. But as the ranking member on the subcommittee dealing with Homeland and being on the border quite a bit, I always talk to the Border Patrol and they tell me at least one of the draws for people coming here illegally is promises to pick up their health care. Obviously, nothing is free.

Ms. Turner, maybe you could comment a little bit on the effect on health care costs in the private sector as more and more people come here illegally and who is paying for their health care?

And, again, I will remind you that the Border Patrol have told me that they feel that some people are coming into this country not just because the administration, obviously, has somewhat of an open door policy but because they feel they are getting free health care. Who is paying for that health care?

Ms. TURNER. A number of different programs are paying for their health care. They are disproportionate share hospital payments to hospitals that have more patients who cannot pay for their care. You actually see employer plans paying more for coverage because private—because public plans and uncompensated care drives up the cost. So in many cases, it is taxpayers and it is also people with coverage and private plans.

Mr. GROTHMAN. Right. How many of these people are paid for by a government program and how many directly have to be eaten by the providers?

Ms. TURNER. You know, I was interested to see when I was looking at the CBO study on the uninsured that about half of the uninsured actually—of illegal immigrants actually have coverage. So I think there are different ways for people to get coverage than through——

Mr. GROTHMAN. Right. If somebody comes here and, I suppose, to get coverage from an employer, right?

Ms. TURNER. I would presume employer but they may have actually some private plans that they buy—short-term limited duration plans, other private plans.

Mr. GROTHMAN. OK. When people don't have plans and the number of illegal immigrants in this country—different people argue about 10 million, 20 million, we don't know.

Let us say there are 15 million people here illegally. Obviously, that is going up every month considerably and it is particularly going up in significance if the Border Patrol is right in telling me that some people come here specifically for the free insurance.

Does that cause private insurance or insofar as individual hospitals bill out their billing to go up to compensate for the people that they are—that they have to pay for health care that they are not being compensated on?

Ms. TURNER. Yes, and they—price negotiations are very opaque and complex among hospitals and plans and private payers.

Mr. GROTHMAN. Right, but somebody has got to eat it, right?

Ms. TURNER. Yes. Somebody pays for it.

Mr. GROTHMAN. At the end of the day, the hospital, to pay their mortgage, to pay their employees, if people are coming into that hospital and they don't have insurance but they have to have something being taken care of, and at least I am told that if they have a serious problem at the border we will deliver them to the local hospital and, of course, other people are being shipped all around the country. Those costs are being eaten by the private sector or the individuals who are being billed on an individual basis. Isn't that true?

Ms. TURNER. Correct.

Mr. GROTHMAN. Do you know—does that happen in other countries? Do you know—do you have any idea, like, in European countries where they have——

Ms. TURNER. Actually, other countries have very different ways. There is really no one way that you can say other countries deal with it. But that is—it is a problem everywhere and it rises cost— increases cost for those who do pay for those from those who don't pay or cannot pay.

Mr. GROTHMAN. OK. And I want to talk a little about pharmacy benefit managers. I am under the impression right now a lot of times there are rebates. A lot of times the pharmacy benefit managers wind up eating those rebates.

Could you comment on the fairness and the kind of who is getting the benefits and who is the intended beneficiaries of the rebates offered by the pharmaceutical companies?

Ms. TURNER. Yes. There are large rebates that go through the pharmaceutical benefit managers and they say that that reduces insurance costs across the board. But there are policy proposals that would have those rebates go directly to patients at the pharmacy to actually reduce their costs. I think that would be better policy.

Mr. GROTHMAN. I have a bill like that. So you think that would be a good idea if we care about the individual to make sure that the—and the rebates are intended to go to the consumer, right? Not the pharmacy benefit manager. Is that true?

Ms. TURNER. And we need more transparency so people understand that those rebates are going to the PBMs—and because of the transparency—lack of transparency we don't know where— rather than to the patient.

Mr. GROTHMAN. Thank you.

Chairwoman MALONEY. The gentleman yields back.

The gentleman from Maryland, Mr. Raskin, is now recognized for five minutes.

Mr. RASKIN. Madam Chair, thank you so much. This is an extraordinary and surpassingly important hearing and I hope it will be an historic one. I want to thank you and Representative Bush and Representative Tlaib for your leadership in bringing this forward.

Dr. Sachs' remarkable testimony shows that we are first in health care costs in America, first in administrative costs, first in CEO salaries, and last in access to care, last in equity, and last in health care outcomes, and our colleagues across the aisle just don't want to deal with any of these realities and are now trying to blame the systemic failures of our health care arrangements on undocumented immigrants, which is just an absurd and irrelevant distraction from the real nature of the problem.

Another sign of the sickness of our system is the staggering levels of medical debt that our constituents have, not just constituents of Democratic members but constituents of Republican members, too.

Americans, collectively, owe an astonishing $195 billion in medical debt and this is a leading and, in many places, the foremost reason for bankruptcy that persons and families go into.

Dr. Collins, let me start with you. What are the leading factors that cause patients and their families to fall into this extraordinary abyss and quicksand of medical debt?

Dr. COLLINS. First, being uninsured is the primary risk factor. So people who are uninsured have the highest rates of medical bill and debt problems.

Second, being underinsured—having a health plan that face really high deductibles or maybe you have a non-ACA compliant policy that doesn't protect you from catastrophic health care costs. That is a second major source of medical debt. But we just have a lot of cost exposure in this—in our health system both through uninsurance and also through underinsurance.

Mr. RASKIN. Around one in five American families are struggling with serious levels of medical debt, and for many people with lower incomes their fear of coming under crushing medical debt becomes a major deterrent to their obtaining critical medical care or even just normal regular checkups.

How does medical debt pose a threat to the health as well as the economic security of families that are working to make ends meet?

Dr. COLLINS. Now, I do find that people who have faced high out-of-pocket costs whether or not they have medical debt or just face really high deductibles make decisions that are not in the best interest of their health.

So they tend to delay care, delay filling their prescriptions, just not getting care until it is—until it becomes very, very serious. And when they do get care they have—incur a lot of debt and have a lot of downstream financial problems like ruined credit ratings.

Mr. RASKIN. My family lived in France for a year, and just in our first month there our youngest daughter came down with just a piercing earache. She began to scream and we called some French friends and asked what to do. They told us to call a service that is connected to their national health care program.

In 20 minutes, somebody knocked on our door. It was a doctor. Came in, diagnosed Tabitha as having strep throat, wrote a prescription that we were able to fill downstairs. And asked if we were citizens. We said no. Asked if we were a member of the national health care plan. We said no.

They said they would have to charge us as strangers and that would be 20 euros that we had to pay. And they had a certain number of pediatricians assigned to each neighborhood that worked with us.

So when people talk to me about universal health coverage it sounds pretty good. But what are the statistics? What do they show about whether millions of people in France and other countries are facing crushing medical debt the way tens of millions of our people are facing crushing medical debt? Does that exist in countries with the dreaded universal health care, or what our colleagues are denouncing as socialized medicine?

Dr. COLLINS. No. People in other high income countries have— face much lower out-of-pocket costs. Just a striking difference between here and—there and the United States.

Mr. RASKIN. So, Dr. Sachs, let me ask you about this. You know, they called Social Security socialism. They called Medicare socialism. They called ACA socialism. So, of course, they are calling universal health coverage socialism. So but hasn't the progress of our system been about taking public responsibility, for making sure that everybody has access to health care?

Dr. SACHS. Every other high income country, Congressman, has found the solution to the problems that we are grappling with, and all of the stories that we hear avoid the most basic point, which is all the other countries have solved these problems. We have not.

The reason we have not is that we have a system that is geared toward not just private profits, massive profits of the hospital system, the pharmaceutical system, and massive waste of administrative costs unmatched by any other country in the world by far.

We are wasting hundreds of billions of dollars of billing time, of churning, of not in the network, in the network, can't cover this, dispute this. Nobody does this.

And I would say to Congressman Grothman we are spending $4.1 trillion right now. How much is that—is undocumented aliens on the border? A pittance. It has nothing to do with that.

It has to do with prices that are out of control in the U.S. And with all the benefits of ACA, which brought people in, it did not create a system of cost control. We need a system of cost control.

And, Congressman, I have had the same experience——

Mr. RASKIN. And thank you so much, Dr. Sachs.

Thank you, Madam Chair. This system is irrational. It is costly. It is unjust. We should move forward with——

Mr. HICE. Madam Chair, his time has expired.

Chairwoman MALONEY. Thank you for your Statement. His time has expired.

The gentleman from Texas, Mr. Cloud, is now recognized.

Mr. CLOUD. Thank you. We keep saying we are having a national discussion on health care and the truth is over the last few years we haven't really had a national discussion on health care.

Too often health care and health insurance get conflated as if they are the same thing. Indeed, the chair, in her opening remarks, claimed that Obamacare expanded health care to 30 million people. That is not exactly true. You could maybe make the case that it expanded health insurance coverage to 30 million people.

But anytime you mandate something by law and say you are going to fine them if they don't have it, there is a probably good chance you are going to see an uptick in the usage of whatever that product is.

But that doesn't mean that it was better. We saw some people who were over insured who didn't need that much insurance. For most Americans, we saw over—a steady decline in what health insurance covers.

Meanwhile, premiums have gone up. Too many times families would even not be able to afford the health care because they are paying for mandated health insurance.

And so it is important for us to remember that health insurance is the middleman in the process and health insurance never—a middleman never decreases a cost. It always increases it. Now, in isolated incidences, it, certainly, should save money and everybody should have some sort of health insurance.

But when we are looking at systemic ways to save money, we probably need to go a different approach than what we have been doing, and what happens too often here in Congress is we, first, pass a program that breaks a system and then we come up behind it and try to be the solution to what we already broke. We definitely need a discussion but the discussion should center on how we provide actual care, how do we open access to care as opposed to mandating insurance for everybody.

Ms. Turner, I would like to ask you why are health care costs increasing in the United States?

Ms. TURNER [continuing]. That.

Mr. CLOUD. I am sure there is a few of them but if you could touch on—

Ms. TURNER. A lot of reasons for that. A lot of it has to do with the lack of transparency. Nobody has any idea how much somebody else is spending on their care and Americans, they want to know those questions.

But to—just to take the ACA as an example, the recent increase in subsidies through the American Rescue Plan put $17,000—every newly insured person in the American Rescue Plan costs about $17,000 for—in taxpayer dollars.

But many of those people are dropping private coverage because the subsidies are more attractive to go on the public—to go in the public plan. So I think that we need to look at what are the incentives in the system. Are there incentives for people to get better care, better coverage, more affordable care, get higher quality?

But we don't do that. We run it through rules and regulations, through Federal and State and local spending programs, rather than really trying to engage the same forces that work in the rest of the economy to give people more choices and more affordable products and services.

Mr. CLOUD. It is interesting. You mentioned—we talked about regulation in this committee hearing being a major driver of healthcare costs, but it is interesting you mentioned price transparency in the sense that for elective procedures, for example, we see technology being a driver and when costs are transparent and people are able to price compare, we actually see those procedures in the market actually decreasing over time, where we see, by and large, most of the industry increasing over time because, as you said, what makes capitalism work is the fact that you can shop. And then so we have removed that ability—that accountability metrics—from the system. And so I would agree that anything we could do to put accountability back in the system would help.

We talked about some of the ways that health care costs are increasing. What are some of the ways, maybe some technological breakthroughs, different ways that prices could be lowered in healthcare—that we could lower the costs and, thus, provide access to more people?

Ms. TURNER. I have reported in my testimony about several States that have used a provision in the Affordable Care Act called Section 1332 to be able to repurpose some of the money that is going through the ACA to be able to figure out how can we do a better job of taking care of the most expensive patients who need the most care but they are not able to see the physicians they need because of—everybody is a one-size-fits-all plan.

They make this a much more—a much more focused plan, doing a better job of taking care of the vulnerable. What that has done is reduced prices across the board for everybody else and that brings more people into the market, just as one example.

Ms. CLOUD. One other thing I would like to ask your opinion on in the short time I have left is what nation produces the most medical innovations?

Ms. TURNER. That would be the United States of America.

Mr. CLOUD. So we definitely have some issues we have to fix. But if we were to adopt the same system that does not lead to innovations, the world at large would really suffer.

Ms. TURNER. The world relies on us for innovation—for medical innovations.

Mr. CLOUD. OK. Thank you. I yield back.

Chairwoman MALONEY. The gentleman yields back.

The gentlelady from Ohio, Ms. Brown, is now recognized for her questions.

Ms. BROWN. Thank you, Chairwoman Maloney and Ranking Member Comer, for holding this important hearing. Most—across the United States, most people of color are most likely to be uninsured and live in communities with higher rates of uninsurance or underinsurance.

As a result, people of color are more likely to be able to afford critical medical care and more likely to go into medical debt trying to pay for it.

Dr. Michener, let me begin with you. How does uninsurance and underinsurance put people of color at elevated risk for adverse health outcomes and what does this mean for health equity in the United States?

Dr. MICHENER. Yes. So uninsurance and underinsurance through many different mechanisms put people of color at risk. One mechanism is through delayed care, through inadequate care, because not only is care delayed but when you do receive care without insurance it is difficult to adhere to care protocol and regimens. It is difficult to get prescriptions and so on and so forth.

One of the things that I think is important to point out in some of the conversation that has emerged around things like choice and innovation is that when we are talking about disproportionately people of color and people who don't have insurance, in fact, they lack choice in a profound way, and to the extent that we are innovating they are the very people who are not benefiting from any of those innovations.

So if we can have the latest technology and the best procedures but you lack health insurance, you are not able to have access to those procedures or to have access to that technology, and those kinds of circumstances are disproportionately encountered by people of color.

And so when we are thinking about choice, innovation, and other things like that, the question is who will have the choice and who won't? Who will be excluded from that? Who will benefit from the innovation and who will not?

And I think that when we take equity into account it really, I think, undermines the overemphasis on some of these things and, at the very least, point out the importance of balancing that with an emphasis on equity so that we actually have full inclusion.

Ms. BROWN. Thank you very much. So achieving universal coverage is necessary to address those structural inequities in our current health care systems that have historically afflicted communities of color.

So, Dr. Blackstock, how would achieving universal coverage help ensure that patients of color receive high quality care before they become seriously ill?

Dr. BLACKSTOCK. Thank you so much for that question. You know, as I mentioned in my earlier testimony, there are other social determinants of health that are very key in influencing the health of communities of color, but lack of access to health care is so incredibly important because we need our patients to be able to access primary and preventive health care services.

They need to be connected with primary care physicians and other types of health care providers so that initial diagnoses are made so that they are placed on the proper protocols and medications and so that they are really cared for and managed in a way so that they don't develop these significant chronic medical problems that will impair, really, their ability to live a full life.

Ms. BROWN. Thank you very much. It is clear throughout the testimony today that universal coverage will help eliminate the entrenched health inequities experienced by people of color in this country and, importantly, it will help eliminate many of the barriers to care for people of color that they so often face because of their employment or immigration status.

So universal coverage will create healthier communities so that every person in the United States can thrive and that is what excites me most.

And so with that, I yield back.

Chairwoman MALONEY. The gentlelady yields back.

The gentleman from Pennsylvania, Mr. Keller, is now recognized for his questions.

Mr. KELLER. Thank you, Madam Chair, thank you, Ranking Member Comer, and thank you to the witnesses for being here today.

Socialized medicine is not only the wrong approach, it would be detrimental to our healthcare system and the patients who rely on it. Americans are the ones who are best equipped to make health care decisions for themselves as well as for their families, not the government.

I want to talk a little bit about a personal experience. But before I do that, two names—Alfie Evans and Charlie Gard, a toddler and an infant in the U.K., whose doctors said they would not survive.

So the doctors took the parents to court and were forced to remove their children from life support. One child could have gone to Italy and one could have come to the United States for care. But their government didn't allow them to do it.

I want to talk about 1994 when my son had a brain injury, and he was life-flighted to Geisinger Medical Center, and they performed brain surgery and he came out of the surgery and the doctors told us—they said kids in his condition aren't a 50 percent mortality rate. It is not a 98 percent mortality rate. It is 100 percent mortality rate. And over the coming weeks, we were told to remove him from life support because he was not going to survive.

But we had control of our health care decisions, not the government, and because of that the following year it says Freddie Keller of Kramer is Geisinger's poster child for 1995 in northeastern and central Pennsylvania. He is now 31 years old and works for the health care industry in supply chain, because we had choices over his care, not the government.

So that is socialized medicine. That is universal health care. That is someone, a bureaucrat from the government, deciding what is best for you and your family, not you, and that should never happen in the United States of America. Never.

So I did want to just ask a question to Ms. Turner. Might these policies affect patient wait times for treatment in which patients would suffer most from the increased wait times?

Ms. TURNER. Very powerful story, Congressman. Thank you for sharing that.

We do have evidence of what happens when systems operate under a global budget in other countries and, as you say, you wind up with government making decisions about whose life matters and they do that in sometimes very subtle ways, something called quality adjusted life year, where they decide whether or not your life is worth getting a new medication that may be on the market.

So I think the choice and control issue is profoundly important because it also focuses the system on the patient rather than on bureaucrats making decisions about people's lives.

Mr. KELLER. Just another question. In addition to restricting choices and access to care, would a single-payer public health option truly lower health costs for Americans?

Ms. TURNER. My colleague, Merrill Matthews, from the Institute for Policy Innovation actually looked at the administrative cost savings, and when he made an apples to apples comparison, he said it is not going to save any money administratively because the government is still going to have to make sure that a procedure was provided.

The documentation will have to be there. The person will still have to be paid. There will still have to be all of the paperwork that we have now. It just runs through a different system.

So it is not clear to me to see how it would save, and Chuck Blahous from Mercatus Center says that it would actually cost $32 trillion over 10 years.

Mr. KELLER. OK. Thank you. You know, this is something that I always say—changing who pays the bill does not make something affordable. All it does is remove choices from people.

Not only would socialized medicine offer patients fewer medical options, limited number of qualified medical personnel in the midst of a healthcare worker shortage, and discourage medical innovation, proposals like Medicare for All would cost the taxpayers an estimated $32 trillion over 10 years. The cost of government-mandated universal health coverage is simply too huge.

And I tell you what, the cost of my son's life under a system like that that had to be endured by the parents of Charlie Gard and Alfie Evans, I don't want to see that happen to any family in America. The government should not be telling you whether or not your child can receive life-saving medical attention.

And thankfully, here in the United States of America, I didn't have to face that choice in 1994 when I was 28 years old, struggling to make ends meet, and my son is still alive today.

Thank you and I yield back.

Chairwoman MALONEY. The gentleman yields back. The gentleman from California, Mr. Khanna, is recognized for five minutes.

Mr. KHANNA. Thank you, Madam Chair. Thank you for your leadership on Medicare for All and holding this historic hearing.

Let us be very clear that private health care insurance is a crushing tax on working families in this country and on businesses. Working families have to pay a tax of almost $12,000, if not more, on the premiums that they pay to private health care insurance and on their out-of-pocket costs.

And businesses in this country are competing with one arm tied behind their back. What is the tax that private health insurance is putting on businesses? Sixteen thousand dollars for a family that businesses are having to pay. That is why they are having to compete in a total disadvantage to many companies and businesses and manufacturers overseas.

In fact, if you talk to CEOs they say the biggest burden on their payroll often is this tax that they are paying to private health insurance. On top of that—and I want to just talk about the economics here—on top of that you have over 23 million Americans in medical debt because of the tax that they are paying to private health insurance.

You have 78 million Americans not able to get the health care they need, not able to treat their kids for the medicine they need or get, in certain care, life-saving treatment—68,000 Americans every year dead because they aren't able to have health care that they need.

This is the current system, and what we are saying is have a tax cut for working families. Have a tax cut for businesses by eliminating the excessive profits of the insurance companies, of the pharmaceuticals, and off the hospital facility fees.

Let us get those deadweight costs out to cut taxes, cut the private insurance tax for working families at a time of inflation. Bring the costs down, bring the costs down for businesses. This would be actually deflationary and it would be one of the largest tax cuts in putting money back in the pockets of working families and businesses.

Dr. Sachs, let me ask you. You are an economist. Can you just explain from a commonsense perspective, if you take out of the system the excessive insurance costs, the excessive pharmaceutical costs, the excessive hospital facility fees, aren't you going to reduce the amount that ordinary Americans are paying and the American businesses are paying, from an economic perspective, into the system?

Dr. SACHS. Congressman, of course you are. It is just bizarre, this discussion that it would be too expensive to lower the health care costs through universal coverage. We just heard it would be an extra $32 trillion.

This is phony numbers because it doesn't count the saving that comes from eliminating the private premiums, which, as you say, that is a tax on household income. It is all verbiage. The United States is paying twice what any other country pays for health care.

I wish there was some—I wish the opposition—the ranking members would ask me some questions, not just their witness some questions, so we could actually have a discussion.

We are paying nearly 20 percent of GDP. We are paying $12,000 per person, more than twice what other countries are paying. Shame. It is just absurd. And where is that? It is procedure by procedure, it is hospital stays, it is doctor's appointments, it is devices, because our system is rigged.

From all the campaign contributors that make this the No. 1 lobbying sector in this country, it is rigged for an overpriced health care system. We could save about a trillion dollars a year for our country to do other useful things.

Mr. KHANNA. Dr. Sachs, I totally appreciate that and, you know, this is why I strongly support Bernie Sanders' Medicare plan, which is a very reasonable plan.

I guess my last point is this. I am not a Ph.D. economist like you but I don't think you have to be a Ph.D. economist understand that if you are—if you have a system where everyone can go to any doctor they want because everyone now is in network under Medicare and you eliminate the middle people—you eliminate the people who are charging the insurance fees, you eliminate the pharmaceuticals who are making their profits in terms of having to negotiate with Medicare, and you eliminate hospitals from just being able to charge whatever they want because they have to negotiate with Medicare, that as a common sense perspective you are going to bring costs down because you are going to not have all those profits.

Am I missing something in that simple explanation?

Dr. SACHS. No. Not only are you not missing something, it is not even hypothetical. It is proven. It is proven in France, in Germany, in Norway, in Denmark, in Netherlands, in Sweden, in Finland. Go look at the data. I live in these countries. I see these countries day by day. It is the demonstrated daily reality.

So it is not theory. It is proven, and the United States is the single outlier because we are driven by greed and by a system of lobbying that imposes this completely overpriced system, which is not a system actually.

And what you said, Congressman, is exactly right. The hospitals charge whatever they want, and we all know that the pricing is a game, completely nontransparent. They charge what they can charge because they are discriminating monopolists. They charge what they can get away with where they can get away with it. There is no market here at all.

Mr. KHANNA. Thank you, Dr. Sachs.

Madam Chair, I yield back.

Chairwoman MALONEY. The gentleman yields back.

The gentlelady from North Carolina, Ms. Foxx, is now recognized for her questions.

Ms. FOXX. Thank you, Madam Chair, and I want to thank our witnesses for coming today.

I have to say that listening to this last interchange, there are some people on this committee and some of our witnesses who live in a Never Never Land—a Never Never Land.

Ms. Turner, today, we have heard a lot about government-run health care such as Medicare for All but we have not heard much about the quality of care. This is not surprising, though. I cannot think of one thing the government does that is both affordable and of high quality.

What would Medicare for All do to employer sponsored insurance and how would this affect the 155 million Americans currently enrolled in employer-sponsored coverage, something that Americans overwhelmingly support?

Ms. TURNER. Well, the Medicare for All would abolish employer-based health coverage and all other current health care programs so that we would all be under one single plan. And you see—you know, you see employers trying so hard to innovate—providing wellness programs.

Wal-Mart, before the Affordable Care Act was implemented, had computer rooms to help their employees tailor a plan that worked best for them. That is the kind of innovation that we would lose, the kind of patient focus, the kind of energy from the private sector that leads to innovation.

Ms. FOXX. How would Medicare for All affect the nearly 64 million seniors who are currently on Medicare? Would they receive better coverage?

Ms. TURNER. Sixty-four million seniors and disabled patients on Medicare, 26 million of them have chosen Medicare Advantage private plans. That shows that they believe that there is more value to having a private plan that can manage their care. They can pick the plan that provides the best network in their area.

So they are—and some, we believe, could be focused care. If you have diabetes or heart disease, you will get the specialist in that care. So I think that there would be a lot of innovation lost and I don't think seniors would be nearly as happy as they are now.

Ms. FOXX. Yes. As I understand it, our friends on the other side of the aisle want to do away with Medicare Advantage and the kinds of things you have described.

Also, under Medicare for All or another universal health care system would Americans have wait times to seek care that are similar to those in Canada and the U.K.?

Ms. TURNER. Absolutely, because you—there are lots of different ways for people to pay for systems and one of them is in care that they don't get and, oftentimes, they don't even know the care that they are not getting.

I talked with a physician from the U.K. and he saw both private sector patients as well as those on the National Health Service Plan. And he said, I can't even tell my public patients about new medications that would be better for them because it is not covered under the system. Patients who are going to have to wait for two years to get a knee replacement surgery pay out of pocket, if they can, to go to the Mayo Clinic if they live in Canada or someplace else. So they—patients pay in other ways, especially those most in need of serious medical care.

Ms. FOXX. Thank you.

Ms. Turner, another question. The Mercatus Center calculated the costs of Medicare for All and found that under the best case scenario it would increase Federal budget commitments by $32.6 trillion over the first 10 years of implementation.

Thirty-two point six trillion is triple what the Federal Government spends on our defense and domestic discretionary programs over 10 years. Even doubling the corporate income tax could not cover that.

Since our government is consistently overspending and running large deficits each year, is a massive new government spending program like Medicare for All financially feasible or sustainable?

Ms. TURNER. It is really hard to see how that could work. As I said in my testimony, that Colorado, Vermont, and, most recently, California have tried to figure out how they could do just on a State basis a single-payer system.

In California—even California saw the price tag of $450 billion a year and they said that is really not something we can afford.

Ms. FOXX. Thanks. And my last question—what lessons can we learn from the implementation of Affordable Care Act, or Obamacare, and how should that inform our expectations for further government involvement in health care?

Ms. TURNER. Running a top-down system is really difficult, especially from Washington, in a country as diverse as this one is, and one of the reasons there have been so many changes to the ACA is because some things worked for some States and others didn't work for other States, and for different sectors of the economy you need to have local control bottom-up decision, making not top-down decisionmaking that could have the same catastrophic effects as healthcare.gov did.

Ms. FOXX. Thank you, Ms. Turner.

I yield back.

Chairwoman MALONEY. The gentlelady yields back.

The gentlelady from Michigan, Ms. Tlaib, is recognized for her questions.

Ms. TLAIB. Thank you so much, Chairwoman, and thank you so much to my good colleague from St. Louis, Congresswoman Bush, for really leading us to making sure that we bring our residents to Congress and make sure that they are seen and heard.

As Bishop Starghill from my district said in his testimony, and it was very clear, lacking access to health insurance not only causes financial hardships but it puts millions of Americans' lives at serious risk every single day.

I represent the third poorest congressional district in the country. Very limited choices when folks talk about choices when it is convenient. But today, whether or not a person has access to high-quality medical care depends, largely, on whether they are insured or whether—what their income is, whether or not they are wealthy enough to pay for it.

Medicare for All will guarantee access to high-quality health care for every person in our country, regardless of their ability to pay, and we have heard a lot of misleading claims from my colleagues on the other side.

But Medicare for All—what we are talking about and what they are saying is simply not true. But what we are saying in regard to making sure it is accessible and making sure folks are covered is true. It simply says you don't have to be rich to have access to quality health care.

So my question to my good friend, Mr. Barkan—and, you know, thank you so much for being here today and getting up so early— your activism has helped put a face to so many people that really don't lack—lack the access to being here but also the fear that comes with being this vulnerable and talking about not being able to access health care.

So I want to hear from you and whether or not you believe we would have universal health care today if we didn't allow those who profit by our broken health care system to make political contributions.

[Pause.]

Voice. Mr. Barkan is writing.

Mr. BARKAN. I think it is crystal clear that we have a corporate corrupted system and it needs to change.

Ms. TLAIB. Thank you, Mr. Barkan. Do you believe in the work and the advocacy work that you are doing that our system is rigged? If yes, how have you seen it so clearly in your advocacy work?

Voice. One moment.

[Pause.]

Mr. BARKAN. Medicare for All boils down to the simple question of whether or not you believe that health care is a human right. Those against Medicare for All will call this policy various names to distract the public from the truth that you and me, nurses and small businesses, all of us, would fare far better under a system that guarantees comprehensive, high-quality, affordable health care to all.

The only people who benefit from our for profit system are the multimillionaire healthcare executives who profit off our illness, their corporate lobbyists, and the elected officials who take campaign contributions from health care corporations and, therefore, their policy views from them.

Ms. TLAIB. Thank you so much, again, for your courage and for helping, again, put a face to this broken health care system. I know I have said it over and over again, and Chairwoman, you have probably heard me, corporate greed does kill in our country and Medicare for All would address the disparity and reduce the health inequities associated with our current broken system while preserving patients' ability to make the best medical decisions for themselves and their families no matter their income.

So for those reasons, I am incredibly proud to support Medicare for All, and, again, thank you so much, Chairwoman Maloney, for your courage in having this hearing.

I yield back.

Chairwoman MALONEY. The gentlelady yields back.

The gentleman from Arizona, Mr. Biggs, is now recognized for his questions.

Mr. BIGGS. Thank you, Madam Chair.

You know, preventing individuals from making personal health care decisions, and then we have heard a lot about how important that is, and ceding those decisions to government bureaucrats is really the violation of fundamental human rights, and one must acknowledge that inherent in President Obama's Statement that if you like your health plan you can keep it was that recognition of that human right to make your personal choices. I mean, that is why he said that, because he knew that is what we want. We want to be able to choose our health plans.

But that was a lie and he told that lie because he wanted to get his Obamacare, ACA, whatever you want to call it plan out there. Which is interesting to me because repeatedly I have heard colleagues across the aisle say today the system is broken.

This is the system you designed. This is the ACA. We are all living under it now one way or the other. It is your system. Dr. Sachs said it is broken. It is unfair. It is too expensive. There is too much administrative costs.

I agree with everything you said there. You are exactly right. But this is the system that my colleagues across the aisle made. Even in the private industrial sector—in the private plans, the administration costs are too high.

They are way too high, and part of that is because of the regulatory environment that mounted on the previous unworkable regulatory environment that was imposed through the ACA.

The good doctor repeatedly mentioned peer countries. But when you talk about single-payer systems or socialized systems, although we don't—apparently we are not supposed to call it that—there really isn't a peer to the United States. Just the size of the United States mediates against that.

The peer countries in population size or cost of health care and expenses paid are not comparable. There is no peer country on the charts that you were putting up there. Go back and take a look.

The scale of a Medicare for All plan will be unlike anything you have seen in the history of the world. And, you know, scalability is a problem but the inherent problems can be even in small States.

I mean, so when Vermont tried to implement its single-payer experiment that failed under the cost. Now, we all say, hey, yes, everybody should be able to have access to their health care. We want it to be affordable.

But Medicare for All would make our ability to buy private insurance even more difficult than it is to buy private insurance in Canada, and it wouldn't necessarily guarantee that you are going to reduce cost. I mean, let us take a look at Medicare and pharmaceutical costs. They are way up. They still remain high, even under Medicare.

So I think so much of what I have heard today is talking around the issue for political purposes. If you want to solve problems, I am willing to talk and let us solve problems.

But I am told today that all the other countries have solved their problems and I don't know that I believe that. There are lots of studies and science that indicates that is not true.

Dr. SACHS. Congressman, could I respond?

Mr. BIGGS. Let us take a look at one specific—let us take a look at one specific issue. And I don't know who is interrupting me.

Dr. SACHS. That was me, Professor Sachs. I was wondering whether I could respond.

Mr. BIGGS. Yes. Yes. I am not asking you a question, sir. I am not asking a question. Please don't interrupt me.

Dr. SACHS. OK.

Mr. BIGGS. In 2009, Medicare cut payments to independent cardiologists. This is what we call—this is what we call an unintended consequence, for people who don't understand economics.

2009, Medicare cut payments to independent cardiologists for common tests but left untouched their payment for cardiologists employed by hospitals. So what do you think what happened? Some imaging services Medicare paid hospitals nearly twice as much as they paid independent physicians for the same service.

The effects were predictable—were predictable. The percent of cardiologists employed by hospitals rocketed. People received many more cardiac imaging from hospital outpatient departments and less from freestanding physicians' offices. That is an unintended consequence.

So I will turn to you now, Ms. Turner. What effects would Medicare for All have on patients' ability to receive care in a timely, affordable fashion?

Ms. TURNER. I can't agree with you more about the comparison. The Swiss system works fine for Switzerland. It is the size of Massachusetts. That is not something that we can impose on this whole country.

We must have diversity, and I think people value not only diversity of places to get care but they also—they value diversity of how that care is going to be paid for and giving people more options than they have today.

As we see, fewer and fewer because so much of the spending is controlled by government—Federal and State government—rather than by patients and rather than seeing what innovations could come to provide people with more options of portable coverage that they own and take with them and that they can afford to keep with a strong safety net for the vulnerable.

Chairwoman MALONEY. The gentleman's time has expired.

Mr. BIGGS. Thank you.

Chairwoman MALONEY. Thank you. I now recognize the gentlelady from California, Ms. Porter. She is recognized for her questions.

Ms. PORTER. Dr. Collins, what percentage of revenue do private insurance companies spend on administrative costs?

Dr. COLLINS. Between—about 17 to 18 percent of spending in private insurance plans.

Ms. PORTER. So if I pay my insurance company $100, 1, 2, 3, 4, 5, 6, 7, 8, 9, 10, 11, 12, 13, 14, 15, 16, $17 go to administrative costs. What about Medicare? What do they spend on administrative costs?

Dr. COLLINS. That range is about, you know, 3 to 5—3 to 5 percent of Medicare spending.

Ms. PORTER. 3 to 5—3 to 5 percent. About 3 to 5 percent right here, and if we look at just billing costs, just billing in insurers' costs, Medicare is at one percent. Private companies spend 17 times more on administrative costs than Medicare?

What are private insurance companies spending on that Medicare is not? Does Medicare spend hundreds of millions of dollars on television advertisements like private insurance does?

Dr. Collins?

Dr. COLLINS. No.

Ms. PORTER. Does Medicare spend millions of dollars on stock buybacks to shareholders?

Dr. COLLINS. No.

Ms. PORTER. Does Medicare spend money on marketing? Private insurance likes to put its name on stadiums and PGA tournaments? Is there a Medicare Arena?

Dr. COLLINS. No.

Ms. PORTER. Does Medicare spend $23 million on executive pay like private insurance companies do?

Dr. COLLINS. No.

Ms. PORTER. We know how much it costs to run a high-quality health insurance program—one dollar. Out of $100, research shows that Medicare spends 1.1 percent on administrative costs.

We spend $4 trillion on health care every year. We could save $200 billion dollars on administrative costs with Medicare for All and those savings, they could go to expand Medicare. We could spend that money to let patients see dentists.

We could spend that money and let patients pay for hearing aids, to help older adults afford eyeglasses, to bring down the cost of prescription drugs, to finally pay mental health professionals for the work they do.

Instead, all this money is wasted. We are not talking about paying to keep the lights on in operating rooms or improving the quality of care. All this money is used to pay big insurance to push paper. It is death by 200 billion paper cuts.

Dr. Sachs, what is it about the U.S. market that leads to these sky-high administrative costs?

Dr. SACHS. Congresswoman, there is no market. These are local, concentrated providers that have tremendous power to set their prices and to set extraordinary salaries. We should contemplate that the so-called not for profits in this country pay their hospital directors $5 million.

This is unbelievable, and so this is why these costs are—why the prices are so high. The administrative costs are so high because we don't have a system because we spend 20 percent of our spending just to funnel money between organizations, which is something that other countries don't spend. And I would like to say—I would like to——

Ms. PORTER. Dr. Sachs, I wanted to ask you——

Dr. SACHS. Sure.

Ms. PORTER. Reclaiming my time for one second, Dr. Sachs.

I wanted to ask you specifically about standardization and what role that might play in reducing some of this waste that we could reallocate to health care costs.

Dr. SACHS. Well, when you go in for billing there is no standardization on anything, on the information technology, on the systems, who is in, who is out, what is going to be reimbursable.

Everything is completely opaque. Everything is completely discriminatory depending on who is being involved. So standardization is a big part of all of this because when you lack standardization you put in resources to suck out whatever rents you can and we end up, as you counted those $17 out of every $100, basically, lost—basically, wasted.

Ms. PORTER. Reclaiming my time. Reclaiming my time, Dr. Sachs.

We heard today about the cost of Medicare for All but there is a cost to letting insurers paperwork patients and providers to death and that cost of inaction is $200 billion on administrative costs.

Now, administrative costs waste money but they also waste health care workers' time. A recent study found that a majority of doctors—56 percent—support a single-payer health care program.

Why? Because today doctors spend only one quarter of their time with patients. What are they doing with the rest of their time? Paperwork.

Ninety—and I want to also—I want to add not only would 56 percent of doctors support Medicare for All but patients would have the most choice under Medicare for All. The health insurance coverage with the biggest network is Medicare. No private insurance comes close. Ninety-nine percent of pediatric—nonpediatric doctors participate in Medicare.

So I want to recap. Medicare for All would save money on administrative costs, $200 billion a year. Medicare for All would give patients the most choices, 99 percent of nonpediatric providers, and Medicare would let doctors practice medicine.

Not surprisingly, given these three things, what do we get with Medicare for All? Better health outcomes, and that is why I support Medicare for All because they support patients over paperwork.

I yield back.

Chairwoman MALONEY. The gentlelady yields back. But before we continue, as mentioned at the beginning of the hearing, Dr. Sachs has a hard stop at 12 o'clock. We thank you for your participation, Dr. Sachs. You are excused. Thank you.

Dr. SACHS. Chairwoman?

Chairwoman MALONEY. Now the gentleman from Kansas, Mr. LaTurner, is recognized for five minutes.

Mr. LATURNER. Thank you, Madam Chair. I appreciate it. Dr. Sachs, I will give you—we don't agree on this but I will give you 30 seconds. I can see that you wanted to say something.

Dr. SACHS. Thank you very much. I want to say there is no economic cost to Medicare for All. It is pure saving. The $32 trillion reference is about the increase of Federal finance.

But there is a larger decrease of private finance. The net is a large saving. We need to take that talking point out of the discussion so that we can solve the problems. We also need to understand we do have a peer. It is the European Union. Life expectancy is 81.3 years for their 440 million people.

Mr. LATURNER. I am going to have to reclaim my time.

Dr. SACHS. Congressman, thank you. Thank you very much for letting me say those words.

Mr. LATURNER. You are welcome. In the name of bipartisanship, Madam Chairwoman.

Dr. SACHS. I appreciate that very much. Thank you.

Mr. LATURNER. Yes. My questions are for Ms. Turner. Much of the money that Americans pay for health care is going toward its administrative costs, whether that is for hospitals, pharmacy benefit managers, or insurance companies.

Many proponents of Medicare for All strategies say that administrative savings would offset some of the costs of the governmentsponsored health care program.

Do you agree that Medicare administrative costs are or would be significantly less burdensome that administrative costs for private insurers? If not, where do you think that misconception comes from?

Ms. TURNER. Thank you, Congressman. I quoted in my written testimony a study by Dr. Merrill Matthews of the Institute for Policy Innovation in Texas, who is saying that when you compare apples to apples, when you compare the actual cost of making sure a procedure was performed, deciding who your—what your patient population is, making sure the doctor gets paid, all of the other procedures, you wind up with about equal cost.

One of the things that the Federal Government is able to do is to be able to shove the cost of collecting payments off to other agencies or not do the kind of due diligence that many of the private plans do to make sure that the revenues are connecting and premiums from the customers are able to be—are spent properly.

So you see much—you see less waste in private programs because they are spending some part of that administrative money on due diligence. We need to see more of that in the Federal Government.

Mr. LATURNER. I am going to stick with you, Ms. Turner.

Committee Republicans have discussed how the expansion of Medicaid and the elimination of eligibility checks have contributed to government waste through improper payments. According to CMS, total improper payments for Kansas in 2021 amounted to nearly $290 million.

Can you provide any further insight into why 20 to 25 percent of all Medicaid payments are disbursed improperly and whether fixing these improper and wasteful payments would change how you feel about a Medicare for All policy?

Ms. TURNER. Well, I already don't think that a Medicare for All policy is the right approach for such a diverse country as this is that values innovation. If you wind up with standardization you get rid of a lot of the innovation.

My colleague, Brian Blase, who—with Paragon Health Institute, also a senior fellow at the Galen Institute, has done a deep dive into the study that you referenced about Medicaid waste, and he assumes—says that in one year Medicaid had improper spending of about $100 billion that was, largely, for people who were on the program and weren't eligible.

There are a number of other ways in which people are taking advantage of the system and it is not being properly monitored. The inability of the Federal Government to be able to contain hundreds of billions of dollars in wasteful spending with a program that would cover 330 million Americans seems to me an in comprehensible task.

Mr. LATURNER. You highlight the burdensome Federal regulatory demands that providers must respond to. Often it is at the expense of their patients. Can you describe further how increased government involvement in the health care sector reaches a point of diminishing return when it comes to addressing patient needs specifically?

Ms. TURNER. Well, writing one more regulation to solve one more problem is when we are going to add more paperwork to a physician's backlog.

The former head of the Mayo Clinic one time looked up the—had his staff look up the number of regulations that the Mayo Clinic— had pages of regulations the Mayo Clinic had to comply with in order to treat Medicare patients. He said, we lost track at 100,000 pages, and that was two decades ago.

So the more regulatory compliance—and we are not going to get rid in this country of demands that taxpayer dollars are spent on this service that is promised. We are going to have to have paperwork trails. People are going to have to follow those trails.

That money is going to have to then go to the provider after it goes through other administrative checks. That—we are not going to get rid of that with Medicare for All. The only way we can get rid of that is through innovation, to give people more choices so that they are—the marketplace is responding to those needs rather than complying with all these hundreds of thousands of pages of rules and regulations.

Mr. LATURNER. Thank you, Ms. Turner.

Madam Chair, I yield back.

Chairwoman MALONEY. The gentleman yields back.

The gentlelady from Missouri, Ms. Bush, is now recognized for her questions.

Ms. BUSH. St. Louis and I thank you, Chairwoman Maloney, and to the committee for this—for convening this critically important hearing, which represents our steadfast commitment to achieving universal health care coverage in the United States.

For my colleagues on this committee, you have a choice in front of you today. It is a choice to save lives or a choice to let people die. Disproportionately low income people, Black people, brown, indigenous people, die. Because you are a human, you deserve health care. Because you are a human, you deserve health care.

In my community, Black mothers die at three to four times the rate of white women. In my community, Black babies are nearly twice as likely to die prematurely. I came to Congress because enacting Medicare for All, it is not a choice for me. It is a moral imperative.

When I worked as a nurse, I cared for uninsured and underinsured patients every single day. I am reminded of one patient with diabetes who was failed by our healthcare system because she could not afford all the aspects of her care.

Technically, she had primary—she had insurance and a primary care provider but she could not afford her insulin prescription, her needles, her test strips to track her blood sugar levels. The patient—this patient, she was forced to ration her insulin and she skipped appointments due to transportation, making it difficult to follow treatment plans. This patient ended up losing a limb and eventually she died.

One health condition, if left untreated, can be deadly. For me, after I turned 18 years old, I became an uninsured low wage worker. I could not afford to retain a primary doctor so I went to the emergency room for treatment for conditions like asthma, sinus infections, and tooth aches.

My asthma was exacerbated by environmental pollution and degradation and continued to worsen without proper medical care.

During the Ferguson uprising, toxic tear gas filled my lungs, leaving me gasping for air and it worsened my condition.

Even though I was working as a nurse, I was forced to pay a $900 monthly premium, a $4,600 deductible, and struggled to treat my asthma.

Dr. Michener, can you please describe the relationship between health care coverage—a healthcare coverage status and economic mobility in the United States? How would Medicare for All reduce poverty and stimulate economic growth in the United States?

Dr. MICHENER. Representative Bush, thank you for the question. I think this is a key dimension.

Oh, I thought it was on. Oh, OK.

Yes, I think this is a key dimension of the—of this discussion that we, I think that on some fronts has been willfully ignored, which is that there are gross inequities not just in our health system but in our economic and social and political systems, more broadly, and the inequities in the health system are exacerbating the inequities in other places.

So if we look at all of our anti-poverty programs that we have in this country, the largest effect on poverty—child poverty in particular but poverty more generally—comes from our Medicaid program. Addressing healthcare disproportionately addresses some of the other core and fundamental challenges we have around economic inequality in this country. And so what happens when you provide people with healthcare? We have seen it through Medicaid. They are less likely to be evicted. They are less likely to recidivate and go back to prison. They are more likely in the long term to have positive financial outcomes.

Ms. BUSH. Yes.

Dr. MICHENER. Less likely to be living in poverty, less likely to have medical debt, more likely to have positive educational outcomes, more likely to have employment. We want to say, "socialized medicine," scare people away with the scary phrases, right? Oh, the government is going to be making the decisions.

Ms. BUSH. Right.

Dr. MICHENER. If the government is not making the decisions, who is? The market, and that is not democratically controlled.

Ms. BUSH. Thank you.

Dr. MICHENER. It is not something that people can influence.

Ms. BUSH. Thank you. If not three years into the pandemic, when will we actually address the fundamental flaws and structural inequities present in our healthcare system, in our privatized healthcare system? Dr. Blackstock, using your extensive experience as an emergency physician, can you please describe what the implementation of Medicare for All would look like for healthcare providers, particularly those who interact with insurance companies?

Dr. BLACKSTOCK. So what it will do is it will enable us as health providers caring for our patients to more efficiently care for our patients, to prioritize the primary and preventive services that we provide them. It will not result in more administrative effort and cost. In fact, it will do the reverse. And so it will help remove barriers for our patients to seek care, and doing so will enable us to buy the best care and to do so even more efficiently than we could that now.

Ms. BUSH. I will say "yes" to that as the nurse that actually worked the bedside. That is true. Thank you, and I yield back.

Chairwoman MALONEY. The gentlelady yields back.

The gentleman from Texas, Mr. Sessions, is now recognized for his questions.

Mr. SESSIONS. Madam Chairwoman, thank you very much. For those members that are here, I only see one other in the room that was here in 2008, 2009, 2010 as we went through this exact same type of hearing about how great the Affordable Care Act would be. And yet you notice no one Democrat that I see talks about how great the Affordable Care Act was because it wasn't. It took $800 billion out of Medicare. Democrats actually took $800 billion away from seniors to pay for this. Now we have Medicare for All like it is their newfound answer. Oh, by the way, I heard one of our persons just a minute ago giving testimony about how Medicaid works so well. I wonder why we are not doing Medicaid for All.

Well, ladies and gentlemen, the bottom line is that both the House bill and the Senate bill under Section 107, "Beginning on the effective date as in Section 106(a), it shall be unlawful for a private insurer to sell health insurance coverage that duplicates the benefits under this act, and it is unlawful for an employer to provide benefits." Well, Mrs. Turner, I recall it took President Obama several election cycles before they could even tell us "what was in the bill." And it took them a long, long time, only to discover that their drawings on a board did not equal success for patients. Why would they want everybody to go into this system that is designed for seniors? It is designed for seniors. It is not designed for children. It is not designed for disabled young adults. As a matter of fact, I have a disabled, at least one in my family, a Downs syndrome young man who is my son. They are trying to take all of America and make it to where we would be at the same place two years later of trying to say, my gosh, what did we do.

Ms. Turner, I know the gentleman, Dr. Merrill Matthews, well. I know the gentleman, Dr. John Goodman, well, and they have spoken about the excessive impact that this would have. Do you agree with me?

Ms. TURNER. I do, Congressman, and I also agree that we really have to figure out what the problem is we are trying to solve since two-thirds of people who are uninsured today have access to coverage. They are just not enrolled. So I think we need to look at specifically how do we help get people into the system who, for a number of different reasons, are not participating. And we also need to figure out how can we do a better job of delivering specialty care to people with special medical needs rather than a one-size-fits-all standardization, which is ultimately going to work for very few people.

Mr. SESSIONS. Yes. Mrs. Turner, when I came to Congress, I had spent 16 years at a small telecommunications company called AT&T. AT&T was prohibited by the law that was passed by Democrats and President Obama that said that they would not allow employers to deduct benefits, money spent on employer-provided healthcare to retirees. That is against the law. They wanted to move everybody off of an employer-provided model, which seemingly everybody was happy with, and to move to a Medicaid model.

The question I would ask you is, do you think that a system, let us say, American Airlines or AT&T, that that would be the model that we want everybody to move to just like employer-provided healthcare? Because as I read this, I am a political science major. When the government competes against somebody, free market that is called socialism. When the government dictates who can be in the marketplace that is communism. What do you think this is, given that as a choice?

Ms. TURNER. Well, I believe that Medicare for All definitely is a socialized healthcare system.

Mr. SESSIONS. Why is it socialized? It doesn't allow anybody to compete against it.

Ms. TURNER. Everybody would——

Mr. SESSIONS. Wouldn't that be communism? You may not have been a political science major.

Ms. TURNER. I don't have a term for it, but certainly it is a one-size-fits-all program.

Mr. SESSIONS. It outlaws anyone else from providing coverage.

Ms. TURNER. Right.

Mr. SESSIONS. That is communism. I thank the gentlewoman for being here, and I thank the chairman of the committee for this hearing today. Thank you.

Chairwoman MALONEY. The gentleman yields back.

The gentleman from Illinois, Mr. Davis, is now recognized for his questions.

Mr. DAVIS. Thank you, Madam Chairman, and thank you so much for calling this very important hearing. And I guess I would say one thing: Pete, I was in the room. I am a strong supporter of the Affordable Care Act. I was then. The 30 million people who got an opportunity to get healthcare coverage, I am sure they are all supportive of it as well.

I believe in a single-payer system of Medicare for All, and I have spent many years advocating for universal healthcare. As a matter of fact, I am pleased to know that I come from an area in Chicago Metropolitan where we have 120 clinic sites for federally qualified health center clinics. But also, we know that for many individuals living with less income, being uninsured and underinsured makes accessing healthcare untenable and unaffordable. People with less income or more likely to be uninsured in every State, but most especially in those States that have refused to expand Medicaid.

Dr. Collins, let me ask you, how has the failure of certain States to expand Medicaid under the ACA affected uninsurance rates in the United States?

Dr. COLLINS. Thank you, Congressman. That is a great question, and I agree that the Affordable care Act has put us on a path to universal coverage. And there are things that are preventing us from getting there right now, and one of them is the fact that 12 States haven't expanded eligibility for Medicaid. People are entitled to Medicaid by law, but States have chosen not to expand. About more than 2 million people are caught in the so-called coverage gap and unable to be enrolled in their State's Medicaid program or enroll in the marketplaces.

Mr. DAVIS. And people with low income or people who don't have the resources, for example, to purchase prescription drugs and pay the rent, they may have a different opportunity. Dr. Blackstock, let me ask you. You are an emergency room physician. What differences have you observed in the health of patients who come to the hospital with health coverage and those who come without?

Dr. BLACKSTOCK. Thank you for that question, Congressman. I have worked in two different types of hospitals. I have worked in hospitals where people have insurance, and their health status and health outcomes are far more superior than patients I have cared for in public hospitals with patients who were uninsured and underinsured. I have seen patients who are uninsured coming in with uncontrolled chronic medical conditions that compromise their quality of life and that lead to an early mortality. And we don't see that in the same way in an insured population.

Mr. DAVIS. Thank you very much, and, Mr. Barkan, let me end with you. What can we do and how can we get rid of the barriers that people without resources have to being able to obtain healthcare for what their needs are?

Voice. OK. Ady is writing.

Mr. DAVIS. Yes, I think we are just waiting for Mr. Barkan.

Mr. BARKAN. We need to build the social movements to transform this reality. Thank you.

Mr. DAVIS. Thank you very much, Madam Chairman. Again, thanks to this very important hearing, and I certainly want to commend those who generated the enthusiasm and the need to hold it and to have it, and I yield back.

Ms. BUSH.

[Presiding.] The gentleman from Florida, Mr. Donalds, is recognized for five minutes.

Mr. DONALDS. Thank you, Madam Chair. To the witnesses, thanks for being here.

Look, here is the deal. We already run a single payer health system in the United States. It is called the VA system. The VA system has been plagued with backlogs. It has been plagued with long lines. It has been plagued with shortages of care. It has been plagued with overspending. It has been plagued with fraud and abuse. We have never fixed it. We choose not to fix it. But what we are going to say is, is that the VA system, which we know has not provided the best outcomes for the men and women who have served our country with honor and distinction, we are going to say instead of fixing that system, we are going to create a much larger system for every American where our own experience with the VA system has already proven what happens when you have universal coverage.

We have another system. It is called Medicare. By and large, it is one of the most popular systems that the Federal Government has in the United States. It goes insolvent in somewhere between 5 to 7 years. I was actually just in the Budget Committee, and director for Office of Management and Budget, in the President's own budget, which he just released yesterday, does not show any slowing down of benefits with respect to Medicare, but then also no proposals about how you are going to keep this situation going in Medicare because we are spending significant amounts of money, providing care to the elderly who paid in through payroll taxes over decades in the United States. But there are no reforms to actually make sure that the benefits can be paid, which means that we are just going to have to dig into the pockets of every American to continue benefits when the money that was actually allocated for those benefits is not even enough to pay the burden going forward. But yet in his hearing, we are talking about universal healthcare.

I remember a video. It was a YouTube video from years and years ago. This was back when I was a fledgling political watcher, and it was from a member of our body who still serves here today, who talked about how the Affordable Care Act, effectively referred to as s Obamacare, was just the first step toward universal healthcare. What Obamacare has done, what the Affordable Care Act has done, however you want to call it, it has led to higher deductibles, and it has led to higher premiums in the United States bar none.

Of course I am a Member of Congress right now. I am on Obamacare. I have never paid higher insurance premiums than I am paying right now. I have never paid higher deductibles that I am paying right now. And everybody I know in my district and throughout the State of Florida, and, frankly, across the United States, their deductibles are higher. Their premiums are higher. Their access to care is actually less than it was before the Affordable Care Act. But the answer from the Democrats in our body is universal healthcare or Medicare for All, or whatever the amalgam is going to be.

Ms. Turner, you said in your opening testimony that undertaking universal healthcare in the United States, according to CBO, would be "complicated, challenging, and disruptive." The complicated, challenging, and disruptive would apply to all Americans whether you are Black, or White, or Hispanic, whether you are rich or whether you are poor. You know, it doesn't matter. When you unleash a system that is complicated, challenging, and disruptive, that affects everybody, and where are they going to go?

Ms. Turner, I have a question for you. Because of all these situations that we are talking about, can you provide some specific examples of potential stalled innovation in the medical field? What products will be most at risk if America adopted a single payer healthcare structure?

Ms. TURNER. What are the advantages today and what would be most adversely affected, Congressman?

Mr. DONALDS. Yes, ma'am.

Ms. TURNER. The world relies on the United States for medical innovation. We saw it in pharmaceutical research with the vaccines just last year. And when you see the Federal Government working together to support the private sector and the incredible resources it has in research and technology, innovation, flexibility, that is when you get results. When you have the Federal Government coming in and saying, this is how we are going to do it that is when you get the CDC with its failure to be able to come up with a test. We have to have the private sector if we are going to have innovation, and if we are going to have innovation, that is what leads to progress. That is what leads to the miracle cures that we see today, new surgeries that would have been impossible to envision 30 years ago.

So having private sector innovators who are rewarded, through ownership of patents oftentimes, but rewarded adequately for their investment in that research is what will solve these problems to give people more choices of more affordable care and coverage. The Surgery Center of Oklahoma is a perfect example. It doesn't rely on government funding to be able to provide the high-quality care it does. It relies on being able to make the procedures that they do as efficient as possible with the best procedure, with the best physicians, the best nurses, and the best outcomes. That is what we need more of.

Mr. DONALDS. Thank you so much, Ms. Turner. Madam Chair, I know I am over my time. The one thing I would say is this. I have long said to a lot of students across the country when I go and speak with them, if the Federal Government was in charge of the telecommunications industry, we would not have iPhones and Samsung Droid phones. We would still be on the Motorola StarTAC, and their response is, what is a Motorola StarTAC, and I am like that is my exact point. It is that funky phone that had the orange buttons and the orange screen. There is no innovation when it comes from the Federal Government. It only comes from private markets. This is the exact wrong way to go. And health outcomes in the United States would actually be worse, and if you don't believe me, look at the VA system. I yield back.

Ms. BUSH. The gentleman from Georgia, Mr. Johnson, is recognized for five minutes.

Mr. JOHNSON. Thank you, Madam Chair. For decades, Democrats have fought to protect and expand access to healthcare, and at every step, Republicans try to gut our efforts. Ms. Turner, do you believe that every American has a right to access America's healthcare system, or is access to healthcare just a privilege reserved only for those who can afford it?

Ms. TURNER. Congress decided in the early 1980's that anyone who needs care and shows up in a hospital emergency room is going to get care. Beyond that, we have just a plethora of government programs to offer coverage to people——

Mr. JOHNSON. But do you believe healthcare is a right or is it a privilege only for those who can afford it?

Ms. TURNER. I think we have a system that allows people who cannot afford it to be able to get care and coverage, but you don't have a right——

Mr. JOHNSON. OK. And you are fine with the system as it is now. I get it.

Ms. TURNER. No.

Mr. JOHNSON. You have been involved in the debate over healthcare reform since President Clinton proposed healthcare reform in 1995. Isn't that correct, Ms. Turner?

Ms. TURNER. That is correct. That was in 1992.

Mr. JOHNSON. And you opposed the Clinton healthcare legislation, correct?

Ms. TURNER. I did not believe then, nor do I now, that the government should be in charge of making all decisions in our health sector.

Mr. JOHNSON. And since 1995, you have headed up an outfit called the Galen Institute. Isn't that correct?

Ms. TURNER. That is correct, that I founded.

Mr. JOHNSON. And the Galen Institute is a right-wing operation funded by right-wing foundations and corporations opposed to healthcare system reform. Isn't that correct?

Ms. TURNER. We work closely with people from both sides of the aisle, and we advocate policies that put doctors and patients at the center of our health sector rather than bureaucrats.

Mr. JOHNSON. OK. Well, let me ask you this. How many times have you testified before Congress on the issue of healthcare reform?

Ms. TURNER. Oh, dozens.

Mr. JOHNSON. And each time you testified, that you spoke in opposition to healthcare reforms proposed by Democrats. Isn't that correct?

Ms. TURNER. Not always. I am sure that there were policies that——

Mr. JOHNSON. You have spoken in favor of some Democratic policy proposals? Is that what you are asking us to believe?

Ms. TURNER. There are some really interesting proposals, like cash for counseling, that were proposed by Democrats to give people in Medicaid the option to be able to get——

Mr. JOHNSON. OK. Well, let——

Ms. TURNER. Absolutely, we support it. We are not partisan.

Mr. JOHNSON. OK. All right. Well, let me ask you this, Ms. Turner. Let me ask you this. For 27 years, you have made a handsome living protecting corporate profits while opposing reforms that would make access to healthcare affordable for all. Isn't that correct?

Ms. TURNER. Our logo of the Galen Institute actually is designed to focus on those who are marginalized and left out, people who don't have access to public programs.

Mr. JOHNSON. And how do you propose for those people to gain access to the healthcare system?

Ms. TURNER. As I said in my testimony, we need targeted solutions. Who is uninsured?

Mr. JOHNSON. Tell me——

Ms. TURNER. Who is being left behind?

Mr. JOHNSON. Tell me your targeted solutions to enable people who can't——

Ms. TURNER. Not one government program.

Mr. JOHNSON. Tell me your solutions targeted toward those who cannot afford access to the healthcare system.

Ms. TURNER. I would like to see States be able to repurpose some of the ACA money to provide care for people who are not covered under Medicaid.

Mr. JOHNSON. So you are in favor of the ACA?

Ms. TURNER. And give people the option to use those resources——

Mr. JOHNSON. Are you in favor of the ACA?

Ms. TURNER. I am in favor of having no one who has coverage today losing it, but I believe many more people could get better coverage——

Mr. JOHNSON. OK. Well, what about those who don't have coverage? What about those who don't have coverage? That is what I am trying——

Ms. TURNER. What I am saying, if you——

Mr. JOHNSON [continuing]. Trying to get you to tell us about.

Ms. TURNER. Repurpose——

Mr. JOHNSON. What proposals do you have that would ensure that folks who cannot access to the healthcare system can have access to the healthcare system?

Ms. TURNER. If States had more flexibility, they would be able to use the existing resources——

Mr. JOHNSON. What about the Federal Government? What is the Federal Government role?

Ms. TURNER. As President Biden said recently, the Federal Government is really out of its element in dealing with something as local and private as healthcare.

Mr. JOHNSON. So you don't believe that the Federal Government should have any role in the delivery of healthcare, do you?

Ms. TURNER. That is not absolutely what I said. I believe that States could do a better job.

Mr. JOHNSON. But I am asking you, you don't believe that the Federal Government should be at all involved in helping poor people access the healthcare system. Isn't that true?

Ms. TURNER. That is not what I said. Absolutely not true. I believe that we need a strong safety net, and we need a strong safety net especially for the vulnerable who find it most difficult to get care and coverage in a system when they are competing with people who are dropping private coverage in order to get onto publicly supported programs. I oppose that.

Mr. JOHNSON. Well, you are not talking about poor people. You are talking people who are paying for insurance premiums. I think the public can see right through your testimony and can see that you support corporate profits over access to the healthcare system for all——

Ms. TURNER. Absolutely not true.

Mr. JOHNSON [continuing]. Including those who cannot afford it.

Ms. TURNER. That is not true.

Mr. JOHNSON. And with that, Madam Chair, I yield back.

Mr. COMER. Madam Chair, that is not what she said. He needs to be on one of Adam Schiff's committees if he is just going to make stuff up. That is not what she said. It is very disappointing——

Ms. BUSH. You are not recognized right now.

Mr. COMER [continuing]. That he would badger the witness like that.

Ms. BUSH. You are not recognized right now. The gentleman from Georgia, Mr. Clyde, is recognized for five minutes.

Mr. CLYDE. Thank you, Madam Chair, for holding this hearing regarding our Nation's disastrous healthcare system. It is long past time that we address this growing crisis, and I commend my Republican colleagues and the Healthy Future Task Force for working on solutions that prioritize innovation and competition to reduce costs and improve quality of healthcare for our constituents.

While many of my Democrat colleagues believe a Medicare for All Program would lower healthcare costs, unfortunately, that couldn't be further from the truth. Reports estimate a Medicare for All Program would increase Federal budget commitments by another $32.6 trillion. That is more than the total of our growing national debt. As the Nation faces continued inflation rates, which are now the highest we have seen in 40 years, one thing is clear:

our current healthcare system is inadequate to meet the needs of Americans. One does not need to look long before realizing the Federal Government is ill-equipped to manage a large-scale healthcare program, as my friend from Florida, Mr. Donalds, pointed out.

It has been 12 years since the passage of the Affordable Care Act, and the Federal Government still fails to provide affordable quality coverage for millions of Americans in rural areas, leaving many communities with only one or two eligible insurers from which to choose. In fact, Obamacare was so disastrous that many States, including my home State of Georgia, filed Section 1332 waivers to exit the ACA marketplace. In addition, the Congressional Budget Office's outlook for major Federal trust funds indicates that the Medicare Hospital Insurance Fund could be exhausted by 2024, and that is in this particular document, the 2020 to 2034 report from September 2d, 2020, right here. If our government cannot even ensure the solvency of Medicare for our seniors and eligible participant recipients which comprise less than 20 percent of our population, there is no feasible way for the Federal Government to provide Medicare for All.

So, Ms. Turner, knowing the current State of the Medicare program, do you believe the Federal Government is equipped to manage a Medicare for All Program?

Ms. TURNER. No, Congressman, I do not. I believe that it has shown over and over that it is very good at spending money. It is not very good at spending money wisely, and it is not very good at all at innovating. When you see the Medicare program, 26 million seniors are voluntarily opting out of fee-for-service Medicare into private plans——

Mr. CLYDE. Wow.

Ms. TURNER [continuing]. Because they say this provides more and better coverage. People want choices. Innovation comes from the private sector and not from government.

Mr. CLYDE. Right.

Ms. TURNER. And that is what our health sector needs to be able to be more affordable and provide more people with coverage.

Mr. CLYDE. Thank you. As a followup, as you know, our rural communities already face problems with limited insurers and lack of access to quality care. In your opinion, would Medicare for All improve or worsen these struggles for patients in rural communities, like mine in Georgia 9?

Ms. TURNER. The CBO has actually shown that it would significantly reduce access to care because a Medicare for All Program would pay physicians and hospitals so much less than they do now, and you would not have the private sector, particularly employer-based plans, picking up the slack in order to be able to make these practices and hospitals solvent. So it is very hard to see how they could provide the same quality, the same access to care by the numbers that they are talking about, the savings that they purport to be able to achieve.

Mr. CLYDE. OK. Thank you. Not only is the Federal Government ill-suited to run a nationwide healthcare program as we just heard, but we must not forget that it is the poor policy decisions of law-makers and executive officials that add to the problem by continuing to overburden our healthcare system, stifle innovative technologies, and raise prescription drug prices. While I am glad that we are holding this hearing to begin addressing our failing healthcare system, simply pointing out a problem is not enough. Our constituents need reliable solutions, not only to ensure the quality healthcare, but also to address the economic crisis, the hyperinflation crisis that is causing prices to currently surge. And I strongly urge my colleagues to abandon a universal healthcare proposal and work toward competitive market-based solutions that are truly in our constituents' best interest.

And in the few seconds I have remaining, Ms. Turner, would you like to respond to anything that my colleague from Georgia asked of you? Is there anything that you want to add to that as you were badgered?

Ms. TURNER. He is putting words in my mouth, things that I am not saying. Can I just make a comment?

Mr. CLYDE. Yes, ma'am.

Ms. TURNER. I really commend you in Georgia and Governor Kemp for the innovative proposal that you have offered to try to repurpose some Federal funds to do a better job of taking care of the vulnerable patients in the State and make care more affordable and efficient by giving them a wider choice of plans. So congratulations. I hope that the Biden administration allows that waiver request to go through.

Mr. CLYDE. Thank you, and I yield back.

Ms. BUSH. The gentlewoman from Illinois, Ms. Kelly, is recognized for five minutes.

Ms. KELLY. Thank you, Madam Chair. Thanks for holding this hearing. One thing I wanted to say really quickly, yes, when the Affordable Care Act was passed, I wasn't here, but it was just the beginning. It wasn't the end. And through the years I have been here, we have been trying to improve it but could not get cooperation from the other side. And the other side always talked about repealing the Affordable Care Act, and when they had a Republican President,

Republican Senate, and a Republican House of Representatives, they did not get it done. So I digress.

Home-and community-based services give older Americans and people with disabilities a chance to live freely and independently in their homes and remain contributing members of their community. Mr. Barkan, I am just going to tell you my question, but I am going to move on to others to give you a chance to prepare to answer. But I wanted to know from you, I would love to hear about the ways in which home-based services have impacted your life, but I am going to move on and come back to you.

The Biden administration significantly expanded access to Medicaid home-and community-based services to the American Rescue Plan. The number of people in the U.S. will need home-and community-based services is projected to more than double by 2050. At the same time, direct care and home service workers are in increasingly short supply. Dr. Collins, what work force investments do we need to make now to prepare for those projected increases in demand, and how can we make sure that these investments are equitable?

Dr. COLLINS. Thank you, Congresswoman. This is a huge burden for families, and everybody is experiencing it both with elderly parents and also with disabled children. It has come up repeatedly in this hearing today. We do need to improve the wages that people are paid who work in these jobs. These need to be living jobs that pay people well enough give people the care they want and the security that people and these families that need them so much need.

Ms. KELLY. Thank you. Dr. Blackstock, let me turn to you. Forty percent of family caregivers identify as Black, indigenous, or people of color. The higher prevalence of family caregiving occurs in Hispanic and Black families. We also know that it is much easier to establish trust with a provider that looks like you, and according to the National Academy of Medicine, this improves health outcomes. I am a person that has worked for the last six years on maternal mortality and morbidity and luckily got some bills passed. Why is it important that we consider health equity in expanding home-and community-based services in America?

Dr. BLACKSTOCK. As you mentioned, by having racial concordance in terms of who the caregiver is or who the healthcare provider is, we know that that will result in better health outcomes overall. So we need to make that investment in making sure that home caregivers receive the funding and support they need to do their jobs.

Ms. KELLY. Thank you. We need to build on the successes of the American Rescue Plan and provide a permanent expansion for home-and community-based services. That is why I support Rep. Debbie Dingell's Better Care, Better Jobs Act, which would invest $150 billion into funding for home- and community-based services through Medicaid and the development of care infrastructure and labor force. Mr. Barkan, I will now conclude with you to respond to the earlier question.

Mr. BARKAN. Thank you for your question and for giving me time to prepare. I get to live a beautiful and full life because of home care. Home care saved my marriage as my wife, Rachel, and I got to be partners and co-parents again instead of patient and caregiver. It is the reason why I get to wake up every morning to my wife and two kids and be an active participant in their lives, but my reality is the exception. Home care is prohibitively expensive, and so when home care is not accessible, which is the reality for most, patients are forced into nursing homes.

Nursing homes are unsafe institutions where patients are merely warehoused and isolated from their loved ones. Since the pandemic began, over 150,000 disabled people have died in nursing homes due to the coronavirus. Many of these deaths could have been prevented if they had the opportunity to receive care safely at home. The loss of these lives are a moral failure and a direct result of the for-profit system of care that corporate lobbyists, like those hired by the nursing home industry, work hard to maintain. It is not exaggeration then to say that the difference between being able to receive care at home surrounded by the love of family and community and living at a nursing home is a matter of life and death.

Ms. KELLY. Thank you so very much for your response. Thank you for being here. Thank you to all the witnesses. Congress must act to ensure that older adults and the disability community are able to access high-quality care in an affordable and inclusive way. Thank you so much, and I yield back.

Ms. BUSH. The gentleman from Kentucky, Mr. Comer, is recognized for five minutes.

Mr. COMER. Thank you, Madam Chair, and, again, I want to thank our witnesses for being here.

Just to begin with, Ms. Turner, we talked about Medicaid, and it has been mentioned many times by those on our side of the aisle that Obamacare was supposed to be the solution for people that couldn't afford healthcare. It was supposed to be the great equalizer and solve all of our healthcare problems. So with Obamacare, many States had the option to expand Medicaid. My home

State of Kentucky was one of those States that expanded Medicaid to the tune of about a third of the State is on Medicaid now.

Now, you talk to medical professionals and providers all over the State, and they will tell you they don't want to see Medicaid patients because the reimbursement rates are so low. That is because the slice of the pie is a certain size of what the States get for Medicaid. The more people that get on Medicaid, the thinner they slice the pie. They have more slices, so the reimbursement rates continue to go down, so a lot of people on Medicaid in Kentucky have trouble finding providers who will get them in. Would something like this happen with Medicare? If we greatly expand Medicare, which is already, as Representative Donalds pointed out, facing financial insolvency, would greatly expanding Medicare have the same negative impact on Medicare patients that expanding Medicaid has had on Medicaid patients?

Ms. TURNER. According to the CBO study, there would be a significant reduction in the number of physicians and hospitals that could afford to take those payment rates. Either they would have to cut back or some of them would even close their doors. So you would have fewer providers, which is the situation that too many people on Medicaid today face that they can't find a provider that can afford to take Medicaid's low payment rates. Many do so out of charity, but then they still have to go through all the ridiculous paperwork to get paid——

Mr. COMER. Right.

Ms. TURNER [continuing]. As I said earlier, six cents for a complicated pulmonary patient. Very few of them would be able to keep their doors open to do that, and I think it would be really a decimation of the medical profession.

Mr. COMER. I have to note I have 29 hospitals in my district. I would go out on a limb and say I have more hospitals than n just about any Member of Congress. Every one of my hospital administrators will say the same thing, and these are, by the way, very rural hospitals for the most part. They say that they lose so much money on Medicaid. Anyone who goes in private pay or has private health insurance, they have to really spike the price up on them to cover the cost for Medicaid. So many of the arguments that my friends on the Democrat side have been making for Medicare for All, I just don't buy because a lot of these policies were tried with Obamacare, and they have failed.

Representative Porter mentioned how efficient the government was in administrative work. That is a joke. The VA is a perfect example of government-run healthcare, and you can talk to my case workers in my office in Tompkinsville, Kentucky, about how inefficient and unresponsive the VA is to the VA patients. Very few VA patients in my district in Kentucky are satisfied with government-run healthcare of the VA. It was also mentioned by several Democrats about the numerous times that Republicans have tried to repeal Obamacare. Can you talk about any of the 60 or so times that Republicans have tried to repeal Obamacare?

Ms. TURNER. Thank you for that question, Congressman. We actually tried to track the number of changes that were being made to the ACA as it was happening, and we gave up, over at the Galen Institute, 70 changes, 43 of which were made by the Obama Administration, some with legal authority, some not. Twenty-four were passed by Congress and signed into law by President Obama, and three were made by the Supreme Court. So the allegation that Republicans have been trying for 60 to 70 times to repeal and replace Obamacare, the law didn't work, and it had to be changed even to marginally work, and still we see that it is not nearly serving the patient population that they had expected, and millions of people are having to pay such high premiums and such high deductibles, that they basically don't feel they are insured.

Mr. COMER. Other thing, and I will close by this, Madam Chair. Rho Khanna made a Statement that I actually agree with. He said we need to eliminate the middle people, and that is why Republicans, with respect to healthcare, we requested a hearing on PBMS—pharmacy benefit managers—that I feel like is an unnecessary level of bureaucracy in the healthcare system. This is something that I believe this committee should have a bipartisan hearing on. Republicans had a hearing. We published a report from our hearing, and I think that is a very good place to start looking if we are talking about trying to make prescription drugs more affordable to people, which is a significant cost of healthcare for people.

So I think the Republicans are serious on this committee about trying to solve the healthcare problems we have in America, but bigger government and government-run healthcare is not the solution to the problem. Madam Chair, my time has expired.

Ms. TURNER. Transparency would be very helpful.

Ms. BUSH. The gentleman from California, Vice Chair Gomez, is recognized for five minutes.

Mr. GOMEZ. Thank you, Chair. First, being uninsured in this country is daunting, and I know that because most of my life I was uninsured until I got a job after college as a child of working class immigrants who had no access to employer-sponsored health insurance, despite them working 4, 5, 6 jobs a week to make ends meet. It is something that it is not only daunting, but it takes a toll on the family. It takes a toll on the children. And when you are uninsured, preventative care is definitely out of the question. You only go to the doctor when it is the absolute last result resort, and that has devastating health and financial consequences that are disproportionately borne by low-income individuals, particularly those of color.

In 2019, the uninsured rate for non-elderly Black Americans was 1.5 times higher than it was for white Americans. For Hispanics and Native Americans or Alaska Natives, it was nearly triple. When people don't have health coverage, they can't get regular checkups and screenings, which leads to preventable and tragic outcomes, such as Black women succumbing to breast cancer at a rate of 42 percent higher than white women, even though the incidence of breast cancer is higher in white women.

The Affordable Care Act helped narrow this coverage gap through premium tax credits that have allowed working families to purchase quality coverage through the marketplaces. The American Rescue Plan built on this key reform through provisions in the Health Care Affordability Act, which I introduced with Congresswoman Lauren Underwood. We expanded eligibility for premium tax credits, which has, on average, lowered existing premiums like 40 percent. Over one-third of the consumers who have taken advantage of the new lower rates provided by the American Rescue Plan have joined plans with monthly premiums of $10 or less. Many individuals have seen their medium deductible fall as much as 90 percent.

Dr. Collins, how have the ACA premium tax credits helped individuals and families get covered, and how has the expansion of the premium tax credit in the American Rescue Plan enhanced the program?

Dr. COLLINS. We know from our survey data that affordability is the main reason people decide to take a coverage or not, and so the premium subsidies in the marketplace has helped millions of people gain coverage through a market that did not work for most people prior to the Affordable Care Act. The American Rescue Plan's subsidiaries have done what is needed and enhanced the affordability of those premiums by decreasing the amount of money people have to contribute to them.

Mr. GOMEZ. And since the American Rescue Plan has passed, since it has passed, more than 1.5 million Americans have enrolled in coverage, while an additional 2.5 million people who were previously enrolled in ACA Marketplace plans have seen their premiums fall by 40 percent on average. And despite this success, this relief is temporary and it will expire soon. Last year, I introduced the Choose Medicare Act with Senator Murphy and Merkley, which would give all Americans the choice of buying Medicare as their health insurance plan, and makes reforms to improve affordability, including expanding eligibility for the premium tax credit, while making it more general.

Dr. Collins, how would changes like these put us on the path to universal healthcare?

Dr. COLLINS. So I think that we can get to universal coverage by building on the Affordable Care Act. It has been modeled and demonstrated that we can do it even at lower cost, particularly if we add a public option to the marketplaces, and also, importantly, develop an auto enrollment mechanism to help people get easily enrolled. People who are not currently enrolled would have a much easier pathway to get covered.

Mr. GOMEZ. Thank you so much for that response, Dr. Collins. And as somebody who has been both uninsured and insured and seen my parents who were uninsured and insured, even in the best scenarios with individuals who have healthcare coverage navigating the healthcare system and ensuring that people who have language barriers who can't get necessarily access to certain types of care, we see that the disparities exist. And even under the current system, we need to work on making that disparity less and making sure that those who are left behind oftentimes by our healthcare system, our education system, and so many different systems, that we try to make changes that improve their health outcomes so that people of color or people who live in certain zip codes are not discriminated against because of where they live or the color of their skin.

So this is something that we need to work on. I believe that the ACA and the American Rescue Plan have given thousands of families a little peace of mind. I know that it is not permanent, but the more we work at improving coverage, the better people will be able to access quality healthcare.

So with that, I yield back. Thank you for the time, Madam Chair.

Ms. BUSH. The gentleman from California, Mr. DeSaulnier, is recognized for five minutes.

Mr. DESAULNIER. Thank you, Madam Chair. Nicely done on the pronunciation. And I want to thank the chair of the full committee for having this hearing.

For too many Americans in need of mental and behavioral health, they have been unable to access services for a variety of reasons. It was hard fought in the Affordable Care Act to make sure we had equity for behavioral health. We are learning so much about how the brain works, the impacts of stress, and trauma, poverty. That access is a real problem, and I wanted to ask a couple of questions about that, also just the capacity. I am told that there is a 75-percent increase in requests for behavioral health services by Americans since the ACA passed, but there are 25 percent fewer young people going into the field.

So access and getting universal healthcare for many medical conditions is extremely important, but also for behavioral health. This is personal for me. I am a survivor of suicide. On April 20th of this year will be 33 years since my father took his life, and largely because of that, myself, my family, my sons have access to great professionals. But it has been a challenge for us, so I can imagine what it is, particularly for poor people and people of color as they try to access healthcare for behavioral and mental health.

The Kaiser Family Foundation has studied and said that more than half of American adults coming out of COVID report experiencing symptoms of anxiety or depression disorder within the past two years. Dr. Collins, I want to ask you, how does our current coverage system present obstacles to people, particularly poor people, seeking mental and behavioral healthcare, especially for uninsured? Dr. Collins?

Dr. COLLINS. Yes. Particularly for uninsured, if you don't have health insurance coverage, it is very difficult to get care of any kind, including mental health, behavioral health, care for substance abuse problems, so that is one issue. Another, if you have insurance, you can't access providers, so there is an increased demand that hasn't necessarily been met by the available capacity in the system, particularly in the wake of the COVID pandemic.

Mr. DESAULNIER. Thanks. How would, Dr. Collins, moving to universal healthcare help with that access, I think, for people who are uninsured and are completely without that access?

Dr. COLLINS. I think for people who are uninsured and are completely without access, particularly in States that haven't expanded Medicaid, expanding Medicaid expansion would clearly help address the problems in those States. Making overage more affordable for people through the ARP subsidies have dramatically increased the affordability of marketplace plans. Mental health is part of the essential benefit package for marketplace coverage. But I think we also need to think about integrating different ways to increase capacity, integrating behavioral health and substance abuse into primary care, for example, expanding and diversifying the behavioral health work force by engaging a wider variety of providers to meet people's unique needs, and also thinking about leveraging current health technology to help improve access.

Mr. DESAULNIER. Dr. Michener, how about disadvantaged communities and communities of color? Clearly, as I said, my experience, although different than poor communities in my district and the Bay Area where I represent, have even larger challenges. So how would universal healthcare and getting at these disparities, even though the law says that it should be open and we should have equity for behavioral health, how might that help? And I will mention I have a bill that allows for money for primary care physicians because for people who commit suicide, over 60 percent of them see a primary care physician within a few months of them attempting to commit suicide or being successful at it. Doctor?

Dr. MICHENER. Yes. So I think there are few different pathways here. One is clearly through providing people who don't have insurance presently with insurance, and that means that they can see mental health specialists, but they can also see primary care providers. And I do think that primary care providers are an important sort of first stop, first base, and they can screen and, in many ways, direct people toward more specialized care that is appropriate for them given their mental health challenges and/or conditions. So I think that that is critical, and I think it is especially critical in communities of color where there are already stigmas around mental health and mental healthcare, and where people face systems and processes, like discrimination and racism, that create even more mental health stressors in their lives and in their communities. So I think that there are hardly any places where these problems are more acute and more imperative than in communities of color, and universal coverage is a primary pathway for getting there.

And I would reinforce this point about the healthcare work force. I think one of the places where we see the most potential and opportunity for growth in the healthcare work force is among people of color and communities of color. And I think investing in resources for education and training in those communities so that the very communities where these struggles exist can be equipped to participate in the work force to address them, a work force that can only be robust under a system where the maximum number of people have health insurance.

Mr. DESAULNIER. Thank you, Doctor. I yield back.

Ms. BUSH. The gentlewoman from Massachusetts, Ms. Presley, is recognized for five minutes.

Ms. PRESSLEY. Thank you, Madam Chair, and thank you to all the witnesses who have shared their testimony today. I do want to just take a moment to offer special recognition for something that, at least to my knowledge, this is the first time in three years that it has occurred while I have been a Member of Congress. And I would like to acknowledge our ASL interpreters. I thank you for joining us today.

Mr. Barkan, my forever local progress brother and my sibling in the work of healthcare justice, I appreciate you so very much, and Rachel and your beautiful children, Carl and Willow, for all that you give to the movement. Like Leslie Templeton from my district, who testified on the previous panel of patients, you have highlighted how universal coverage and Medicare for All specifically is a healthcare justice issue and a disability justice issue.

The life and death consequences of our current healthcare system have been made tragically clear over the course of this pandemic, and it was the disability community, in fact, that sounded alarms early on, warning that this crisis would be a mass disabling event. With millions now suffering with the impacts along COVID, it is clear that they were right. There is simply no way we can return to the pre-COVID status quo normal because that normal was fundamentally unjust to begin with. Across the United States, folks with disabilities and chronic conditions, who are disproportionately people of color, are more likely to be uninsured and underinsured, creating a barrier to critical care. This, in part, is a result of how our current healthcare system frequently ties one's healthcare coverage to their employment status. For many disabled people, in particular, maintaining a full-time job with health insurance may not be feasible. And even if you have insurance, sky-high co-pays and out-of-pocket costs can keep people with disabilities in perpetual poverty.

Mr. Barkan, how does a system that ties health coverage to employment perpetuate deep inequities for people with disabilities, and how would Medicare for All help to address this?

Voice. He is writing.

Mr. BARKAN. Thank you. As of August 2021, 1 in 5 workers with disabilities lost employment during the pandemic, which does not include the 1.2 million newly disabled adults the coronavirus has created. For many in the United States, health insurance is tied to employment. If you change or lose your job, you are likely to lose your health insurance or have to start over again and build a new team of providers that exist in network. Patients who have medically complex conditions rely on continuity and their medical teams to monitor their health. The disruptions that result from our patchwork system not only inconvenience patients but endangers those of us who most need uninterrupted, high-quality care.

And as you heard from the patient panel this morning, critical health needs can make it difficult or impossible to work, leaving the people who need the care the most to either navigate being uninsured or too often work in jobs that are inaccessible or damaging to their health. Additionally, despite the ability to and interest in working, disabled people are often employed at much lower rates than people without disabilities, in part because of discrimination. Barriers like ableism in hiring, inaccessible workplaces, and pay discrimination all contribute to the lower rates of employment for disabled people. By disconnecting healthcare from employment, disabled people, who are already burdened by ableism and discrimination, would not have to worry for their healthcare at the same time.

Ms. PRESSLEY. Thank you so much, Mr. Barkan. Congress must stop enabling a predatory health insurance system, one that repeatedly fails our most vulnerable communities. Today in America, if you are poor, Black, brown, indigenous, or disabled, your ability to live, to survive is jeopardized by a broken healthcare system that puts profit over people. We must stop allowing the greed of insurance companies to outweigh the health of our constituents, of our community members. We must ensure that every person has access to quality care when they need it and where they need it.

Babies with heart conditions ending up with parents in bankruptcy is not healthcare justice. A grandmother working the night shift so she can scrape together cash for insulin is not healthcare justice. These are moral failures and policy choices, violent ones. In fact, Coretta Scott King reminded us that, "Ignoring medical need is violence. Contempt for poverty is violence." Healthcare is a human right, and we need Medicare for All. Thank you, and I yield back.

Voice. Excuse me. I am sorry, Congresswoman Pressley, but Mr. Barkan was going to add a little more.

Ms. PRESSLEY. Oh yes.

Mr. BARKAN. One in 4 Americans live with a disability, and this number is growing exponentially due to those who have become recently disabled because of the long-term effects of the coronavirus. Only a single payer system can possess the scale and resources necessary to guarantee care for all, detached from employment. As one example, Medicare for All covers home- and community-based services for all who need it.

The Federal Government currently requires States to fund nursing home care for everyone eligible. This is not the case with regards to home-and community-based services. And because States manage their own home care programs through Medicaid eligibility requirements, the services available vary widely across States. It is by default and design that so many Americans who require care are forced into unsafe institutions like nursing homes. Patients overwhelmingly favor the option to receive care at home, but these services are prohibitively expensive and, therefore, inaccessible to most.

The government would actually save money covering the cost of home- and community-based services instead of covering nursing homes. Under a single-payer system like Medicare for All, home- and community-based services would be prioritized over institutional care, giving patients the safe and dignified care they prefer and deserve.

Voice. Thank you so much.

Ms. PRESSLEY. Thank you.

Ms. BUSH. The gentleman from New York, Mr. Jones, is recognized for five minutes.

Mr. JONES. Thank you, Madam Chair, for your leadership. I represent a district that people often think of as very affluent, and yet there are still too many people who cannot afford healthcare. I think of my grandmother, for example, who, like so many seniors throughout this country, worked well past the age of retirement just to pay for the high cost of prescription drugs, dental care, and other medical procedures that are not fully covered by Medicare as we know it today. Other of my constituents who lack healthcare coverage are working middle-class people who make too much money to qualify for Medicaid or other subsidies under the Affordable Care Act but not enough to afford the high cost of healthcare on their own.

The price of premiums and deductibles is simply too high for many families. Still others have experienced gaps in coverage at critical times due to job loss. In fact, we saw millions of Americans lose their jobs during the COVID–19 pandemic, and with that, their healthcare. The pandemic made it clear that the employer-based healthcare system just does not work in our modern economy.

Mr. Barkan, thank you for your testimony and for your dedication to making America a Nation that treats every person with dignity and with compassion. You are a leading voice in our push to finally realize universal healthcare coverage, our push for Medicare for All. We have heard a number of misleading claims from my colleagues on the other side of the aisle today, so now I would like to give you the opportunity to correct the record on what we have heard today.

Mr. BARKAN. Thank you for your comment and your leadership. There has been a lot of misleading information today about how Medicare for All would take away our freedom of choice, but the reality is our for-profit system does exactly this by inhibiting our ability to make choices for ourselves and by dictating and limiting our experience of care. As I told you this morning, my health insurance provider denied the ventilator that I needed to survive until I forced him to cover it.

Right now, multi-millionaire healthcare executives already make unilateral decisions about our health coverage. There is no freedom to be found in a system that tells us who we can or cannot see or which services we can or cannot access. Medicare for All would ensure that all of us have the freedom to choose our healthcare providers and hospitals without worrying about whether a provider is in network. It would mean that patients would have uninterrupted access to care and that we would be able to build long-term relationships with our providers. It would mean that seniors and disabled people have the option to live safely and with dignity at home instead of being warehoused in unsafe nursing homes. Medicare for All would mean that Americans would be free of medical debt. Health insurance companies and their multi-millionaire executives do not belong in the intimate decisions we make about our health. Medicare for All is a system designed to empower the people by placing the power of choice back in the hands of patients and providers.

A single payer system is, in fact, the only system that would allow us the true freedom to make our own decisions about our lives. When it comes to waiting times, we already have incredibly long wait times for every element of our healthcare system. Even prior to the pandemic, which has deeply exacerbated this issue, the wait time for the ER takes hours. Wait times for specialists can take months or years, and that doesn't include the people who have to ration their own care because they cannot afford this. With a Medicare for All system, the system would expand. There would be more providers, and care would not need to be rationed in this way.

Mr. JONES. Thank you, Mr. Barkan, for your leadership. Madam Chair, I yield back.

Ms. BUSH. The gentlewoman from New York, Ms. Ocasio-Cortez, is recognized for five minutes.

Ms. OCASIO-CORTEZ. Thank you so much, Chairwoman Bush, and to all of our witnesses for being here today. But I have to underscore how grateful we are for Representative Bush's leadership and determination in securing such a historic and unprecedented hearing, not just for this committee, but for the country, so thank you.

We know that private insurance is the primary health coverage for two-thirds of Americans, with the majority of private insurance being employer sponsored. But what I think most people in the U.S., most working-class people need to contend with is the fact that the money employers spend on health benefits, and particularly for-profit private health insurance, comes from the money that they would have otherwise spent on our wages.

Dr. Collins, in 2020, the standard company-provided health insurance policy totaled over about $7,000 a year for single coverage and over $21,000 a year for family coverage. Is that correct?

Dr. COLLINS. Yes.

Ms. OCASIO-CORTEZ. And with employer-sponsored insurance, your employer pays a large portion, and you pay a smaller portion, correct?

Dr. COLLINS. Yes.

Ms. OCASIO-CORTEZ. So in the case of individual coverage, if the total cost is around $7,400 and your employer pays, say, $6,200, and you pay for around $1,200, now that is thousands of dollars more that everyday people could be saving per year if it weren't going directly to insurance companies' private profits, correct?

Dr. COLLINS. Yes.

Ms. OCASIO-CORTEZ. Interesting. So one of the things that we are really seeing here is that the potential to moving to a Medicare for All system could actually give people a raise in many circumstances. Now, a common rebuttal to that and a common rebuttal to Medicare for All that you will hear from conservatives and the right is that we would merely just change the way in which that same premium is charged, and that those same dollars that are coming out of our paychecks now would then just be coming out in the form of taxes. But the truth is that Medicare for All actually lowers the overall cost of healthcare as well.

Dr. Collins, isn't it true that Medicare for All would also reduce the average total costs for lower-and middle-income families by eliminating more medical expenses than they would pay in taxes?

Dr. COLLINS. How it was structured is there is that possibility, particularly in terms of getting provider prices down which drive these cost that people are paying.

Ms. OCASIO-CORTEZ. Mm-hmm. Thank you. And you don't even have to take just our word for it. In fact, that conclusion has been confirmed via thorough research by the Center for a Responsible Federal Budget. We also know that Medicare for All is much cheaper than private insurance. Dr. Collins, public options like Medicare actually pay hospitals and service providers less than private insurance companies have to for the same service. So a single-payer public option would drive down costs additionally through its ability to negotiate on health services and drug prices. Isn't that right?

Dr. COLLINS. That is very true.

Ms. OCASIO-CORTEZ. And, in fact, I think the evidence for that isn't just theoretical, it isn't just calculated by think tanks, but we see it in everyday life. Another case in point right here comes from my district. Almost everywhere in the world, health outcomes are correlated with a person's income, but one of the only places in the world that that doesn't apply is in Queens, one of the handful of zip codes where your income does not determine the quality of healthcare that you have. And the reason for that is our crown jewel of the public hospital, Elmhurst Hospital in Queens.

Years ago, we as a community made a commitment that we would never turn anybody away based on their health insurance status, their documentation status, their housing, or their income. Every single person who enters Elmhurst Hospital gets treated regardless of their ability to afford care. And what we have found is that it is more affordable to treat everybody, it is possible to treat everybody, and people can get higher-quality care than they ever could under our current privatized for-profit system.

And with that, I yield back to the chairwoman. Thank you very much.

Ms. BUSH. The gentleman from Vermont, Mr. Welch, is recognized for five minutes.

Mr. WELCH. Thank you very much, Madam Chair. I appreciate it. I am a co-sponsor of Medicare for All as well, and the incredible challenge we have with healthcare, as many of my colleagues have said, it is too expensive. We pay the most and we get the least, and we still have 30 million folks who are uninsured, and it is unconscionable. It is unconscionable because it is not necessary. It is not as though we don't have the capacity to provide care, and it is not as though we don't have the capacity to save money. But we have a healthcare system that is so fragmented, both in the delivery system in the payment system that we end up paying the most and getting the least. And how we are not all shocked by that from a fiscal standpoint, but from a moral justice standpoint, is astonishing. It really is. So, Congressman Jayapal, I want to thank you for the carrying the torch on this.

The public option is something a lot of us advocate for. The Medicare for All is something we all advocate for. A major reason I do is that I think we do have to get the costs down, and what we have seen in this pandemic is our frontline providers, folks hands-on like our nurses, they haven't been paid enough, and they are getting hammered with work responsibilities. On the other hand, you have private equity finding those seams in the healthcare system where they can take over an emergency room physician practice, and then, through double billing, make an immense amount of profit. And it is exploitation of the fragmentation of the healthcare system that is helping to lead to these high costs and low access. So that is just a little background.

The things we have done, I think, that are good is telehealth has really worked. That has been incredibly beneficial. We have got to bring down the cost of prescription drugs, and the House, of course, passed the legislation to do that. We have got to have mental health that has parity.

Just a couple of questions. Dr. Michener, I want to have you focus on rural communities because so much of my district is rural, but that is true for so much of America. What are the particular challenges that rural America has in accessing affordable, highquality medical care?

Dr. MICHENER. Yes, this is an appropriate question given that I hail from UpState New York. So I think a lot about the rural communities there, and I am actually a part of a collaborative that focuses specifically on health equity in rural communities, and I think there are a range of challenges. So one is the basic challenge that we have been talking about today, which is access, and I think that because in rural communities we see higher rates of poverty and we see more difficulty and challenges around having health insurance, having just access to being insured, that is a primary and an initial barrier. And then I think there are some specific barriers that are particularly challenging in rural areas. Transportation is one.

Mr. WELCH. Right. Yes, very much.

Dr. MICHENER. And that that is an important problem and one that is, in part, addressed through a program like Medicaid, which has a transportation benefit. We don't see that same benefit available in the private sector, and we know that that benefit is correlated with all sorts of positive health outcomes.

Mr. WELCH. Thank you. Thank you. And I will ask Dr. Collins, how would universal coverage improve healthcare options in rural communities, and as we work to ensure that all in America can prosper, how would universal coverage foster economic growth in rural areas?

Dr. COLLINS. Well, I think we have seen in Medicaid non-expansion States, as a case in point, rural hospitals have closed. They just haven't had the financing that they need to serve people in their communities. And so having a universal financing mechanism to make it possible for these hospitals to stay in business would be one of the benefits of universal coverage in every State.

Mr. WELCH. You know, one final point I am going to make, and I will ask you, Dr. Collins, to just respond to it, if you have universal coverage, then the challenges that each of us faces in access to healthcare become the challenges that all of us face. It is not as though having Medicare for All necessarily solves all problems. It just means we are all in it together to try to solve the problems we face. Does that make some sense to you?

Dr. COLLINS. That is right, and insurance is the most important and it is a necessary condition for people getting access to care, but it is not the only factor. And so we also need to work at making sure people have adequate provider networks, that providers are paid well enough to participate in the networks, and we have good transportation systems so people in hard-to-reach areas are able to get the healthcare that they need.

Mr. WELCH. I yield back. Thank you, Madam Chair.

Ms. BUSH. The gentleman from Maryland, Mr. Sarbanes, is recognized for five minutes.

Mr. SARBANES. Thank you very much, Madam Chair. I appreciate the opportunity to join the hearing today.

We know that the research shows very clearly that there is a correlation between uninsurance or underinsurance and poor patient outcomes, and we saw that during the coronavirus pandemic, in particular. More than 40 percent of Americans who contracted coronavirus in the first year of the pandemic were either uninsured or underinsured. And a recent study found that a 10-percent increase in the number of uninsured residents per county was associated with a 70-percent increase in coronavirus cases and a nearly 50 percent increase in deaths from the coronavirus. Dr. Blackstock, I would like to ask you, what inequities in our healthcare system could explain this correlation?

Dr. BLACKSTOCK. Yes. So, you know, we have to think about when people lack access to care, they are lacking access to primary and preventive services, mammograms, colonoscopy screenings, proState cancer screenings, and so that will cause an exacerbation of these inequities. And then with the pandemic, we saw that our systems were under even increased stress, so people, when they lost their jobs, they also lost their insurance and were not able to access care. We also have seen that, as our government has picked up the slack in terms of vaccines and testing, that those gaps actually in terms of COVID mortality rates have closed. So we see what happens when we are able to provide communities and people to services that they need.

Mr. SARBANES. You know, the threat from the pandemic, we spoke often and we continue to about how that combines with underlying conditions to pose a great risk to patients. And if underlying conditions are persisting and not being addressed in certain communities and populations that is obviously going to increase the risk. Can you talk about how universal coverage could have improved the experiences of patients during the coronavirus pandemic? Let's look at it from the positive side.

Dr. BLACKSTOCK. Right, absolutely. We know that people who carry a higher burden of chronic disease were more at risk for the more severe outcomes of COVID–19. So if people have access to care, if they have access to, you know, care that prevents their diabetes, and their high blood pressure, and their asthma from worsening, then that could ultimately improve their outcomes from COVID–19. So it is really about investing in health, investing in people from the beginning to prevent these worse outcomes later on.

Mr. SARBANES. Dr. Michener, I would love to get your perspective as well. How would universal coverage ensure more equitable outcomes in the case of a future public health crisis because we want to learn our lessons obviously, and adapt, and make clear-headed decisions going forward? So if you could speak to that that would be wonderful.

Dr. MICHENER. Yes, I think universal coverage, in addition to providing people with access to care, they get to go to the hospital. They get to go to the doctor. They get to get the treatments in the medications that they need. They don't have to delay. They don't have to forego care. The other thing to recognize is that uninsurance and underinsurance are concentrated in particular communities, that there are zip codes and there are neighborhoods that have disproportionately high levels of uninsurance and underinsurance. So when we address those problems, we don't just address them among individuals. We address them at the community level, which means that the solutions and the benefits can really amplify.

For example, we have research that shows that when you insure parents, they are more likely to take their children to well care visits. Even if the children were already insured, if the parents weren't, they weren't socialized into the habit of going to the doctor. And so you see families, and you see social networks, and you see communities, and the benefits of insurance ripple throughout these levels so that we can see amplified positive effects if we have universal insurance.

Mr. SARBANES. You know, there are so many connections here that aren't necessarily intuitive, but when it is brought to your attention, it makes perfect sense. So a lot of the adults with less income in our society experienced coronavirus-related job loss or pay cuts at the beginning of the pandemic, and then had consequential coverage laws that went with that. In Maryland, we saw 200,000 people enroll in healthcare coverage through our State-based health exchange during the special enrollment period that we extended during COVID–19, and nearly two-thirds of those people enrolled in Medicaid.

I am running out of time, but, Dr. Michener, what does it tell us about how Federal healthcare programs can support people and the ability to lift up communities during times of crisis and volatility?

Dr. MICHENER. I will quickly say, mindful of time, given all that has been said about the government, and Big Government, and government inefficiency, this is a really important point. There was a time before Medicare, there was a time before Medicaid, and it was a dark and dismal time where many more people had much worse outcomes. The private side of the market could not address the fundamental needs of the American people, and that is why we developed these public programs. And they are not perfect, but they are absolutely saving lives, and the science around that is quite incontrovertible.

Mr. SARBANES. Thank you, and I will just note as I yield back, their administrative costs tend to be much lower than what we see in the private sector and other arguments for the universal healthcare coverage that we are talking about today. Thank you, Madam Chair.

Ms. BUSH. The gentlewoman from Washington, Ms. Jayapal, is recognized for five minutes.

Ms. JAYAPAL. Thank you, Madam Chair, and thank you for your incredible leadership in making this hearing happen, and to all my sisters in service that were part of it, and to all the colleagues who have been talking about the various aspects of universal healthcare. Also, thank you for the powerful testimoneys that we have heard.

My Medicare for All act would provide healthcare to everyone in the United States without the financial, racial, or demographic barriers that exist in our current system. My bill creates a comprehensive, universal single-payer healthcare system that provides all the medically necessary care that someone needs. Imagine that: a comprehensive care that includes dental, vision, and hearing, and for the first time when we introduced this bill two Congresses ago, long-term care, something that Mr. Barkan has spoken extensively on.

The bill eliminates insurance premiums, co-pays, deductibles, and all other out-of-pocket costs, and removes the for-profit insurance companies from the doctor-patient relationship, while controlling medical costs to bring down overall spending. That is a very important piece of this. And I think at the end of the day, I have heard people arguing against Medicare for All by saying it takes away choice. I would just argue that Medicare for All would actually allow people to make choices, like being able to go see a doctor or a hospital without worrying about out-of-network costs that come later when there are tens of thousands of dollars that people can't afford; or the choice to be able to have healthcare even when you lose your job instead of 27 million people losing healthcare because they lost their jobs during COVID; or the choice to start a small business because you don't have to worry about your healthcare, it is covered already; or, most importantly, the choice to live and not die.

Researchers have found that Medicare for All will save over 68,000 lives per year. That means 68,000 more birthdays, 68,000 more anniversaries, 68,000 more loved ones alive every year simply because we transitioned to a Medicare for All system. And under Medicare for All, those 68,000 lives saved would also see a drastic increase in quality of life.

Mr. Barkan, you have been an incredible patient advocate your entire life, and even now you are still. How would your life be different if Medicare for All were enacted? And I am going to give you a few moments because I know you have to get your answer prepared, and I will come back to you for your answer.

Dr. Blackstock, as a physician and expert in health inequities, you have seen firsthand who the winners and losers are in our forprofit healthcare system, and we often forget the crucial role that Medicare actually played in beginning the desegregation of hospitals. We sort of overlook that, but there is a lot more to do. So tell me, who do the 68,000 lives that Medicare for All would save, the lives that are lost in our current healthcare system, who do those lives belong to?

Dr. BLACKSTOCK. Thank you, Representative Jayapal, and thank you for mentioning that because I think we often forget that Medicare was probably one of the greatest civil rights achievements in terms of desegregating hospitals and providing or advancing health equity. But the 68,000 lives are people who matter, people who deserve humanity. They are mostly and disproportionately people of color. They are also low-income families. They are predominantly located in the Southern part and the Western part of this country. They are people who aren't able to afford the out-of-pocket costs, you know, to purchase medication or to access insurance. So this is giving people with families, low-income families with children, the opportunity to have a choice to access the care that they need.

Ms. JAYAPAL. Dr. Michener, you have spoken so eloquently about racial inequity. Tell us how a Medicare for All system would help alleviate those racial health inequities that people are facing right now.

Dr. MICHENER. One of the main benefits of a Medicare for All system is that it is not a tiered system. It is not a system that is rationed based on where you live. We know that rationing based on geography leads to racial inequities, so that people who live in the South or people who live in what we call hospital or our public health deserts, have less access. We don't have rationing based on income. We know that causes racial disproportionalities because people of color are more likely to be living in poverty. We don't have rationing based on a range of other factors that all bake in racial discrimination. Instead, we have access that is equally available to all.

Ms. JAYAPAL. Thank you so much. Let me go back to Mr. Barkan before my time expires and ask you for your answer. Mr. Barkan.

Mr. BARKAN. Thank you so much for your leadership. It is an honor to be in the struggle with you. I am not the only one whose life has been upended, first, by illness and then by the moral abomination that is our healthcare system. Right now, about 30 million people in this country are uninsured, and even more get necessary care denied every year by their insurance company. We are richest Nation in the history of the world, and yet Americans regularly go bankrupt from their medical bills and cut their pills in half because they can't afford the cost of prescription drugs. It reveals much about our country that we see spikes in cancer diagnoses for Americans aged 65 once they become eligible for Medicare. Too many go far too long without care because they cannot afford it.

By securing Medicare for All, we can save thousands of lives and free mourning families from the lingering pain of asking themselves, what if we had caught this sooner. Americans across the Nation and across the political spectrum have been harmed by corporate greed. I believe we can overturn our for-profit system because our power lies in our solidarity. Our movement for Medicare for All isn't slowing down any time soon. We intend to win our due rights, and we will continue to organize for our collective freedom until all of us are free from this corrupt system of corporate greed.

Ms. JAYAPAL. Thank you so much, Mr. Barkan. We are not giving up until we pass Medicare for All. Thank you, Madam Chair. I yield back.

Ms. BUSH. The gentleman from New York, Mr. Bowman, is recognized for five minutes.

Mr. BOWMAN. Thank you so much to Chairwoman Maloney and Rep. Bush for holding this historic hearing, and thank you to all the members of this committee for allowing me to join you today. Thank you also to Rep. Jayapal for her incredible leadership on this issue.

More than 27 million adults in the United States today are uninsured. Millions more are underinsured. As a Member of Congress, I am more than adequately covered. I can get a checkup any time I want. If something is wrong, I can get treated on the spot. Those of us who support Medicare for All believe that every single person who lives in this country should have that level of care. It is very simple. If people knew they had exemplary healthcare, they would go to the doctor more, but as it stands, millions of people often skip preventive and routine care, instead waiting until they are severely ill to seek treatment.

Dr. Blackstock, how do these delays in seeking care affect patients?

Dr. BLACKSTOCK. So delays in care result in late or misdiagnoses. They also result when a condition is diagnosed that is more difficult to treat, it results in higher mortality rates. We know that people who are uninsured have about a 40-percent higher age-specific mortality risk. And so, you know, access to care is equivalent to your mortality risk, so we need to give people access to care through health insurance so that we can reduce their risk and so they can lead full, healthy lives.

Mr. BOWMAN. Thank you, Dr. Blackstock. My next question is for Dr. Michener. As you have mentioned already today, people of color are more likely to be uninsured than white people. They are more likely to experience severe medical events or suffer from catastrophic medical debts. As a Black man, I am acutely aware of the specific care needs that Black men have in our society. It is well known, for example, that Black Americans have the highest rates of hypertension, and Black men are least likely to have their high blood pressure controlled. Lack of trust in our current healthcare system is one of the reasons they are not seeking treatment. Dr. Michener, how could we rebuild that trust under a Medicare for All system with universal access to comprehensive healthcare? How could Medicare for All strengthen communities of color generally and improve other social determinants of health?

Dr. MICHENER. I think that Medicare for All contributes to and can contribute to precisely this problem of lack of trust. We can think about lack of trust as sort of an individual attitude, right, but it is rooted in experiences with structures. So when you go to the doctor or you try to go to the doctor and you are not able to get access, or when you are worried about whether when you show up you will be able to see someone given your health insurance status, when you are worried about the cost, these are experiences that are disproportionately in communities of color, and they all erode trust.

Over and above that, Medicare for All, a universal coverage system, is going to strengthen the healthcare system more generally. It is going to allow us to make investments in the healthcare work force. Again, this will increase access and increase access in ways that, if designed right, can disproportionately benefit the very communities of colors that are disproportionately harmed by the current system. All of these things contribute to repairing what, frankly, is broken and has always been broken.

Mr. BOWMAN. Thank you so much for those responses. I want to briefly share a personal story. Just recently, maybe a month or so ago, I was feeling unwell in my office on the Capitol. I literally took a 10-minute walk to the healthcare unit on the Capitol, was seen immediately, treated immediately, and sent on my way to go home and take care of myself. It made me think of all the Black men, and people of color, and uninsured and underinsured people in this country who do not have that privilege and do not have that access. When they don't feel well at home, they have to just deal with it in whatever way they can using home remedies, which is OK. But imagine if they can walk right downstairs or take a 5-to 10-minute walk to a doctor right down the street, get seen on the spot, be treated on the spot, and be sent on their way with the medication or care that they needed, and also, by the way, have unlimited access for followup. I can call a doctor on the Capitol 24 hours a day and weekends to followup on the care that I received.

Everyone in this country deserves that level of care. Thank you, and I yield back.

Ms. BUSH. The gentlewoman from Minnesota, Ms. Omar, is recognized for five minutes.

[No response.]

Ms. BUSH. We can't hear you.

Ms. OMAR. My apologies. Thank you, Madam Chairwoman, for having me on your committee today, and thank you to all of our witnesses for your excellent testimoneys.

When a person needs healthcare, they should not have to worry about whether their coverage status will be a barrier, but unfortunately, that is not the case for millions of marginalized gender identities in the in the United States. Across the United States, transgender people are uninsured at a greater rate than their cisgendered counterparts. When trans folks who are covered seek care, they experience denials of medically necessary services at higher rates.

Dr. Blackstock, can you speak to how these trends perpetuate stigma against trans folks and the broader LGBTQ+ communities in healthcare settings?

Dr. BLACKSTOCK. Yes. Yes, Representative Omar. So, you know, one thing that we know is that the healthcare system is not sensitive enough to the needs of the LGBTQA+ community, and that many of our healthcare providers are not trained in a way that is needed to provide the best care. But access is so incredibly important, especially for these communities, because we know that these health inequities exist, and they are perpetuated because people from these communities are unable to access care. So I think Medicare for All will provide an opportunity for members from stigmatized communities to engage in access with the healthcare system, and the healthcare system also needs to be equipped to provide the resources and services in a culturally sensitive way, in a culturally responsive way to these communities.

Ms. OMAR. Dr. Michener, what steps can Congress take to ensure that people of marginalized gender identities are able to access medical that are necessary care and free of stigma and financial barriers?

Dr. MICHENER. I think the sorts of policies, the commitment to universal coverage that we have been talking about here today, is the first and critically important step. I think that there are barriers that are really concrete around simply being able to have access, and that is a sort of first point to address. Over and above this, though, I do think that we need to think about interventions that are sort of tailored to these uniquely marginalized populations. And so we need to be aware of what the unique challenges are in those populations, and I think part of what that means is talking to those folks, understanding better their perspectives and barriers, and connecting that information with the policy choices that we make going forward.

So I guess the broad point I am making is to really think about how we can improve voice in addition to access so that the people who are most affected, who have really unique stakes around these particular kinds of barriers, can really help us to understand how to engage and move forward in a way that is going to address their particular vulnerabilities.

Ms. OMAR. And I wanted to also ask you, you know, as someone who supports Medicare for All and serves as the vice chair of the Medicare for All Caucus, oftentimes we hear how universal access to care can lessen the quality of care that is available to people. Can you respond to that sort of critique as an advocate for universal access?

Dr. MICHENER. I appreciate the opportunity to address that. So one of the things that I always emphasize is that quality of care, just like access to care, is a choice. It is a political choice, and so many of the critiques that we have heard around quality to care— look at the VA and its weaknesses, or look at Medicare and its weaknesses—those are a reflection of political choices: choosing to under fund those services, choosing to create administrative burden and barriers, choosing to make life for people on those programs more difficult. And if we make different choices, we can have government programs that are just as well run, just as efficiently run, actually more so than private options, and the reason is because there is no profit motive.

We are not trying to maximize what we can gain in exchange for what we give in the context of a government program. We are trying to maximize what we can give in exchange for improving people's lives, saving their lives, and helping them to thrive. That is the best context for both efficient and effective programs that are going to help people. And to the extent that that is not what we have, it is because we are choosing not to put the pieces and the resources in place to achieve it.

Ms. OMAR. Thank you. Thank you so much for that response. I will just say as someone who has been fully insured for the first time in my life here in the United States, I know just how much my healthcare has improved, not just having the anxiety of worrying about whether I could access, you know, what Congressman Bowman was talking about, being able to pick up the phone, walk 10 steps to a medical professional to care for you. That is the kind of access that we want for everyone, and that is the kind of access everyone deserves. So, again, thank you all for the opportunity to have this conversation.

Chairwoman, I yield back.

Ms. BUSH. Before we close, I want to offer the ranking member an opportunity to offer any closing remarks he may have. Ranking Member Comer, you are now recognized.

Mr. COMER. Well, thank you, Madam Chair, and I just want to reiterate the fact that the Oversight Committee's role is to determine waste, fraud, abuse, and mismanagement in the Federal Government and try to provide solutions to those problems with waste, fraud, and abuse. This hearing, like just about every other hearing this committee has had this year, hasn't touched upon that. In fact, not only does it not save money and reduce waste, fraud, and abuse, it increases the size of government significantly, and this is a pattern that we have seen with this committee.

We had an energy hearing where many of the members on the Democrat side asked the energy CEOs to pledge to decrease production. Now, think about that: decrease production. Now we have President Biden going to OPEC, Venezuela, and begging them to increase production. I say that because we don't believe that the government can efficiently run healthcare. We believe that the solution to healthcare problems is with innovation, is with competition, and that is where Republicans will continue to work to try to find solutions when we talk about healthcare.

Madam Chair, thank you for the time, and I yield back.

Ms. BUSH. Thank you. I now recognize myself.

The choice before the committee today, the choice is saving lives or increasing profits. It is the quality of life or the quantity of yachts. Medicare for All would guarantee high-quality healthcare to every person in America in the prioritizing of Big Pharma over human life and health, and, more importantly, it would save lives.

To the 30 million people in this country who are uninsured, to those who are underinsured, and to the Black, brown, indigenous, disabled, low-income, and trans people who are burdened under the various inequalities of our healthcare system, we see you, we know, and you matter. We are fighting for you. You deserve life. You deserve care.

I am grateful to Chairwoman Maloney and to our sisters in service for their partnership in this hearing. In closing, I want to thank our panelists for their remarks. I want to commend my colleagues for participating in this important conversation.

With that, without objection, all members will have five legislative days within which to submit extraneous materials and to submit additional written questions for the witnesses to the chair, which will be forwarded to the witnesses for their response. I ask our witnesses to please respond as promptly as you are able.

This hearing is adjourned.

[Whereupon, at 1:52 p.m., the committee was adjourned.]

Index

I

K

L

M

N